Dietary Habits and Metabolic Health

Dietary Habits and Metabolic Health

Guest Editors

Guowei Le
Xue Tang
Bowen Li

MDPI

Basel • Beijing • Wuhan • Barcelona • Belgrade • Novi Sad • Cluj • Manchester

Guest Editors
Guowei Le
School of Food Science and Technology
Jiangnan University
Wuxi
China

Xue Tang
School of Food Science and Technology
Jiangnan University
Wuxi
China

Bowen Li
College of Food Science
Southwest University
Chongqing
China

Editorial Office
MDPI AG
Grosspeteranlage 5
4052 Basel, Switzerland

This is a reprint of the Special Issue, published open access by the journal *Nutrients* (ISSN 2072-6643), freely accessible at: https://www.mdpi.com/journal/nutrients/special_issues/152X9KV52G.

For citation purposes, cite each article independently as indicated on the article page online and as indicated below:

Lastname, A.A.; Lastname, B.B. Article Title. *Journal Name* **Year**, *Volume Number*, Page Range.

ISBN 978-3-7258-4917-8 (Hbk)
ISBN 978-3-7258-4918-5 (PDF)
https://doi.org/10.3390/books978-3-7258-4918-5

Contents

nutrients

Editorial

Dietary Habits and Metabolic Healt

Bowen Li [1,2,*], Xue Tang [1,2] and Guowei Le [1,2]

1 State Key Laboratory of Food Science and Resources, Jiangnan University, Wuxi 214122, China; tangxue@jiangnan.edu.cn (X.T.); lgw_jiangnan@163.com (G.L.)
2 School of Food Science and Technology, Jiangnan University, Wuxi 214122, China
* Correspondence: lbw1965841356@gmail.com; Tel.: +86-15651519190

Dietary habits refer to the long-term dietary patterns and habits that an individual forms and maintains in their daily life. Dietary behavior is an essential and ongoing activity in daily life, which involves internal, external, and conscious activities related to eating. With a deeper understanding of nutritional science, people are increasingly aware of the complex relationship between dietary habits and health outcomes.

Exploring the variations in nutrient composition in food contributes to the formation of proper dietary habits. Positive dietary behaviors are important strategies for individuals to ensure their health. Eating regular meals, moderating the intake of fats and sugars, consuming an adequate number of fruits and vegetables, paying attention to nutritional labels and calorie content, practicing good hygiene, and choosing foods based on principles of nutrition and health are all considered behaviors that promote physical well-being. However, as the pace of life accelerates, various fast-food products and the rapid development of the ultra-processed food industry have flooded the market. Ultra-processed foods refer to foods that have undergone packaging, processing, and the addition of numerous additives, preservatives, seasonings, and added sugars. These foods often lack a variety of nutrients such as fiber, vitamins, and minerals, while containing excessive amounts of sugar, salt, and unhealthy fats [1]. This leads to nutritional imbalance and can contribute to metabolic health problems such as obesity, diabetes, and cardiovascular disease. In these processed foods, significant changes have occurred in the nutritional composition, including the presence of protein oxidation products, lipid oxidation products, and advanced glycation end products [2]. These products not only stimulate the appetite center, making individuals more prone to excessive intake of these unhealthy components, but they also potentially have a negative impact on the gut microbiota, disrupting the balance of beneficial bacteria and compromising gut health.

In addition to reducing the intake of harmful substances in food, dietary patterns with nutrient interactions and synergistic effects, or specific food combinations, have become popular dietary strategies for the prevention of metabolic diseases. A whole grain diet refers to a dietary pattern that primarily relies on grains as the main source of food. Compared to refined grains, a whole grain diet is rich in dietary fiber, vitamins, minerals, and antioxidants, which can improve blood glucose control, insulin sensitivity, and lipid levels. This dietary habit is associated with lower risks of cardiovascular diseases, diabetes, cancer, and mortality [3]. Energy restriction refers to limiting energy intake and is commonly used for weight control or weight loss. An energy-restricted diet can reduce body weight, fat content, and body fat percentage. This dietary habit can improve insulin sensitivity, reduce insulin resistance, lower the risk of cardiovascular diseases, and improve lipid levels [4]. Specific amino acid restriction refers to limiting the intake of specific amino acids, such as methionine, phenylalanine, etc. This type of diet can be used to treat certain genetic metabolic diseases, such as phenylketonuria [5]. Recent studies have shown that methionine restriction helps in improving neurological disorders and extending lifespan [6]. A diet with specific amino acid restriction can reduce the accumulation of pathological products, improve pathological symptoms, maintain amino acid balance in the body, and reduce the generation of harmful metabolic by-products.

Changes in dietary habits can affect the structure of the gut microbiota, and alterations in the gut microbiota can also regulate the development of metabolic diseases [7]. The gut microbiota is involved in the breakdown and metabolism of food, aiding in the digestion and utilization of nutrients. When the gut microbiota is imbalanced, the activity of digestive enzymes and other related enzymes may be inhibited, leading to the incomplete digestion and absorption of food. This can increase the risk of malnutrition and related diseases. Changes in the gut microbiota can also disrupt energy balance. Microbes can convert prebiotics in food into different metabolites, providing energy to intestinal cells and participating in the regulation of energy balance. This may result in excessive energy absorption and storage, thus increasing the risk of obesity and metabolic syndrome when the gut microbiota is imbalanced. In addition, an imbalanced gut microbiota can also affect toxin metabolism, leading to the accumulation of toxins in the body and adversely affecting metabolic health. Probiotics, prebiotics, and postbiotics are currently the most widely used methods to regulate the gut microbiota [8]. Probiotics can regulate the gut microbiota in various ways. Firstly, they occupy positions in the gut microbiota and competitively exclude harmful bacteria, maintaining the balance of the gut microbiota. Secondly, specific probiotics can produce beneficial metabolites, such as short-chain fatty acids, which help promote gut health and regulate energy metabolism. Research has also found that certain probiotics, such as *Bifidobacterium* and *Lactobacillus*, can improve metabolic health by regulating immune function, suppressing inflammatory responses, and enhancing the integrity of the intestinal mucosa [9]. Prebiotics are a type of carbohydrate that is not broken down by human digestive enzymes and can promote the growth and activity of beneficial bacteria. Prebiotics, such as inulin, oligofructose, and lactulose, are considered as the "food" for gut microbiota. Prebiotics improve the balance of the gut microbiota by providing nutrients that beneficial bacteria require for their growth. The intake of prebiotics can increase the abundance and diversity of beneficial bacteria, and regulate the gut ecosystem, thereby improving metabolic function and reducing the risk of metabolic diseases [10]. Postbiotics are important intermediates between the gut microbiota and human metabolism. Postbiotics help promote the diversity and balance of the gut microbiota, thereby providing protection against metabolic diseases [11]. Therefore, forming dietary habits that include an adequate supplementation of probiotics, prebiotics, and postbiotics contributes to metabolic health.

Furthermore, individualized dietary interventions for metabolic regulation in special populations are also necessary. Firstly, special populations may face unique health risks. For example, diabetes patients need to control blood glucose levels, hypertension patients need to limit sodium intake, and liver disease patients need to reduce fat intake. Personalized dietary interventions can develop suitable healthy eating plans according to the specific conditions of patients, forming personalized dietary habits, and reducing the risk of related diseases. Secondly, special populations may have specific nutritional needs. For instance, pregnant women need to increase the nutrients required during pregnancy, older adults need to consume adequate protein and vitamin D to maintain bone health, and athletes need to supplement enough protein and carbohydrates to improve sports performance [12]. Personalized dietary interventions can aid in developing specific dietary plans to meet the nutritional needs of different populations, providing the necessary nutrients for their bodies.

In conclusion, dietary habits are closely related to metabolic health. Therefore, it is crucial to explore the regulatory principles and mechanisms of different dietary habits on metabolic health, deepen our understanding of the relationship between dietary habits and health outcomes, promote healthy dietary habits, and prevent metabolic diseases.

Author Contributions: B.L., X.T. and G.L. have contributed equally to this editorial. All authors have read and agreed to the published version of the manuscript.

Funding: This research was funded by National Natural Science Foundation of China grant number No. 31901679 and Standard Foods (China) Co., Ltd., Jiangsu, P.R. China (No. 221388).

Conflicts of Interest: The authors declare no conflict of interest.

References

1. Popkin, B.M.; Barquera, S.; Corvalan, C.; Hofman, K.J.; Monteiro, C.; Ng, S.W.; Swart, E.C.; Taillie, L.S. Towards unified and impactful policies to reduce ultra-processed food consumption and promote healthier eating. *Lancet Diabetes Endocrinol.* **2021**, *9*, 462–470. [CrossRef] [PubMed]
2. Li, B.; Yang, Y.; Ding, Y.; Ge, Y.; Xu, Y.; Xie, Y.; Shi, Y.; Le, G. Dityrosine in food: A review of its occurrence, health effects, detection methods, and mitigation strategies. *Compr. Rev. Food Sci. Food Saf.* **2023**, *22*, 355–379. [CrossRef] [PubMed]
3. Hu, Y.; Ding, M.; Sampson, L.; Willett, W.C.; Manson, J.E.; Wang, M.; Rosner, B.; Hu, F.B.; Sun, Q. Intake of whole grain foods and risk of type 2 diabetes: Results from three prospective cohort studies. *BMJ* **2020**, *370*, m2206. [CrossRef] [PubMed]
4. Teong, X.T.; Liu, K.; Vincent, A.D.; Bensalem, J.; Liu, B.; Hattersley, K.J.; Zhao, L.; Feinle-Bisset, C.; Sargeant, T.J.; Wittert, G.A.; et al. Intermittent fasting plus early time-restricted eating versus calorie restriction and standard care in adults at risk of type 2 diabetes: A randomized controlled trial. *Nat. Med.* **2023**, *29*, 963–972. [CrossRef] [PubMed]
5. Green, C.L.; Lamming, D.W.; Fontana, L. Molecular mechanisms of dietary restriction promoting health and longevity. *Nat. Rev. Mol. Cell Biol.* **2022**, *23*, 56–73. [CrossRef] [PubMed]
6. Wang, D.; Ye, J.; Shi, R.; Zhao, B.; Liu, Z.; Lin, W.; Liu, X. Dietary protein and amino acid restriction: Roles in metabolic health and aging-related diseases. *Free. Radic. Biol. Med.* **2022**, *178*, 226–242. [CrossRef] [PubMed]
7. Hill, J.H.; Round, J.L. SnapShot: Microbiota effects on host physiology. *Cell* **2021**, *184*, 2796–2796.e1. [CrossRef] [PubMed]
8. Li, H.-Y.; Zhou, D.-D.; Gan, R.-Y.; Huang, S.-Y.; Zhao, C.-N.; Shang, A.; Xu, X.-Y.; Li, H.-B. Effects and Mechanisms of Probiotics, Prebiotics, Synbiotics, and Postbiotics on Metabolic Diseases Targeting Gut Microbiota: A Narrative Review. *Nutrients* **2021**, *13*, 3211. [CrossRef] [PubMed]
9. Li, B.; Ding, M.; Liu, X.; Zhao, J.; Ross, R.P.; Stanton, C.; Yang, B.; Chen, W. Bifidobacterium breve CCFM1078 Alleviates Collagen-Induced Arthritis in Rats via Modulating the Gut Microbiota and Repairing the Intestinal Barrier Damage. *J. Agric. Food Chem.* **2022**, *70*, 14665–14678. [CrossRef]
10. Miniello, V.L.; Miniello, A.; Ficele, L.; Skublewska-D'Elia, A.; Dargenio, V.N.; Cristofori, F.; Francavilla, R. Gut Immunobiosis and Biomodulators. *Nutrients* **2023**, *15*, 2114. [CrossRef] [PubMed]
11. Ma, L.; Tu, H.; Chen, T. Postbiotics in Human Health: A Narrative Review. *Nutrients* **2023**, *15*, 291. [CrossRef] [PubMed]
12. De Toro-Martín, J.; Arsenault, B.J.; Després, J.-P.; Vohl, M.-C. Precision Nutrition: A Review of Personalized Nutritional Approaches for the Prevention and Management of Metabolic Syndrome. *Nutrients* **2017**, *9*, 913. [CrossRef] [PubMed]

nutrients

MDPI

Article

Sex-Specific Associations of Red Meat and Processed Meat Consumption with Serum Metabolites in the UK Biobank

Bohan Fan and Jie V. Zhao *

School of Public Health, Li Ka Shing Faculty of Medicine, The University of Hong Kong, Hong Kong, China
* Correspondence: janezhao@hku.hk; Tel.: +852-3917-6739; Fax: +852-3917-9280

Abstract: Red meat consumption has been found to closely related to cardiometabolic health, with sex disparity. However, the specific metabolic factors corresponding to red meat consumption in men and women have not been examined previously. We analyzed the sex-specific associations of meat consumption, with 167 metabolites using multivariable regression, controlling for age, ethnicity, Townsend deprivation index, education, physical activity, smoking, and drinking status among ~79,644 UK Biobank participants. We also compared the sex differences using an established formula. After accounting for multiple testing with false discovery rate < 5% and controlling for confounders, the positive associations of unprocessed red meat consumption with branched-chain amino acids and several lipoproteins, and the inverse association with glycine were stronger in women, while the positive associations with apolipoprotein A1, creatinine, and monounsaturated fatty acids were more obvious in men. For processed meat, the positive associations with branched-chain amino acids, several lipoproteins, tyrosine, lactate, glycoprotein acetyls and inverse associations with glutamine, and glycine were stronger in women than in men. The study suggests that meat consumption has sex-specific associations with several metabolites. This has important implication to provide dietary suggestions for individuals with or at high risk of cardiometabolic disease, with consideration of sex difference.

Keywords: red meat; processed meat; UK Biobank; serum metabolites

1. Introduction

Cardiovascular disease (CVD) is the leading cause of mortality [1]. Diabetes is an established risk factor for CVD. Dietary factors are key components for cardiometabolic disease prevention. In recent years many national dietary guidelines, such as the US the 2020–2025 Dietary Guidelines, have recommended limiting red and processed meat due to their associated detrimental health outcomes [2]. Several observational studies have shown that red meat consumption is linked with increased risks of cardiometabolic disease, including CVD and diabetes [3]. The changes in metabolites, such as lipids and glucose, which occur prior to cardiometabolic events, are predictive of these events. Disentangling the specific metabolic factors that correspond to red meat consumption could provide insights for cardiometabolic disease prevention strategies. In addition, red meat consumption is associated with cardiometabolic deaths with a potential sex disparity; the association is higher in men than in women [4]. However, the sex-specific association of red meat consumption with metabolic factors have not been clarified. The dietary guidelines, including the US 2020–2025 Dietary Guidelines, have not considered men and women separately in the recommendations of meat intake, possibly due to the lack of relevant evidence. Prior studies suggested red meat consumption may be related to higher gut microbiota-generated metabolite trimethylamine *N*-oxide [5], lipoprotein subclasses and lipids [6], ferritin, and lower glycine [7]. However, no studies took account of a wide range of metabolites corresponding to different biological pathways and none of them considered sex disparity.

Given the apparent sex differences in meat consumption and in cardiometabolic disease risk, it is worthwhile to assess the association of meat consumption and metabolic factors in a sex-specific manner. Metabolomics, which is systematic profiling of the small circulating molecules of our body, can reveal metabolic alterations due to changes in diet and lifestyle and provide a way to comprehensively assess the associations [8]. Therefore, we systematically assessed metabolic factors corresponding to red meat and processed meat consumption in men and women with metabolomics. The identification of the sex-specific associations of red meat consumption with metabolic factors may help understand the sex-specific associations of red meat consumption with cardiometabolic diseases. The information can also be applied to health promotion program and provide more references for dietary guidelines.

2. Materials and Methods

2.1. Study Population

This study examined the sex-specific associations of unprocessed red meat and processed meat consumption with serum metabolites in the UK Biobank. The UK Biobank is a population-based cohort study consisting of half a million individuals aged 40–69 years across the UK between 2006–2010 [9]. The UK Biobank participants were registered via National Health Service for on-going follow up.

2.2. Metabolomic Profiling

Metabolomic profiling was conducted using high-throughput proton nuclear magnetic resonance spectrometry (NMR) on plasma samples from approximately 120,000 randomly selected participants between 2019–2020. The samples are stored at a temperature of −80 °C and go through minimal sample preparation by only adding a phosphate buffer to each sample. A sample volume of 100 μL or 350 μL is used for the analysis and the quality-control procedures detect irregularities from potential sample degradation. The measurements of all 249 metabolites, including 14 lipoproteins subclasses, fatty acids, and various low-molecular weight metabolites, such as amino acids, ketone bodies, and glycolysis metabolites and fluid balance related metabolites (albumin and creatinine), were yielded automatically at once [10]. The NMR metabolomics platform has now been applied to large-scale epidemiological studies and in clinical settings. We obtained metabolites quantified in absolute mmol/l units and standardized them before analysis.

2.3. Assessment of Dietary Intake

At recruitment, participants electronically signed consent forms and were invited to assessment centres for verbal interviews, physical measures, biosample collection, and completed various questionnaires. The baseline questionnaires collected information on sociodemographic (i.e., ethnicity, employment status, marital status, education, income etc.), lifestyle (i.e., diet, food consumption, physical activity, smoking and alcohol drinking etc.), as well as a dietary questionnaire [11]. The intakes of processed meat (i.e., bacon, ham, sausages, meat pies, kebabs, burgers, chicken nuggets), and unprocessed red meat (i.e., unprocessed beef, lamb/mutton, and pork) was obtained from the baseline questionnaires. The intakes of unprocessed red meat and processed meat were transformed into weekly frequency of consumption: never eaten = 0, eaten < 1 time/week = 0.5, 1 time/week = 1, 2–4 times/week = 3, 5–6 times/week = 5.5, and ≥1 time daily = 7; 'Do not know' or 'prefer not to answer' were coded as missingness.

2.4. Assessment of Potential Confounders

Information on age, ethnic background, smoking status, Townsend deprivation Index, education, physical activity level, smoking status and alcohol drinking status was collected by baseline questionnaires. Ethnicity was regrouped into 5 categories as: White; Asian or Asian British; Black or Black British; Chinese; mixed; and Other. Acquired qualifications including 'College or University degree', 'A levels/AS levels or equivalent', 'O levels/GCSEs or equivalent', 'CSEs or equivalent', 'NVQ or HND or HNC or equivalent', 'Other professional qualifications' were regrouped as 'with college/university degree' and 'without college/university degree'. Townsend deprivation Index is calculated based on unemployment, overcrowded households, households without car ownership, and non-home owners percentages [12]. Physical activity measurement was taken from the International Physical activity questionnaire at baseline and was classified as low, moderate, and high levels [13]. Smoking status and alcohol drinking status were classified as never, previous, and current users. Body mass index (BMI) is calculated by dividing weight (kg) by standing height^2 (m^2) measured during the baseline assessments according to standard protocol.

2.5. Statistical Analysis

We used multivariable regression to assess the association of unprocessed red meat consumption and processed meat consumption with each metabolite in men and women separately, controlling for age, ethnicity, Townsend deprivation Index, education, physical activity level, smoking status, and drinking status in model 1. As BMI is a potential confounder or a mediator, we further controlled for BMI in model 2. To account for multiple testing, we controlled the false discovery rate (FDR) at 5% [14]. We then selected metabolites significantly associated with red meat consumption in men and women separately, after controlling for multiple testing. For the metabolites which passed the statistical significance in both men and women, we also tested whether the associations differ by sex. Sex differences were estimated using z-test with a statistical significance of $p < 0.05$. All statistical analyses were conducted using R version 4.0.1 (Foundation for Statistical Computing, Vienna, Austria).

3. Results

Baseline characteristics of the included ~79,644 participants (47.7% men) with information of both meat consumption and metabolites measures were shown in Table S1. The mean ages of men and women were 56.7 years, and 56.3 years, respectively. As expected, men consume more meat (2.29 times per week) than women (1.98 times per week), and both men and women eat more unprocessed red meat than processed meat (Supplemental Table S1).

Among 167 metabolites examined, we found 148 significant metabolites in men and 149 in women associated with unprocessed red meat consumption (Figure 1). Majorities of associations remained after controlling for BMI in model 2 (Figures 1 and 2). Among these 148 metabolites in men and 149 metabolites in women, 135 metabolites are shared in men and women. Regarding processed meat consumption, 148 significant metabolites were found in men and 130 in women (Figure 2). Among these, 122 metabolites are shared in men and in women. When testing the heterogeneity by sex, 34 metabolites had sex differences (testing for sex difference with significance of p value < 0.05) corresponding to unprocessed red meat consumption (Table S2), and 45 for processed meat consumption (Table S3).

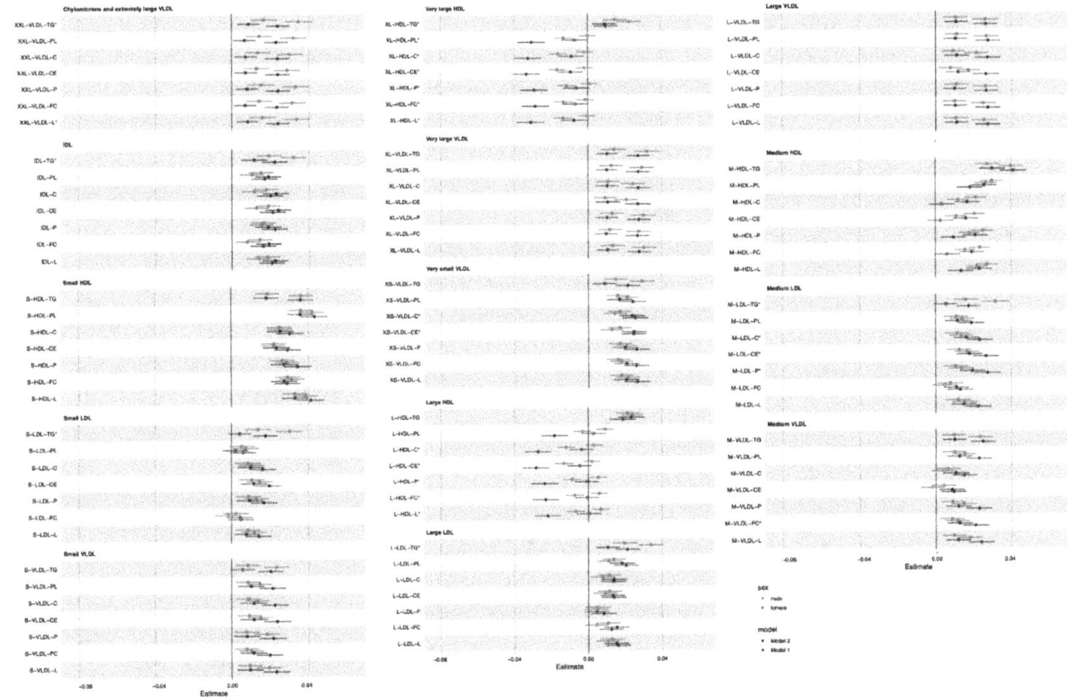

(a)

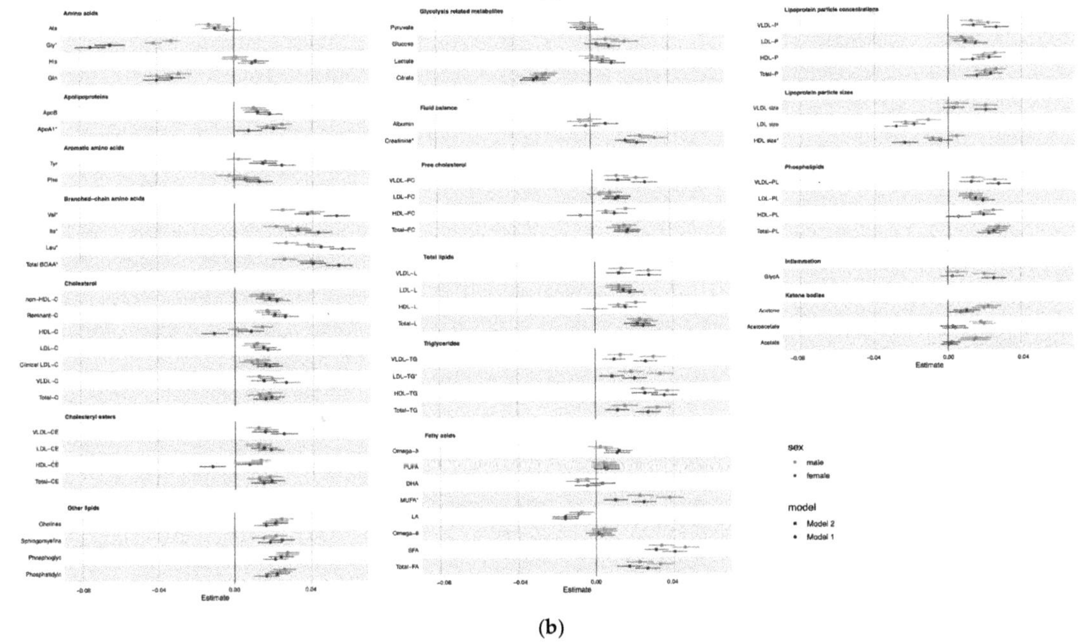

(b)

Figure 1. Associations of unprocessed red meat consumption with metabolites in men and women. (**a**) Associations with lipid subclasses. (**b**) Associations with other metabolites. Footnote: Mode l adjusted for age at recruitment, ethnicity (White/Asian or Asian British/Black or BlackBritish/Chinese/Mixed/Other), Townsend deprivation Index (TDI), education (with/without university degree), physical activity level (low/moderate/high), smoking status (never/previous/current), alcohol drinking status (never/previous/current); model 2 additionally adjusted for body mass index (BMI). Non-significant associations that did not pass FDR < 5% threshold is shown in hollow dot. Metabolites showing significant sex differences after adjusting for minimally adjusted confounders are indicated with *.

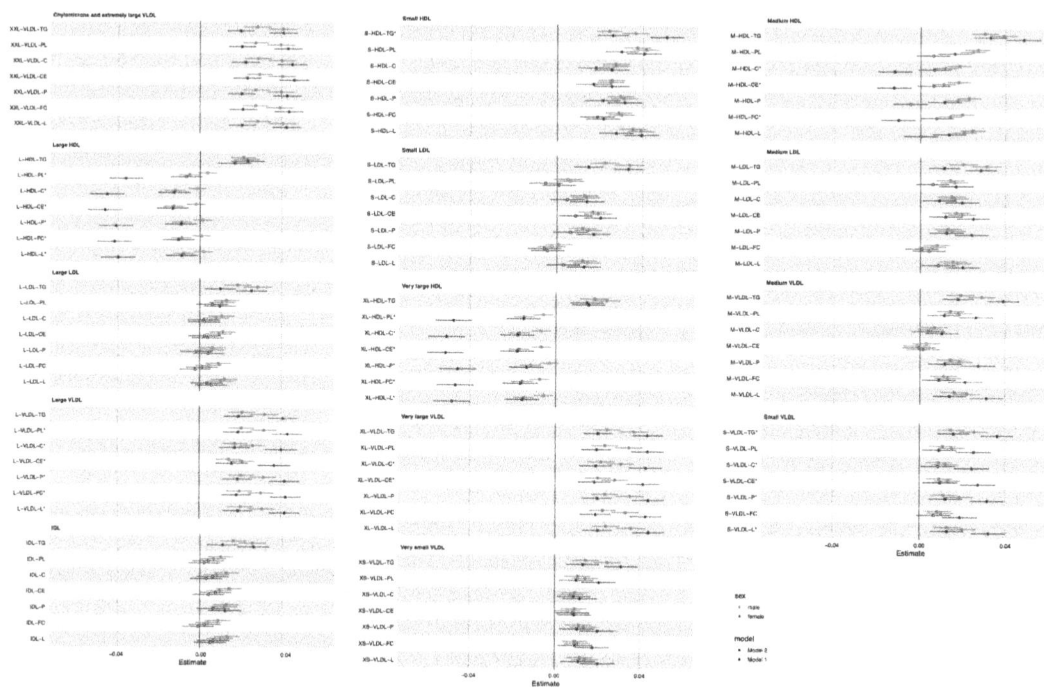

(a)

Figure 2. *Cont.*

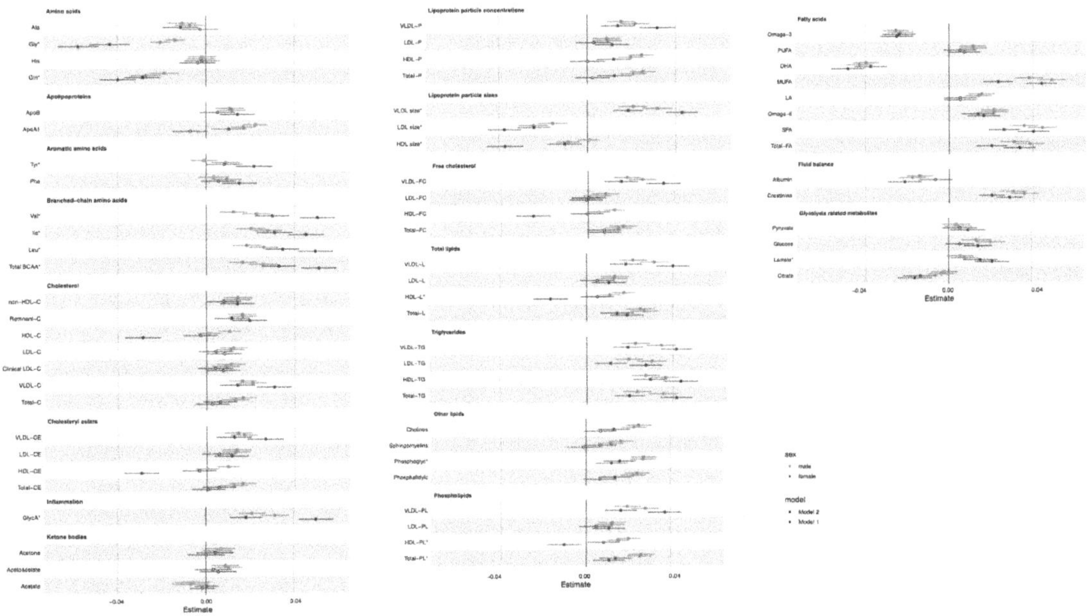

(**b**)

Figure 2. Associations of processed meat consumption with metabolites in men and women. (**a**) Associations with lipid subclasses. (**b**) Associations with other metabolites. Footnote: Mode 1 adjusted for age at recruitment, ethnicity (White/Asian or Asian British/Black or Black British/Chinese/Mixed/Other), Townsend deprivation Index (TDI), education (with/without university degree), physical activity level (low/moderate/high), smoking status (never/previous/current), alcohol drinking status (never/previous/current); model 2 additionally adjusted for body mass index (BMI). Non-significant associations that did not pass FDR < 5% threshold is shown in hollow dot. Metabolites showing significant sex differences after adjusting for minimally adjusted confounders are indicated with *.

For unprocessed red meat consumption, its positive association with branched-chain amino acids and various lipid measures in lipoprotein subclasses including cholesterol and cholesterol esters in very small very-low-density lipoprotein (VLDL), triglycerides, cholesterol, cholesterol esters, and phospholipids in medium low-density lipoprotein (LDL) and free cholesterol in medium VLDL; as well as its inverse association with glycine, high-density lipoprotein (HDL) size, cholesterol, cholesterol esters, phospholipids, free cholesterol and lipids in large HDL and all lipid measures in large HDL is larger in women than in men (Figure 1). More unprocessed red meat consumption is also related to higher apolipoprotein A1, creatinine, monounsaturated fatty acids, triglycerides, and lipids in chylomicrons and extremely large VLDL, as well as triglycerides in small LDL, medium LDL, intermediate-density lipoprotein (IDL), LDL, large LDL, and very large HDL. These metabolites have stronger associations with unprocessed red meat consumption in men than in women (Figure 1).

More processed meat consumption is associated with higher branched-chain amino acids, tyrosine, glycolysis related metabolite lactate, inflammation marker glycoprotein acetyls, triglycerides in small HDL and small VLDL, total lipids, phospholipids, free cholesterol, cholesteryl esters, cholesterol in large VLDL, and large VLDL particles sizes but lower glutamine, glycine, LDL and HDL participle sizes, phosphoglycerides, free cholesterol, cholesteryl esters and cholesterol in medium HDL, and phospholipids in HDL, large HDL, large VLDL, and very large HDL, the associations are generally larger in women than in men (Figure 2).

4. Discussion

This is the first study comprehensively evaluating the sex-specific association of red meat and processed meat consumption with 167 metabolites in the UK Biobank. We added to the limited evidence on sex disparity in association, by showing various metabolites, such as branched-chain amino acids, glycine, monounsaturated fatty acids, lipids in lipoprotein subclasses, apolipoprotein A1, and creatinine were linked to red meat consumption. These sex differences may underlie differential metabolic and cardiovascular risk.

Red meat is rich in essential amino acids, consistently we found red meat and processed meat consumption are associated with higher branched-chain amino acids in both sexes. Previous evidence has shown that branched-chain amino acids may link to higher risk of diabetes [7] and cardiovascular disease [15]. Their stronger positive associations in women are consistent with a previous cohort study suggesting women had a higher risk of ischemic heart disease associated with red meat consumption than men [16]. We also found the inverse associations with glycine in response to both red meat and processed meat consumption are larger in women than in men. Glycine is related to insulin resistance and may be linked to risk of type 2 diabetes [7]. The evidence regarding sex-specific associations with tyrosine and glutamine has not been reported previously, hence, these results need to be replicated.

Cholesterol and triglycerides are the major lipids that are transported in plasma by lipoproteins. The associations of red meat consumption with higher lipids for lipoprotein subclasses are partly consistent with a previous Chinese study [6], that reported increased cardiovascular disease risk with these metabolites. Our findings showed these associations of lipids and lipoprotein metabolites in response to meat consumption were stronger in women than in men. The sex disparity in apolipoprotein A1, the main apolipoprotein of plasma HDL, was also consistent with the patterns for HDL and its subclasses. However, the underlying mechanisms are unclear. A possible explanation is that red meat may alter sex hormones which could play a role modulating lipid and lipoprotein metabolism [17].

Moreover, we found red meat was associated with higher serum creatinine in men than in women. Men have more red meat consumption and more muscle mass that produce creatine than women, which were converted to creatinine that is excreted by the kidneys into the urine [18]. This is consistent with the sex-specific association of red meat consumption with creatinine. Women had more pronounced increase in glycolysis-related lactate with regard to processed meat but not red meat intake, that could be due to the use of lactate in processed meat for antimicrobial and flavoring purposes [19]. Glycoprotein acetyls biomarker could predict risk of cardiovascular and diabetic risk outcomes [20]. Here we showed more elevated inflammation marker glycoprotein acetyls associated with processed meat consumption in women than in men, possibly because processed meat could change female sex hormone estrogen that regulates metabolic inflammation [21]. Whether this biomarker mediates the sex-specific association between processed meat consumption and cardiometabolic risks requires further investigation.

Our study takes advantage of powerful metabolomics data in UK Biobank to study sex-specific associations of meat consumption and metabolic factors. Despite the novelty, there are several limitations. First, self-reported questionnaires for ascertaining dietary intake are susceptible to recall bias. Second, residual confounding may still exist, even if potential confounding factors such as baseline sociodemographic factors, lifestyle factors, and BMI were adjusted in multivariable models. These associations should be confirmed in interventional studies. Third, UK Biobank participants are not fully representative because they are healthier than the general population [22], and results from Europeans may not be generalized to other populations with different dietary habits.

Taken together, our study is in line with the US 2020–2025 Dietary Guidelines regarding the limitation of meat consumption. In addition, our study provides information on the sex-specific associations of red meat consumption with metabolites, which may promote the consideration of sex disparity in the future dietary recommendations. Although in dietary recommendations, red meat is grouped under the category of "protein foods", in our study, a large variety of metabolites including lipids, lipoproteins, fatty acids, amino acids and fluid balance indicator (creatinine), correspond to red meat consumption. This means that people with hyperlipidemia and metabolic dysfunction, such as people with renal failure and Maple syrup urine disease (with excessive accumulation of branched-chain amino acids in the organism) are especially recommended to limit red meat intake. Our finding regarding the sex-specific associations of red meat consumption with metabolites may also be applied to health promotion programs, to advance the lowering of red meat consumption thereby lowering the risk of cardiometabolic diseases (Figure 3).

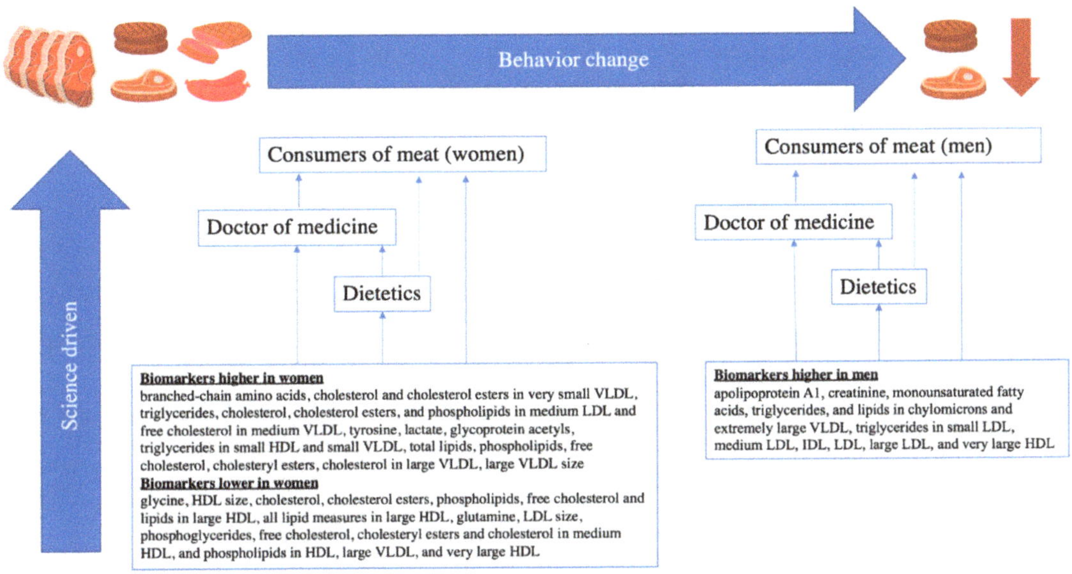

Figure 3. A simple model comprising the key findings of this study, consumers of meat (men and women), doctors of medicine, and dietetics to demonstrate science-based health education strategy.

5. Conclusions

We showed meat consumption was associated with metabolites by sex, which are consistent with differential cardiometabolic disease risk related to meat consumption. The study has important implications in primary prevention and treatment because diet is modifiable that can be incorporated into people's daily life. Our study suggested that people with hyperlipidemia and metabolic dysfunction, such as people with renal failure and Maple syrup urine disease, are especially recommended to limit red meat and processed meat consumption. Given the sex-disparity in the associations with metabolites, our findings also suggested that sex disparity should be considered in dietary suggestions.

Supplementary Materials: The following supporting information can be downloaded at: https://www.mdpi.com/article/10.3390/nu14245306/s1, Table S1: Baseline characteristics of participants included in the study. Table S2: Sex differences for metabolites and unprocessed red meat consumption. Table S3: Sex differences for metabolites and processed meat consumption.

Author Contributions: J.V.Z. conceived the idea and designed the study; B.F. drafted the manuscript with great help of J.V.Z.; J.V.Z. did the data acquisition; B.F. conducted the analysis with double check by J.V.Z.; B.F. and J.V.Z. interpreted the results; J.V.Z. critically revised the manuscript for important intellectual content. All authors have read and agreed to the published version of the manuscript.

Funding: This research received no external funding.

Institutional Review Board Statement: This research has been conducted using the UK Biobank Resource under application number 42468. The UK Biobank has already received the ethical approval from North West Multi-centre Research Ethics Committee (MREC) which covers the UK. It also got the approval from the Patient Information Advisory Group (PIAG) in England and Wales and from the Community Health Index Advisory Group (CHIAG) in Scotland. Ethical review and approval were waived for this study because UK Biobank has approval from the North West Multi-centre Research Ethics Committee (MREC) as a Research Tissue Bank (RTB) approval. This approval means that researchers do not require separate ethical clearance and can operate under the RTB approval.

Informed Consent Statement: Written informed consent was obtained from all participants in the UK Biobank.

Data Availability Statement: Data described in the manuscript will be available upon request and approval by the UK Biobank (https://www.ukbiobank.ac.uk/enable-your-research/apply-for-access, accessed on 10 November 2022).

Acknowledgments: The authors would like to thank the UK Biobank for approving our application (#42468) and shared the valuable data.

Conflicts of Interest: The authors declare no conflict of interest.

References

1. Global, regional, and national age-sex-specific mortality for 282 causes of death in 195 countries and territories, 1980–2017: A systematic analysis for the Global Burden of Disease Study 2017. *Lancet* **2018**, *392*, 1736–1788. [CrossRef]
2. *Dietary Guidelines for Americans, 2020–2025*, 9th ed.; US Department of Health and Human Services, US Department of Agriculture: Washington, DC, USA, 2020.
3. Zhong, V.W.; Van Horn, L.; Greenland, P.; Carnethon, M.R.; Ning, H.; Wilkins, J.T.; Lloyd-Jones, D.M.; Allen, N.B. Associations of Processed Meat, Unprocessed Red Meat, Poultry, or Fish Intake With Incident Cardiovascular Disease and All-Cause Mortality. *JAMA Intern. Med.* **2020**, *180*, 503. [CrossRef] [PubMed]
4. Micha, R.; Peñalvo, J.L.; Cudhea, F.; Imamura, F.; Rehm, C.D.; Mozaffarian, D. Association Between Dietary Factors and Mortality from Heart Disease, Stroke, and Type 2 Diabetes in the United States. *JAMA* **2017**, *317*, 912. [CrossRef] [PubMed]
5. Wang, Z.; Bergeron, N.; Levison, B.S.; Li, X.S.; Chiu, S.; Jia, X.; Koeth, R.A.; Li, L.; Wu, Y.; Tang, W.H.W.; et al. Impact of chronic dietary red meat, white meat, or non-meat protein on trimethylamine N-oxide metabolism and renal excretion in healthy men and women. *Eur. Heart J.* **2019**, *40*, 583–594. [CrossRef] [PubMed]
6. Pan, L.; Chen, L.; Lv, J.; Pang, Y.; Guo, Y.; Pei, P.; Du, H.; Yang, L.; Millwood, I.Y.; Walters, R.G.; et al. Association of Red Meat Consumption, Metabolic Markers, and Risk of Cardiovascular Diseases. *Front. Nutr.* **2022**, *9*, 703. [CrossRef] [PubMed]
7. Wittenbecher, C.; Mühlenbruch, K.; Kröger, J.; Jacobs, S.; Kuxhaus, O.; Floegel, A.; Fritsche, A.; Pischon, T.; Prehn, C.; Adamski, J.; et al. Amino acids, lipid metabolites, and ferritin as potential mediators linking red meat consumption to type 2 diabetes. *Am. J. Clin. Nutr.* **2015**, *101*, 1241–1250. [CrossRef] [PubMed]
8. Soininen, P.; Kangas, A.J.; Würtz, P.; Suna, T.; Ala-Korpela, M. Quantitative Serum Nuclear Magnetic Resonance Metabolomics in Cardiovascular Epidemiology and Genetics. *Circ. Cardiovasc. Genet.* **2015**, *8*, 192–206. [CrossRef] [PubMed]
9. Sudlow, C.; Gallacher, J.; Allen, N.; Beral, V.; Burton, P.; Danesh, J.; Downey, P.; Elliott, P.; Green, J.; Landray, M.; et al. UK Biobank: An Open Access Resource for Identifying the Causes of a Wide Range of Complex Diseases of Middle and Old Age. *PLoS Med.* **2015**, *12*, e1001779. [CrossRef] [PubMed]
10. Würtz, P.; Kangas, A.J.; Soininen, P.; Lawlor, D.A.; Davey Smith, G.; Ala-Korpela, M. Quantitative Serum Nuclear Magnetic Resonance Metabolomics in Large-Scale Epidemiology: A Primer on-Omic Technologies. *Am. J. Epidemiol.* **2017**, *186*, 1084–1096. [CrossRef] [PubMed]
11. Bradbury, K.E.; Young, H.J.; Guo, W.; Key, T.J. Dietary assessment in UK Biobank: An evaluation of the performance of the touchscreen dietary questionnaire. *J. Nutr. Sci.* **2018**, *7*, E6. [CrossRef] [PubMed]
12. Townsend, P.; Phillimore, P.; Beattie, A. *Health and Deprivation: Inequality and the North*; Croom Helm: London, UK, 1988.
13. Craig, C.L.; Marshall, A.L.; Sjöström, M.; Bauman, A.E.; Booth, M.L.; Ainsworth, B.E.; Pratt, M.; Ekelund, U.; Yngve, A.; Sallis, J.F.; et al. International Physical Activity Questionnaire: 12-Country Reliability and Validity. *Med. Sci. Sport. Exerc.* **2003**, *35*, 1381–1395. [CrossRef] [PubMed]
14. Benjamini, Y.; Hochberg, Y. Controlling the False Discovery Rate: A Practical and Powerful Approach to Multiple Testing. *J. R. Stat. Soc. Ser. B* **1995**, *57*, 289–300. [CrossRef]
15. Wang, Y.; Huang, K.; Liu, F.; Lu, X.; Huang, J.; Gu, D. Association of circulating branched-chain amino acids with risk of cardiovascular disease: A systematic review and meta-analysis. *Atherosclerosis* **2022**, *350*, 90–96. [CrossRef] [PubMed]

16. Zhang, J.; Hayden, K.; Jackson, R.; Schutte, R. Association of red and processed meat consumption with cardiovascular morbidity and mortality in participants with and without obesity: A prospective cohort study. *Clin. Nutr.* **2021**, *40*, 3643–3649. [CrossRef] [PubMed]
17. Palmisano, B.T.; Zhu, L.; Eckel, R.H.; Stafford, J.M. Sex differences in lipid and lipoprotein metabolism. *Mol. Metab.* **2018**, *15*, 45–55. [CrossRef] [PubMed]
18. Wyss, M.; Kaddurah-Daouk, R. Creatine and Creatinine Metabolism. *Physiol. Rev.* **2000**, *80*, 1107–1213. [CrossRef] [PubMed]
19. Sebranek, J.G. An overview of functional non-meat ingredients in meat processing: The current toolbox. In Proceedings of the 68th Annual Reciprocal Meat Conference, Lincoln, NE, USA, 18 December 2015; pp. 42–46.
20. Kettunen, J.; Ritchie, S.C.; Anufrieva, O.; Lyytikäinen, L.-P.; Hernesniemi, J.; Karhunen, P.J.; Kuukasjärvi, P.; Laurikka, J.; Kähönen, M.; Lehtimäki, T.; et al. Biomarker Glycoprotein Acetyls Is Associated with the Risk of a Wide Spectrum of Incident Diseases and Stratifies Mortality Risk in Angiography Patients. *Circ. Genom. Precis. Med.* **2018**, *11*, e002234. [CrossRef]
21. Coffey, D.S. Similarities of prostate and breast cancer: Evolution, diet, and estrogens. *Urology* **2001**, *57*, 31–38. [CrossRef] [PubMed]
22. Fry, A.; Littlejohns, T.J.; Sudlow, C.; Doherty, N.; Adamska, L.; Sprosen, T.; Collins, R.; Allen, N.E. Comparison of Sociodemographic and Health-Related Characteristics of UK Biobank Participants with Those of the General Population. *Am. J. Epidemiol.* **2017**, *186*, 1026–1034. [CrossRef]

nutrients

MDPI

Article

Differences in Dietary and Lifestyle Triggers between Non-Erosive Reflux Disease and Reflux Esophagitis—A Multicenter Cross-Sectional Survey in China

Yang Chen [1,†], Xiaohong Sun [1,2,†], Wenjuan Fan [3,†], Jiao Yu [4], Peng Wang [5], Dong Liu [6], Mingwei Song [1,7], Shi Liu [4], Xiuli Zuo [5], Rong Zhang [6], Yuantao Hou [1], Shaomei Han [8], Yanqing Li [5], Jun Zhang [6], Xiaoqing Li [1], Meiyun Ke [1] and Xiucai Fang [1,*]

1 Department of Gastroenterology, Peking Union Medical College Hospital, Chinese Academy of Medical Sciences and Peking Union Medical College, Beijing 100730, China; dr_chenyang@126.com (Y.C.); sunxiaoh2010@126.com (X.S.); songmingwei163@163.com (M.S.); houyuantao2013@163.com (Y.H.); lixiaoqing20060417@126.com (X.L.); kemypumch2006@aliyun.com (M.K.)

2 Department of Geriatrics, Peking Union Medical College Hospital, Chinese Academy of Medical Sciences and Peking Union Medical College, Beijing 100730, China

3 Department of Gastroenterology, Tongji Hospital, Tongji Medical College, Huazhong University of Science and Technology, Wuhan 430030, China; juanwenfan1989@163.com

4 Department of Gastroenterology, Union Hospital, Tongji Medical College, Huazhong University of Science and Technology, Wuhan 430022, China; liusu1982@163.com (J.Y.); 1986xh0568@hust.edu.cn (S.L.)

5 Department of Gastroenterology, Qilu Hospital of Shandong University, Jinan 250012, China; wangpeng_qd@163.com (P.W.); zuoxiuli@sdu.edu.cn (X.Z.); liyanqing@sdu.edu.cn (Y.L.)

6 Department of Gastroenterology, The Second Affiliated Hospital, Xi'an Jiaotong University, Xi'an 710003, China; liudong_doc@163.com (D.L.); zr4056@163.com (R.Z.); jun3z@163.com (J.Z.)

7 Department of Gastroenterology and Hepatology, Tianjin Medical University General Hospital, Tianjin 300052, China

8 Department of Epidemiology and Statistics, Institute of Basic Medical Sciences, Chinese Academy of Medical Sciences & School of Basic Medicine, Peking Union Medical College, Beijing 100005, China; hansm5102@outlook.com

* Correspondence: fangxiucai2@aliyun.com

† These authors contributed equally to this work.

Abstract: The occurrence of gastroesophageal reflux disease (GERD) and symptom onset are closely associated with diet. We aimed to compare the dietary and lifestyle triggers between non-erosive reflux disease (NERD) and reflux esophagitis (RE) in Chinese patients and to provide evidence for development of practical dietary modifications for GERD. A multicenter cross-sectional survey was conducted. A total of 396 GERD patients with typical gastroesophageal reflux symptoms who received upper endoscopy in the previous month were enrolled, including 203 cases of NERD patients and 193 cases of RE patients. All participants completed questionnaires including demographic data, reflux symptoms, previous management, dietary and lifestyle habits, triggers of reflux symptoms, psychological status, and quality of life. There were no significant differences in GERD symptom scores between NERD and RE. RE patients had a higher male proportion and smoking/drinking and overeating rates than NERD patients. In the NERD group, more patients reported that fruits, dairy products, yogurt, bean products, cold food, and carbonated beverages sometimes and often induced reflux symptoms and had more triggers compared to RE patients. The number of triggers was positively correlated to GERD symptom score and GERD-HRQL score in both NERD and RE patients. However, 74.0% of GERD patients still often consumed the triggering foods, even those foods that sometimes and often induced their reflux symptoms, which might be related to the reflux relapse after PPI withdrawal considering NERD and RE patients had similar GERD symptom severity. There were some differences in terms of dietary habits, dietary and lifestyle triggers, and related quality of life between NERD and RE, and these results may provide evidence of different approaches toward the dietary modification of NERD and RE patients.

Keywords: gastroesophageal reflux disease; non-erosive reflux disease; reflux esophagitis; diet; lifestyle; triggers

1. Introduction

Gastroesophageal reflux disease (GERD) is the condition in which the reflux of gastric contents into the esophagus results in symptoms and/or complications [1,2]. Typical symptoms include heartburn and regurgitation. The extra-esophageal symptoms present in about one-third GERD patients, including laryngeal, oropharyngeal, pulmonary, and sleep-related symptoms [3,4]. All these symptoms adversely affect health-related quality of life, especially when complications occur, such as esophageal ulceration, stricture, perforation, metaplasia, and adenocarcinoma. The overall pooled prevalence of GERD is about 14.0% and varied greatly according to region and country. The highest prevalence was in North America (19.6%), followed by Europe (14.1%), and Asia (12.9%) [5]. Over the past two decades, the prevalence of GERD in China has increased from 6.0% to 10.6% [6]. The incidence was approximately 5 and 7 per 1000 person years in the Western world and China, respectively [7,8]. GERD has brought substantial economic and health burdens to patients and society. The annual direct cost of GERD management in the USA is ranging from USD 9.3 to 12.1 billion, especially in patients with extra-esophageal symptom [7,9].

According to esophageal mucosa injury condition under endoscopy, GERD could be categorized into non-erosive reflux disease (NERD), reflux esophagitis (RE), and Barrett's esophagus (BE). The most common subtype is NERD, which accounts for 60–70% of GERD patients, followed by RE (30%) and BE (6–8%) in Western counties [10]. The pathophysiology of GERD is multifactorial, including a poorly functioning anti-reflux barrier, impaired esophageal clearance and motility, decreased salivary production, delayed gastric emptying, and esophageal mucosal integrity and hypersensitivity (especially in NERD) [2,3,11].

The epidemiological studies of Western countries revealed GERD is associated with some dietary triggers, including increased consumption of high fat diet, sweets, chocolate, coffee and caffeine, spicy food, carbonated beverages, and acidic foods, such as citrus and tomatoes, salt, tobacco, and alcohol, while it is inversely associated with consumption of fruit and fiber [12–14]. Eating habits such as irregular meal pattern, large volume of meals, and eating meals just before bedtime may correlate with reflux symptom onset. Obesity is a strong risk factor for GERD [3,12,15]. It was noted there are some differences in the associated dietary and lifestyle risk factors between NERD and RE, which seem to have different pathophysiological mechanisms and clinical characteristics [11]. It is reported that female gender, younger age, low body mass index (BMI), non-smoking, absence of hiatal hernia, psychological distress, and severity of gastric atrophy were positively associated with NERD compared with RE in Japanese patients [16–18]. In Korean subjects, a higher dietary intake of beans, fruits, vegetables, seaweed, fish, milk, eggs, and drinking tea reduced NERD prevalence, but the dietary component had little effect on RE, while RE was associated with men, high BMI, alcohol, hiatal hernia, and total energy intake rather than dietary component [19,20]. Dietary and lifestyle modifications are first-line therapy for GERD patients, including avoidance of the trigger foods above, reducing or quitting tobacco/smoking, weight loss in overweight and obese patients, and elevating the head of the bed at nighttime [2].

Dietary habits and lifestyles differ between regions. There are various dietary cuisines, including food categories and cooking methods in China, which makes it difficult to identify the dietary risk factors of GERD. While GERD has increased over the past few decades, there are few studies on differences in diet and lifestyle triggers between NERD and RE in the Chinese population. Therefore, we aimed to investigate the diet and lifestyle triggers between RE and NERD in a large multicenter cross-sectional survey to understand the comprehensive relationship between the patient's diets and lifestyles and reflux symptoms and to provide more lifestyle advices for GERD patients with similar dietary culture.

2. Materials and Methods

2.1. Study Design and Population

Consecutive adult patients with GERD aged 18–80 years were enrolled in this study from the gastroenterology clinics in four tertiary hospitals from November 2011 to October 2012. All patients had experienced typical reflux symptoms, i.e., mild heartburn and/or regurgitation symptoms, for at least 2 days per week or moderate/severe reflux symptoms for more than 1 day per week [1] during the previous 3 months and had upper endoscopy examinations in the previous month, which was used to classify GERD into NERD and RE as well as the severity of RE graded from A to D according to the Los Angeles classification [21]. Patients with secondary esophagitis, peptic ulcer, malignant cancer, and surgery of upper gastrointestinal tract were excluded from this study. All participants provided oral consent to participate before the enrollment.

The study was designed to consecutively enroll 100 patients with NERD and 100 patients with RE in each hospital.

The study was approved by the Ethics Committee of Peking Union Medical College Hospital (Project identification code I-23PJ1009).

2.2. Questionnaires and Data Collection

"Questionnaire of GERD and diets" consists of demographic data, GERD symptoms and extra-esophageal symptoms, GERD-related tests and previous management, alarm signs and comorbid diseases, psychological and sleeping status, dietary habits and lifestyle, dietary and other triggers for reflux symptoms, and so on. The typical GERD symptoms include heartburn, acid reflux, food regurgitation, and retrosternal chest pain. The severity of each symptom during the previous 3 months was graded as follows: 0 = no symptom, 1 = mild symptoms which can be felt when paying attention and no interference with normal activity or sleep; 2 = moderate symptoms between mild and severe and mild interference with normal daily activities or sleep; and 3 = severe symptoms and marked interference with normal daily activities or sleep. The frequency of each symptom was recorded as days per week and further scored as follows: 0 = none; 1 = <2 days per week; 2 = 2–4 days per week; 3 = >4 days per week [22]. The GERD symptom score was the product of severity and frequency. The extra-esophageal symptoms include swallow related pain or dysphagia, respiratory (chronic cough, asthma, short of breath, and snore), laryngopharyngeal (hoarseness, sensation of a lump in the throat, sore or burning throat), and oral symptoms (toothache, dental erosion). The extra-esophageal symptoms were recorded at the levels of severity mentioned above.

According to Chinese's dietary peculiarities, we asked the following questions concerning diet habits and lifestyle in the questionnaire: the type of staple food, the proportion of staple foods and dishes, the amounts of vegetables/fruits and meat consumed, food preferences (listing eight kinds of common foods), eating habits (degree of satiety and eating speed), association of reflux symptoms and meals in time, and smoking and drinking. Among the factors that may trigger reflux symptoms, 25 dietary and 6 other factors (including lifestyle) were listed for patients to choose and answer with options "never triggered, occasionally, sometimes, and often or never experienced".

The questionnaires also included questions about anxiety, depression, and sleeping disorders, such as "In the last 3 months, have you felt tense or wound up?" and "In the last 3 months, have you felt downhearted and low?". If participants answered these questions with "often" ($\geq$2 days a week) or "most of the time" or "always", they were defined as having self-reported anxiety or depression in this study [8,23]. Sleeping disorders were defined as difficulty in falling asleep, early awakening, shallow sleep, sleep time < 6 h, or daytime drowsiness. The questionnaire was completed by well-trained investigators in face-to-face interviews. The coexisting functional gastrointestinal disease, including functional dyspepsia (FD), functional constipation (FC), irritable bowel syndrome (IBS), and psychological and sleep disorders were recorded, which were diagnosed according to the Rome III diagnostic criteria [23].

The quality of life was assessed by gastroesophageal reflux disease health-related quality of life (GERD-HRQL) and 36-item short-form health survey (SF-36). These two instruments were completed by patients according to the instruction provided, and the total scores were calculated as in the previous publications [24,25].

2.3. Statistical Analysis

All statistical analyses were conducted by SPSS 25 (IBM, Armonk, NY, USA). We used mean ± standard deviation for continuous variables with normal distribution, median (interquartile range) for those without normal distribution, and count with percentage for categorical variables. Univariate analyses were performed using parametric (Student's *t*-test) or non-parametric methods (Mann–Whitney U test) for continuous variables, and chi-square test for categorical variables. NERD and RE patients were compared to assess their differences in demographic data, clinical symptoms, dietary habits, trigger factors, and management. *p*-Values are two-sided and considered significant when <0.05. Pearson's test and Spearman's test were performed to assess correlations between two quantitative variables with normal distribution and without normal distribution.

3. Results

3.1. Demographic Data

In total, 396 GERD patients were enrolled in this study, with an average age of 46.8 ± 12.7 years. There were 238 males (60.1%) and 158 females (39.9%). There were 203 NERD patients (51.3%) and 193 RE patients (48.7%). Among RE patients, 95 patients (49.2%) were classified as LA-A, and 76 (39.4%), 20 (10.4%), and 2 (1.0%) were classified as LA-B, LA-C, and LA-D respectively. Male patients were more likely to present with RE than female patients, and there were no significant differences in age, BMI, and other demographic characteristics (Table 1).

Table 1. Demographic data of RE and NERD patients.

Variable	NERD (n = 203)	RE (n = 193)	p-Value
Age (years)	45.1 ± 12.8	48.5 ± 12.3	0.729
Gender, n of male (%)	94 (46.3)	144 (74.6)	<0.001 *
BMI (kg/m^2)	22.8 ± 3.1	23.7 ± 3.0	0.472
Education level, n of college and above (%)	49 (24.2)	48 (24.8)	0.865
Family economic status, n of well-off and above (%)	94 (46.3)	72 (37.3)	0.070
Marriage status, n of married (%)	179(88.2)	179 (92.7)	0.123
Labor intensity, n of severe (%)	15 (7.4)	16 (8.3)	0.739

Data presented as mean ± standard deviation or number (%). Student's *t*-test and chi-square test. * *p*-value < 0.05.

3.2. Characteristics of Reflux Symptoms

There were no significant differences in general GERD symptom scores and the scores of heartburn, acid reflux, food regurgitation, and retrosternal chest pain between NERD and RE patients (Table 2).

There was no significant difference in extra-esophageal symptom score, including swallowing-related symptoms, respiratory symptoms, and laryngopharyngeal symptoms. The prevalence of oral symptoms of NERD patients was higher than for RE patients (Table 2).

In addition to GERD symptoms and extra-esophageal symptoms, we found NERD patients were more likely to coexist with FD and FC than RE patients. NERD patients had higher prevalence of self-reported anxiety and depression than RE patients, and more NERD patients thought that their reflux symptoms were related to emotion than RE patients (Table 2). NERD patients had a higher prevalence of sleep disorders but without significant difference compared with RE patients.

Table 2. Characteristics of clinical manifestations of RE and NERD patients.

Variable	NERD (n = 203)	RE (n = 193)	p-Value
GERD symptom score	7 (8)	8 (8)	0.277
Heartburn	3 (6)	3 (6)	0.460
Acid reflux	2 (6)	3 (5.8)	0.078
Food regurgitation	0 (0)	0 (0)	0.608
Retrosternal chest pain	0 (2)	0 (2)	0.723
Extra-esophageal symptoms			
Swallowing-related symptoms, n (%)	39 (19.2)	25 (13.0)	0.091
Respiratory symptoms, n (%)	120 (59.1)	122 (63.2)	0.403
Laryngopharyngeal symptoms, n (%)	119 (58.6)	98 (50.7)	0.117
Oral symptoms, n (%)	54 (26.6)	25 (13.0)	0.001 *
Coexisting functional dyspepsia, n (%)	63 (31.0)	32 (16.6)	0.001 *
Coexisting functional constipation, n (%)	19 (9.4)	8 (4.1)	0.040 *
Coexisting irritable bowel syndrome, n (%)	7 (3.4)	2 (1.0)	0.107
Feelings of anxiety, # n (%)	80 (39.4)	42 (21.8)	<0.001 *
Feelings of depression, # n (%)	64 (31.5)	40 (20.7)	0.015 *
GERD symptoms related to emotion, n (%)	50 (24.6)	24 (12.4)	0.002 *
Sleep disorder, n (%)	77 (37.9)	57 (29.5)	0.078
GERD symptoms related to sleep disorder, n (%)	60 (29.6)	40 (20.7)	0.083

Data presented as median (interquartile range) or number (%). Mann-Whitney test and chi-square test. * $p < 0.05$.
Patients with sometimes, often, and always had feelings of anxiety or depression.

We collected the data for pH or pH-impedance monitoring in 26 (12.8%) NERD patients and 15 (7.8%) RE patients, and we collected the data for esophageal manometry in 19 (9.4%) NERD patients and 12 (6.2%) RE patients while they were enrolled in this survey. We did not further analyze the association of dietary and lifestyle triggers and esophageal reflux and motility parameters in NERD and RE patients.

3.3. Characteristics of GERD Management

We summarized GERD management during the whole disease. Sixty-five (16.4%) patients used medications long term to treat GERD. Proton-pump inhibitors (PPIs) were mostly used by 225 (56.8%) patients and the effective rate was 50.2%. The relapse rate after PPI withdrawal was as high as 88.0%. There were no significant differences in patients who mostly used PPIs, H_2-receptor antagonists, or antacids and the effective rate and relapse rate after drug withdrawal between NERD and RE patients. In addition to medications, 93 (23.5%) patients raised the head of the bed, 99 (25.0%) patients stopped smoking and drinking, 96 (24.2%) patients chose a low-lipid and low-sugar diet, 174 (43.9%) patients avoided overeating to relieve symptoms, and 44.4% and 45.7% of NERD patients reported the effectiveness from a low-lipid/low-sugar diet and avoiding overeating respectively. There were no significant differences in the proportions of the above management strategies and effective rates between NERD and RE patients (Table 3).

Table 3. Management of RE and NERD patients.

Variable	NERD (n = 203)	RE (n = 193)	p-Value
Long-term use of medications	36 (17.7)	29 (15.0)	0.467
Proton-pump inhibitor was mostly used	125 (61.6)	100 (51.8)	0.050
Effective rate	63 (50.4)	50 (50.0)	0.952
Relapse after withdrawal	111 (88.8)	87 (87.0)	0.680
H_2-receptor antagonist was mostly used	27 (13.3)	24 (12.4)	0.797
Effective rate	12 (44.4)	10 (41.7)	0.842
Relapse after withdrawal	22 (81.5)	19(79.2)	0.835
Antacid was mostly used	29 (14.3)	19 (9.8)	0.176
Effective rate	11 (37.9)	4 (21.1)	0.217
Relapse after withdrawal	26 (89.5)	16 (84.2)	0.577
Raise the head of bed	60 (29.6)	33 (17.1)	0.354
Effective rate	20 (33.3)	11 (33.3)	1.000
Stop smoking and drinking	45 (22.2)	54 (28.0)	0.182
Effective rate	14 (31.1)	19 (35.2)	0.669
Low-lipid and low-sugar diet	54 (26.6)	42 (21.8)	0.261
Effective rate	24 (44.4)	12 (28.6)	0.111
Avoid overeating	92 (45.3)	82 (42.5)	0.570
Effective rate	42 (45.7)	27 (33.0)	0.087

Data presented as number (%). Chi-square test.

3.4. Dietary Habits

We compared dietary habits between NERD patients and RE patients. The RE group had a higher proportion of overeating than NERD patients (26.4% vs. 17.2%, p = 0.027). There were no significant differences in fast eating, degree of satiety, dominant food type, dish style, and consumption of fruits or meat between the two groups. The rates of patients who often consumed spicy food, greasy food, sweet food, sticky food, cold food, carbonated beverages, coffee, and strong tea had no significant difference between the two groups. In the RE group, more patients had smoking and drinking habits than did NERD patients (Table 4).

Table 4. Comparison of dietary habits between RE and NERD patients.

Variable	NERD (n = 203)	RE (n = 193)	p-Value
Overeating, n (%)	35 (17.2)	51 (26.4)	0.027 *
Fast eating, n (%)	77 (37.9)	91 (47.2)	0.064
Degree of satiety (0–10)	8.9 ± 6.0	8.5 ± 1.2	0.936
Dominant food			0.163
Staple food, n (%)	86 (42.4)	64 (33.2)	
Dish food, n (%)	15 (7.4)	18 (9.3)	
Both equivalent, n (%)	102 (50.2)	111 (57.5)	
Dish styles			0.055

Table 4. *Cont.*

Variable	NERD (n = 203)	RE (n = 193)	p-Value
More vegetables, n (%)	89 (43.8)	63 (32.6)	
More meat, n (%)	17 (8.4)	24 (12.4)	
Both equivalent, n (%)	97 (47.8)	106 (54.9)	
Consumption of fruits			0.319
Seldom, n (%)	51 (25.1)	45 (23.3)	
Moderate, n (%)	137 (67.5)	140 (72.5)	
Much, n (%)	15 (7.4)	8 (4.1)	
Consumption of meat			0.087
Seldom, n (%)	66 (32.5)	44 (22.8)	
Moderate, n (%)	121 (59.6)	138 (71.5)	
Much, n (%)	15 (7.4)	11 (5.7)	
Often consumption of foods			
Spicy, n (%)	33 (16.3)	35 (18.1)	0.145
Greasy, n (%)	25 (12.3)	28 (14.5)	0.386
Sweet food, n (%)	22 (10.8)	16 (8.3)	0.390
Sticky food, n (%)	8 (3.9)	7 (3.6)	0.870
Cold food, n (%)	19 (9.4)	9 (4.7)	0.068
Acid drink, n (%)	6 (3.0)	5 (2.6)	0.238
Coffee, n (%)	2 (1.0)	6 (3.1)	0.280
Strong tea, n (%)	1 (0.5)	1 (0.5)	0.549
Smoking, n (%)	41 (20.2)	67 (34.8)	0.001 *
Drinking, n (%)	42 (20.7)	74 (38.3)	<0.001 *

Data presented as mean ± standard deviation or number (%). Student's t-test and chi-square test. * $p < 0.05$.

3.5. Triggers of GERD Symptoms

We compared dietary and other lifestyle triggers that sometimes and often induced GERD symptoms between NERD patients and RE patients (Table 5). In the NERD group, more patients reported fruits, dairy products, yogurt, bean products, uncooked food, cold food, midnight snacks, sweet food, cold weather, and emotional disturbance sometimes and often induced GERD symptoms than did RE patients. The mean number of triggers was higher in NERD patients than in RE (5 [8] vs. 4 [6], $p = 0.007$). In all of the GERD patients, 346 (87.4%) patients had at least one trigger and 274 (69.2%), 204 (51.5%), 90 (22.7%), and 13 (3.3%) patients had at least 3, 5, 10, and 20 triggers, respectively. The percentages of patients who had at least 3, 5, and 20 triggers in the NERD group were higher than the RE group (74.9% vs. 63.2%, $p = 0.012$; 59.6% vs. 43.0%, $p = 0.001$; and 5.4% vs. 1.0%, $p = 0.014$, respectively). The number of triggers was positively correlated to the GERD symptom score in both NERD and RE patients (Figure 1).

Table 5. Comparison of triggers that sometimes and often induced GERD symptoms between RE and NERD patients.

Triggers	NERD (n = 203)	RE (n = 193)	p-Value
Rice	31/198 (15.7)	26/192 (13.5)	0.554
Cooked wheaten food	30/202 (14.9)	33/193 (17.1)	0.542
Wheat bran	12/139 (8.6)	6/136 (4.4)	0.157
Fruits	43/195 (22.1)	15/189 (7.9)	<0.001 *
Shallot or fragrant-flowered garlic	73/191 (38.2)	58/187 (31.0)	0.141
Dairy products	30/179 (16.8)	15/178 (8.4)	0.018 *
Yogurt	29/174 (16.7)	14/172 (8.1)	0.016 *
Bean products	29/197 (16.2)	5/190 (2.6)	<0.001 *
Meat	34/197 (19.0)	35/189 (18.5)	0.747
Salted food	37/169 (21.9)	32/169 (18.9)	0.500
Spicy food	94/161 (58.4)	95/171 (55.6)	0.603
Greasy food	61/178 (34.3)	65/183 (35.5)	0.803
Uncooked food	51/161 (31.8)	29/175 (16.6)	0.001 *
Cold food	58/161 (36.0)	30/175 (17.1)	<0.001 *
Carbonated beverages	27/126 (21.4)	32/136 (23.5)	0.684
Coffee	14/66 (21.2)	15/73 (20.5)	0.923
Strong tea	20/91 (22.0)	26/105 (24.8)	0.646
Drinking	44/96 (45.8)	62/108 (57.4)	0.099
Dining out	31/155 (20.0)	22/155 (14.2)	0.175
On business	22/120 (18.3)	14/128 (10.9)	0.098
Overeating	80/174 (46.0)	71/168 (42.3)	0.489
Diet food	4/45 (8.9)	2/34 (5.9)	0.617
Midnight snacks	35/117 (30.0)	21/121 (17.4)	0.022 *
Sweet food	76/177 (43.0)	48/177 (27.1)	0.002 *
Sticky food	37/152 (24.3)	28/161 (17.4)	0.130
Cold weather	71/100 (71.0)	40/71 (56.3)	0.048 *
Weather change	54/88 (61.4)	28/59 (47.5)	0.096
Emotional disturbance	77/119 (64.7)	36/84 (42.9)	0.002 *
Sleep disorder	43/99 (43.4)	26/73 (35.6)	0.301
Bedtime meal	42/124 (33.9)	31/109 (28.4)	0.373
Postprandial bending	41/105 (39.0)	35/94 (37.3)	0.793

Data presented as number (%); the number of denominators refers to the number of patients who had this experience. Chi-square test. * $p < 0.05$.

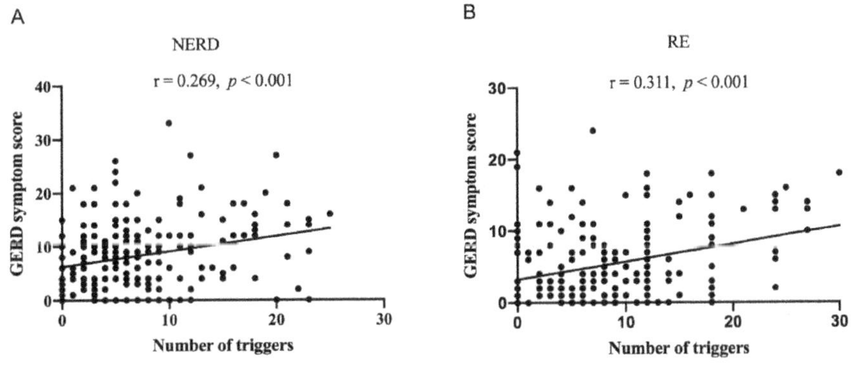

Figure 1. Correlation analysis of the number of triggers with GERD symptom score in NERD (**A**) and RE (**B**) patients.

3.6. Diet Modification Based on Triggers

We analyzed whether patients would avoid their reflux-symptom-trigger foods. We found in patients with rice as a trigger, a higher percentage of RE patients still ate rice compared with NERD patients. While in patients with cooked wheaten food as a trigger, a higher percentage of NERD patients still ate cooked wheaten food compared with RE patients. In patients with fruits, spicy food, greasy food, uncooked food, cold food, carbonated beverages, coffee, strong tea, sweet food, and sticky food as triggers, a considerable number of patients still often ate these foods, especially strong tea, spicy food, sweet food, and cold food (Table 6). In total, 74.0% (214/289) of patients still often consumed the triggering foods, even those foods that sometimes and often induced their reflux symptoms, and RE patients had higher percentage than NERD patients (82.1% vs. 66.4%, $p = 0.002$), while there were no significant differences in the percentage of patients who still often ate any type of triggering food between NERD and RE except the staple foods mentioned above.

Table 6. Comparison of patients who still often consumed foods which sometimes and often induced GERD symptoms.

Variables	NERD ($n = 203$)	RE ($n = 193$)	p-Value
Rice as staple food	5/31 (16.1%)	12/26 (46.2%)	0.014 *
Cooked wheaten food as staple food	21/30 (70.0%)	14/33 (42.4%)	0.028 *
Fruits (often)	4/43 (9.3%)	1/15 (6.7%)	0.754
Spicy food (often)	23/94 (24.5%)	26/95 (27.4%)	0.649
Greasy food (often)	11/61 (18.0%)	15/65 (23.1%)	0.484
Uncooked food (often)	10/51 (19.6%)	2/29 (6.9%)	0.126
Cold food (often)	12/58 (20.7%)	2/30 (6.7%)	0.088
Carbonated beverages (often)	2/27 (7.4%)	3/32 (9.4%)	0.787
Coffee (often)	2/14 (14.3%)	1/15 (6.7%)	0.501
Strong tea (often)	6/20 (30.0%)	8/26 (30.8%)	0.955
Drinking	30/44 (68.2%)	51/62 (82.3%)	0.093
Sweet food (often)	18/76 (23.7%)	11/48 (22.9%)	0.922
Sticky food (often)	6/37 (16.2%)	4/28 (14.3%)	0.879

Data presented as number (%). Chi-square test. * $p < 0.05$.

3.7. GERD-HRQL Score and SF-36 Total Score

NERD patients had higher GERD-HRQL scores than RE patients (Figure 2A), indicating NERD patients had worse GERD-related quality of life. There was no significant difference in SF-36 total score between NERD patients and RE patients (Figure 2B). The number of triggers was positively correlated to GERD-HRQL score (Figure 2C,D) and negatively correlated to SF-36 total score (Figure 2E,F) in both NERD and RE patients.

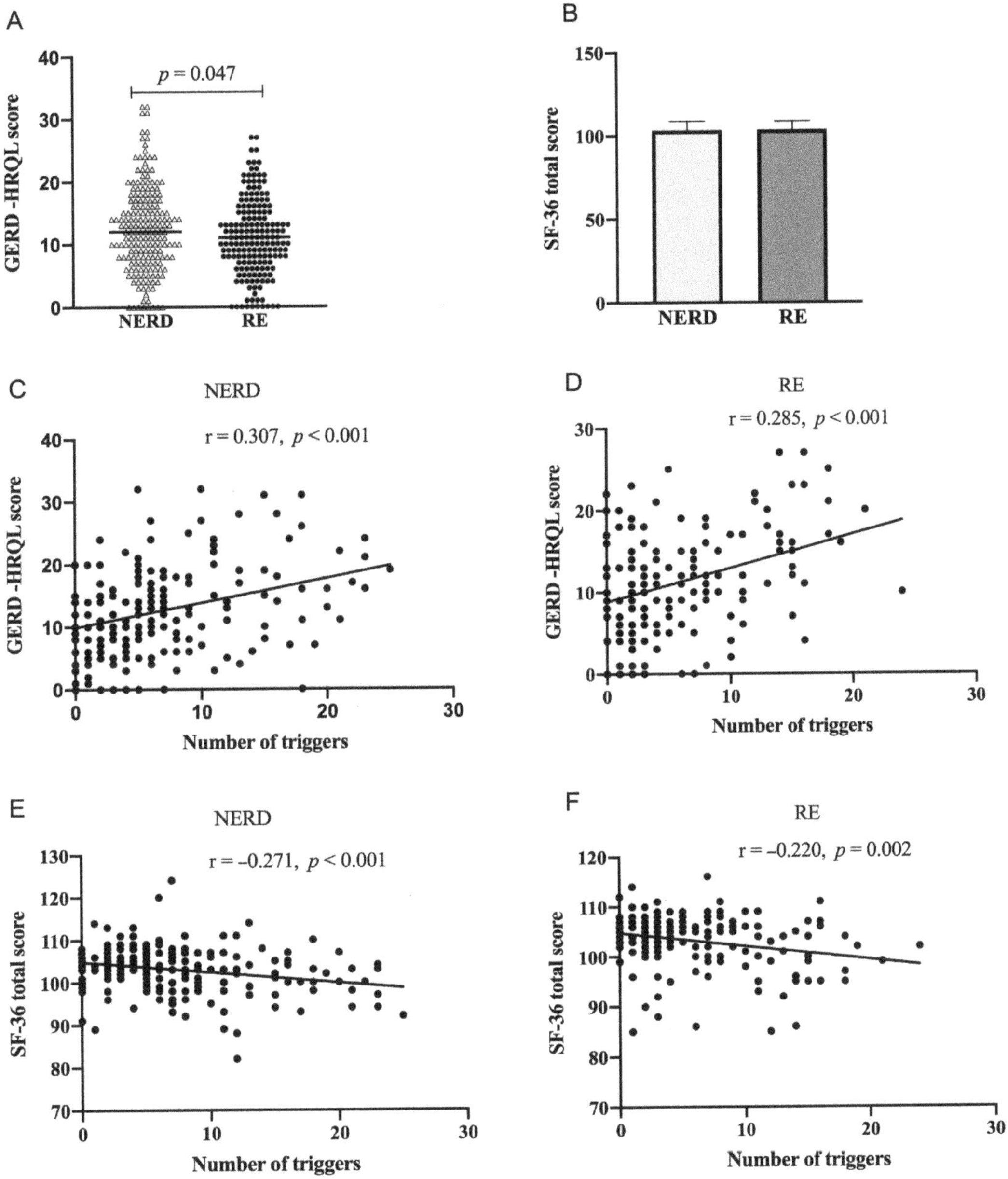

Figure 2. Comparison of GERD-HRQL and SF-36 total score and correlation analysis of the number of triggers with GERD-HRQL and SF-36 total score in NERD and RE patients. (**A**) comparison of GERD-HRQL between NERD and RE patients. (**B**) Comparison of SF-36 total score between NERD and RE patients. (**C**,**D**) Correlation analysis of the number of triggers with GERD-HRQL in NERD and RE patients. (**E**,**F**) Correlation analysis of the number of triggers with SF-36 total score in NERD and RE patients.

4. Discussion

This is a large-scale, multicenter, cross-sectional survey on dietary and lifestyle triggers of NERD and RE patients in China. We found there were no significant differences in GERD symptom scores between NERD and RE, while RE patients had a higher male proportion, smoking/drinking rate, and overeating rate than NERD patients. In total, 87.4% GERD patients had at least one trigger for their reflux symptoms, and NERD patients had more triggers than RE. The number of triggers was positively correlated to GERD symptom scores and GERD-HRQL scores; meanwhile, they were negatively correlated to SF-36 scores. Of those who took dietary modifications, 44.4% and 45.7% of NERD patients reported the effectiveness from low-lipid/low-sugar food and avoiding overeating, respectively, while as high as 82.1% RE patients often consumed triggering foods, even those foods that sometimes and often induced their reflux symptoms.

In our result, we found there was no significant difference in major GERD symptoms and most extra-esophageal symptoms between NERD and RE patients, which was consistent with a previous study [26]. The NERD consensus indicated symptom severity does not allow confident differentiation between NERD and erosive reflux disease [11]. There are many similarities between NERD and RE in the perspective of pathophysiological mechanisms. RE is characterized by excessive esophageal acid exposure and esophageal mucosa injury under endoscopy. Generally, the number of acid reflux episodes and the delay of acid bolus clearance cause excessive acid exposure [27]. RE seemed to have more obvious esophageal motor dysfunctions and injury of the mucosa barrier, and the pathophysiology of NERD was poorly understood. The mechanism of esophageal mucosa injury in RE patients compared to NERD patients with similar symptom severity was not completely clear. In this study, the self-reported effective rate of PPI was about 50%, but the relapse rate after PPI withdrawal was over 80%, which indicated there are some lifestyle and dietary aspects combined with dysmotility of the esophagus to enhance the reflux persistence.

Considering the potential side effects of long-term pharmacotherapy, lifestyle modifications are increasing in popularity. Although dietary manipulation is commonly employed in clinical settings, data are conflicting for definitive recommendations. Various lifestyle factors, such as smoking, alcohol intake, poor dietary habits (large volume of meals, lying down after a meal, meals just before bedtime) and lack of regular physical activity have been reported to be risk factors of GERD occurrence [2]. Studies indicated high-fat and high-caloric-load food; fried, sour, and spicy food; chocolate; and coffee/tea as triggers for GERD symptoms [15,18,28,29]. High-fat meals could significantly increase postprandial esophageal acid exposure in both RE and NERD [30]. Some diets were related to a proposed mechanism of GERD symptoms, coffee, alcohol, chocolate, mint and fats were related to reduction in lower esophageal sphincter (LES) tone, and late-night meals were related to increased gastric acid production [31], but few studies document the benefits of avoiding these foods. Rare data exist regarding the association between diet in RE and NERD, especially in China, where foods and cooking methods are very rich and diversified, which makes it difficult to determine the dietary risk factors for reflux symptoms in clinical practice. In this study, we set as many questions as possible and easy-to-answer options for participants, including the eating habits and triggering factors according to the dietary particularities of the Chinese, and aimed to understand the comprehensive relationship between the patients' diets and lifestyles and reflux symptoms.

With regard to ordinary dietary habits, we found more RE patients reported overeating, smoking, and drinking than NERD patients, and RE patients had a tendency to report higher percentages of fast eating than NERD patients. We found that 87.4% GERD patients had at least one trigger for their reflux symptoms, and NERD patients had more triggers than RE patients. GERD patients seemed to have similar most-common triggers; in NERD patients, the top five triggers were cold weather, emotional disturbance, weather change, spicy food, and drinking, and in RE patients, the top five triggers were drinking, cold weather, spicy food, weather change, and emotional disturbance. Thus, in clinical settings, we recommend GERD patients to avoid the five top triggers. More NERD patients reported fruits, dairy products, yogurt, bean products, uncooked food, cold food, midnight snacks, sweet food, cold weather, and emotional disturbance sometimes and often induced GERD symptoms than RE patients. The percentages of patients who had at least 3, 5, and 20 triggers in the NERD group were higher than the RE group. We assumed that NERD patients were more concerned or sensitive to dietary and lifestyle triggers than RE patients. Indeed, we also found NERD patients were more likely to coexist with FD, FC, and psychological disorders, indicating the important role of visceral hypersensitivity and psychological factors in the pathogenesis and perception of symptoms of NERD [11,32] as well as reporting more triggers for their reflux symptoms.

It is disappointing that 74.0% of GERD patients still often consumed the triggering foods, even those foods that sometimes and often induced their reflux symptoms, and RE patients had a higher percentage than did NERD patients (82.1% vs. 66.4%, $p = 0.002$). Considering that NERD and RE patients had similar GERD symptom severity with the latter group presenting with esophageal mucosal injury, we supposed that dietary habits like higher percentage of overeating, smoking, and drinking and more patients still often consuming the triggering foods were closely related to more severe acid exposure in RE patients than in NERD patients.

NERD patients had worse GERD-related quality of life than RE patients, while both groups have comparable GERD symptom scores and prevalence of extra-esophageal symptoms (except of oral symptom). The number of triggers was positively correlated to GERD-HRQL score and negatively correlated to SF-36 total score. We speculated that NERD patients with more dietary triggers might be more worried about their types of foods and excessive diet avoidance, and anxiety adversely affected their quality of life. Therefore, identification and effective management of the adverse effect of dietary and lifestyle triggers to reflux symptoms and quality of life was significant for NERD patients.

Management of GERD requires a multifaceted approach; PPI and other acid suppression therapy were first-line treatments. We observed the relatively low effective rate of PPI and high relapse rate after PPI withdrawal. A study showed the relapse rate of 4 weeks and 12 weeks after PPI treatment suspension was 48.64% and 17.57%, and they found citrus fruits (OR = 14.76) were independent risk factors of GERD relapse [33]. A Japanese study showed hiatus hernia and past severe erosive GERD (grade C or D) were risk factors for RE relapse during long-term maintenance treatment with PPIs [34]. Diet modification includes manipulation of meal size, avoidance of late-night meals and bedtime snacks, tobacco and alcohol cessation, and cessation of foods that potentially aggravate reflux symptoms, such as coffee, chocolate, carbonated beverages, spicy foods, acidic foods, such as citrus and tomatoes, and foods with high fat content were recommended in the literature [31,35]. Supporting data for these suggestions were limited and variable. According to our study, we recommend trying to avoid cold weather, emotional disturbance, weather change, spicy food, and drinking in all GERD patients. Additionally, we advise GERD patients to avoid smoking, drinking, and overeating, especially in RE patients. Also, we recommend properly avoiding the intake of fruits, dairy products, yogurt, bean products, uncooked food, and cold food, especially in NERD patients. We hope that these recommendations will be useful to patients with GERD who have similar food habits and dietary cultures. More importantly, good education on dietary and lifestyle modification are needed for GERD patients, especially emphasizing the avoidance of the intake of already known symptom-triggering foods, which is basic and important for permanent management of GERD. Further well-designed randomized, controlled trials are still needed to study the effects of dietary modification on GERD management.

There were several limitations of our study. Firstly, this study was retrospective with a food survey that spans three months prior to the survey and therefore requires a mnemonic effort and an important involvement of the subjects. Secondly, less than 20% NERD and RE patients had pH or pH-impedance monitoring tests, and less than 10% NERD and RE patients had esophageal manometry data. NERD was diagnosed with typical symptoms and self-reported response to PPIs, not rigorously distinguished from acid reflux, non-acid reflux, or functional heartburn, and we did not explore the relationship among GERD symptoms, dietary and lifestyle triggers, and pathophysiological mechanisms. Thirdly, we only collected data of GERD management during the whole disease, including PPI use and response, but we did not perform PPI tests after patients' enrollment. Finally, we did not observe the real effective rate of dietary modifications. In addition, the healthcare systems in China permmit for both referral and non-refereral patients to have a registered appointment in the tertiary hospitals when they would like to seek more professional consultation; we hope our results could be referred to those patients in parimary care.

5. Conclusions

GERD is a common gastrointestinal disease which is closely related to diet habits and lifestyles. Of the 87.4% GERD patients who had at least one trigger for their reflux symptoms, the number of triggers had close association to GERD symptoms and quality of life. Both NERD and RE patients had high relapse rates after PPI withdrawal, which could be related to dietary triggers. NERD patients had more dietary triggers and psychological factors than RE patients, indicating the underlying pathophysiology of visceral hypersensitivity, while more RE patients had poor dietary habits and often consumed the triggering foods indicating the potential effect on prolonged esophageal acid exposure. It is important to educate those GERD patients to modify their poor dietary habits and avoid already known symptom triggers based on individual triggers, especially for RE patients in the long-term course of therapy.

Author Contributions: Conceptualization, Y.C., X.S. and X.F.; methodology, X.S. and X.F.; software, X.S. and W.F.; validation, X.S. and X.F.; formal analysis, X.F., S.H. and W.F.; investigation, X.S., J.Y., P.W., D.L., M.S., S.L., X.Z., R.Z., Y.H., Y.L., J.Z., X.L., M.K. and X.F.; resources, X.S. and X.F.; data curation, X.S. and X.F.; writing—original draft preparation, Y.C. and W.F.; writing—review and editing, X.F.; visualization, Y.C. and W.F.; supervision, X.S. and X.F.; project administration, X.S. and X.F.; funding acquisition, X.F. and X.S. All authors have read and agreed to the published version of the manuscript.

Funding: This research was funded by National High-tech R&D Program (863 Program), grant number 2010AA023007.

Institutional Review Board Statement: The study was conducted in accordance with the Declaration of Helsinki, and approved by the Ethics Committee of Peking Union Medical College Hospital (Project identification code I-23PJ1009).

Informed Consent Statement: All participants provided oral consent to participate before the enrollment.

Data Availability Statement: The datasets used and/or analyzed during the current study are available from the corresponding author on reasonable request.

Conflicts of Interest: The authors declare that the study was conducted without any commercial or financial relationships that could be construed as a potential conflict of interest. This manuscript has not been published or presented elsewhere in part or in entirety and is not under consideration by another journal.

Abbreviations and Acronyms

GERD	gastroesophageal reflux disease
NERD	non-erosive reflux disease
RE	reflux esophagitis
BE	Barrett's esophagus
BMI	body mass index
FD	functional dyspepsia
FC	functional constipation
IBS	irritable bowel syndrome
GERD-HRQL	gastroesophageal reflux disease health-related quality of life
SF-36	36-item short-form health survey
PPI	proton pump inhibitor

References

1. Vakil, N.; van Zanten, S.V.; Kahrilas, P.; Dent, J.; Jones, R. The Montreal definition and classification of gastroesophageal reflux disease: A global evidence-based consensus. *Am. J. Gastroenterol.* **2006**, *101*, 1900–1920, quiz 1943. [CrossRef] [PubMed]
2. Katz, P.O.; Dunbar, K.B.; Schnoll-Sussman, F.H.; Greer, K.B.; Yadlapati, R.; Spechler, S.J. ACG Clinical Guideline for the Diagnosis and Management of Gastroesophageal Reflux Disease. *Am. J. Gastroenterol.* **2022**, *117*, 27–56. [CrossRef] [PubMed]
3. Fass, R.; Boeckxstaens, G.E.; El-Serag, H.; Rosen, R.; Sifrim, D.; Vaezi, M.F. Gastro-oesophageal reflux disease. *Nat. Rev. Dis. Primers* **2021**, *7*, 55. [CrossRef]
4. Durazzo, M.; Lupi, G.; Cicerchia, F.; Ferro, A.; Barutta, F.; Beccuti, G.; Gruden, G.; Pellicano, R. Extra-Esophageal Presentation of Gastroesophageal Reflux Disease: 2020 Update. *J. Clin. Med.* **2020**, *9*, 2559. [CrossRef] [PubMed]
5. Nirwan, J.S.; Hasan, S.S.; Babar, Z.U.; Conway, B.R.; Ghori, M.U. Global Prevalence and Risk Factors of Gastro-oesophageal Reflux Disease (GORD): Systematic Review with Meta-analysis. *Sci. Rep.* **2020**, *10*, 5814. [CrossRef]
6. Lu, T.L.; Li, S.R.; Zhang, J.M.; Chen, C.W. Meta-analysis on the epidemiology of gastroesophageal reflux disease in China. *World J. Gastroenterol.* **2022**, *28*, 6410–6420. [CrossRef]
7. Dent, J.; El-Serag, H.B.; Wallander, M.A.; Johansson, S. Epidemiology of gastro-oesophageal reflux disease: A systematic review. *Gut* **2005**, *54*, 710–717. [CrossRef]
8. Fang, X.; Zhu, L.; Wu, D.; Wang, Z.; Fei, G.; Chang, M.; Liu, F.; Xin, H.; Xu, T.; Chen, W.; et al. Natural history of gastroesophageal reflux: A prospective cohort study in a stratified, randomized population in Beijing. *J. Dig. Dis.* **2019**, *20*, 523–531. [CrossRef]
9. Hom, C.; Vaezi, M.F. Extra-esophageal manifestations of gastroesophageal reflux disease: Diagnosis and treatment. *Drugs* **2013**, *73*, 1281–1295. [CrossRef]
10. Fass, R.; Ofman, J.J. Gastroesophageal reflux disease--should we adopt a new conceptual framework? *Am. J. Gastroenterol.* **2002**, *97*, 1901–1909. [CrossRef]
11. Modlin, I.M.; Hunt, R.H.; Malfertheiner, P.; Moayyedi, P.; Quigley, E.M.; Tytgat, G.N.; Tack, J.; Heading, R.C.; Holtman, G.; Moss, S.F. Diagnosis and management of non-erosive reflux disease--the Vevey NERD Consensus Group. *Digestion* **2009**, *80*, 74–88. [CrossRef] [PubMed]
12. Kaltenbach, T.; Crockett, S.; Gerson, L.B. Are lifestyle measures effective in patients with gastroesophageal reflux disease? An evidence-based approach. *Arch. Intern. Med.* **2006**, *166*, 965–971. [CrossRef] [PubMed]
13. Wang, S.E.; Hodge, A.M.; Dashti, S.G.; Dixon-Suen, S.C.; Mitchell, H.; Thomas, R.J.; Williamson, E.M.; Makalic, E.; Boussioutas, A.; Haydon, A.M.; et al. Diet and risk of gastro-oesophageal reflux disease in the Melbourne Collaborative Cohort Study. *Public Health Nutr.* **2021**, *24*, 5034–5046. [CrossRef]
14. El-Serag, H.B.; Satia, J.A.; Rabeneck, L. Dietary intake and the risk of gastro-oesophageal reflux disease: A cross sectional study in volunteers. *Gut* **2005**, *54*, 11–17. [CrossRef] [PubMed]
15. Taraszewska, A. Risk factors for gastroesophageal reflux disease symptoms related to lifestyle and diet. *Rocz. Panstw. Zakl. Hig.* **2021**, *72*, 21–28. [CrossRef] [PubMed]
16. Fujiwara, Y.; Higuchi, K.; Shiba, M.; Yamamori, K.; Watanabe, Y.; Sasaki, E.; Tominaga, K.; Watanabe, T.; Oshitani, N.; Arakawa, T. Differences in clinical characteristics between patients with endoscopy-negative reflux disease and erosive esophagitis in Japan. *Am. J. Gastroenterol.* **2005**, *100*, 754–758. [CrossRef] [PubMed]
17. Minatsuki, C.; Yamamichi, N.; Shimamoto, T.; Kakimoto, H.; Takahashi, Y.; Fujishiro, M.; Sakaguchi, Y.; Nakayama, C.; Konno-Shimizu, M.; Matsuda, R.; et al. Background factors of reflux esophagitis and non-erosive reflux disease: A cross-sectional study of 10,837 subjects in Japan. *PLoS ONE* **2013**, *8*, e69891. [CrossRef]
18. Matsuki, N.; Fujita, T.; Watanabe, N.; Sugahara, A.; Watanabe, A.; Ishida, T.; Morita, Y.; Yoshida, M.; Kutsumi, H.; Hayakumo, T.; et al. Lifestyle factors associated with gastroesophageal reflux disease in the Japanese population. *J. Gastroenterol.* **2013**, *48*, 340–349. [CrossRef]
19. Nam, S.Y.; Park, B.J.; Cho, Y.A.; Ryu, K.H.; Choi, I.J.; Park, S.; Kim, Y.W. Different effects of dietary factors on reflux esophagitis and non-erosive reflux disease in 11,690 Korean subjects. *J. Gastroenterol.* **2017**, *52*, 818–829. [CrossRef]
20. Kim, N.; Lee, S.W.; Cho, S.I.; Park, C.G.; Yang, C.H.; Kim, H.S.; Rew, J.S.; Moon, J.S.; Kim, S.; Park, S.H.; et al. The prevalence of and risk factors for erosive oesophagitis andRnon-erosive reflux disease: A nationwide multicentre prospective study in Korea. *Aliment. Pharmacol. Ther.* **2008**, *27*, 173–185. [CrossRef]
21. Lundell, L.R.; Dent, J.; Bennett, J.R.; Blum, A.L.; Armstrong, D.; Galmiche, J.P.; Johnson, F.; Hongo, M.; Richter, J.E.; Spechler, S.J.; et al. Endoscopic assessment of oesophagitis: Clinical and functional correlates and further validation of the Los Angeles classification. *Gut* **1999**, *45*, 172–180. [CrossRef] [PubMed]
22. Li, X.; Lin, S.; Wang, Z.; Zhang, H.; Sun, X.; Li, J.; Wu, D.; Ke, M.; Fang, X. Gastroesophageal reflux disease and chronic cough: A possible mechanism elucidated by ambulatory pH-impedance-pressure monitoring. *Neurogastroenterol. Motil.* **2019**, *31*, e13707. [CrossRef] [PubMed]
23. Drossman, D.A. *Rome III: Functional Gastrointestinal Disorders*, 3rd ed.; Allen Press, Inc.: Lawrence, KS, USA, 2006.
24. Velanovich, V.; Vallance, S.R.; Gusz, J.R.; Tapia, F.V.; Harkabus, M.A. Quality of life scale for gastroesophageal reflux disease. *J. Am. Coll. Surg.* **1996**, *183*, 217–224. [PubMed]
25. Ware, J.E., Jr.; Sherbourne, C.D. The MOS 36-item short-form health survey (SF-36). I. Conceptual framework and item selection. *Med. Care* **1992**, *30*, 473–483. [CrossRef] [PubMed]

26. Kovács, Z.; Kerékgyártó, O. Psychological factors, quality of life, and gastrointestinal symptoms in patients with erosive and non-erosive reflux disorder. *Int. J. Psychiatry Med.* **2007**, *37*, 139–150. [CrossRef]
27. Lin, S.; Li, H.; Fang, X. Esophageal Motor Dysfunctions in Gastroesophageal Reflux Disease and Therapeutic Perspectives. *J. Neurogastroenterol. Motil.* **2019**, *25*, 499–507. [CrossRef]
28. Festi, D.; Scaioli, E.; Baldi, F.; Vestito, A.; Pasqui, F.; Di Biase, A.R.; Colecchia, A. Body weight, lifestyle, dietary habits and gastroesophageal reflux disease. *World J. Gastroenterol.* **2009**, *15*, 1690–1701. [CrossRef] [PubMed]
29. Mehta, R.S.; Nguyen, L.H.; Ma, W.; Staller, K.; Song, M.; Chan, A.T. Association of Diet and Lifestyle with the Risk of Gastroesophageal Reflux Disease Symptoms in US Women. *JAMA Intern. Med.* **2021**, *181*, 552–554. [CrossRef]
30. Fan, W.J.; Hou, Y.T.; Sun, X.H.; Li, X.Q.; Wang, Z.F.; Guo, M.; Zhu, L.M.; Wang, N.; Yu, K.; Li, J.N.; et al. Effect of high-fat, standard, and functional food meals on esophageal and gastric pH in patients with gastroesophageal reflux disease and healthy subjects. *J. Dig. Dis.* **2018**, *19*, 664–673. [CrossRef]
31. Newberry, C.; Lynch, K. The role of diet in the development and management of gastroesophageal reflux disease: Why we feel the burn. *J. Thorac. Dis.* **2019**, *11*, S1594–S1601. [CrossRef]
32. Xu, C.; Niu, X. Progress on the Mechanism of Visceral Hypersensitivity in Nonerosive Reflux Disease. *Gastroenterol. Res. Pract.* **2022**, *2022*, 4785077. [CrossRef] [PubMed]
33. López-Colombo, A.; Pacio-Quiterio, M.S.; Jesús-Mejenes, L.Y.; Rodríguez-Aguilar, J.E.; López-Guevara, M.; Montiel-Jarquín, A.J.; López-Alvarenga, J.C.; Morales-Hernández, E.R.; Ortiz-Juárez, V.R.; Ávila-Jiménez, L. Risk factors associated with gastroesophageal reflux disease relapse in primary care patients successfully treated with a proton pump inhibitor. *Rev. Gastroenterol. Mex.* **2017**, *82*, 106–114. [CrossRef] [PubMed]
34. Fujimoto, K.; Hongo, M. Risk factors for relapse of erosive GERD during long-term maintenance treatment with proton pump inhibitor: A prospective multicenter study in Japan. *J. Gastroenterol.* **2010**, *45*, 1193–1200. [CrossRef] [PubMed]
35. Ness-Jensen, E.; Lindam, A.; Lagergren, J.; Hveem, K. Tobacco smoking cessation and improved gastroesophageal reflux: A prospective population-based cohort study: The HUNT study. *Am. J. Gastroenterol.* **2014**, *109*, 171–177. [CrossRef] [PubMed]

nutrients
MDPI

Article

A High-Fat, High-Cholesterol Diet Promotes Intestinal Inflammation by Exacerbating Gut Microbiome Dysbiosis and Bile Acid Disorders in Cholecystectomy

Fusheng Xu [1,2,†], Zhiming Yu [3,†], Yaru Liu [1,2], Ting Du [1,2], Leilei Yu [1,2], Fengwei Tian [1,2], Wei Chen [1,2,4] and Qixiao Zhai [1,2,*]

1 State Key Laboratory of Food Science and Resources, Jiangnan University, Wuxi 214122, China; 6210112164@stu.jiangnan.edu.cn (F.X.); 6210113061@jiangnan.edu.cn (Y.L.); 1012200610@stu.jiangnan.edu.cn (T.D.); edyulei@126.com (L.Y.); fwtian@jiangnan.edu.cn (F.T.); chenwei66@jiangnan.edu.cn (W.C.)
2 School of Food Science and Technology, Jiangnan University, Wuxi 214122, China
3 Wuxi People's Hospital Afliated to Nanjing Medical University, Wuxi 214023, China; yuzhimingxinjie@sina.com
4 National Engineering Research Center for Functional Food, Jiangnan University, Wuxi 214122, China
* Correspondence: zhaiqixiao@jiangnan.edu.cn; Tel./Fax: +86-510-85912155
† These authors contributed equally to this study.

Abstract: Patients with post-cholecystectomy (PC) often experience adverse gastrointestinal conditions, such as PC syndrome, colorectal cancer (CRC), and non-alcoholic fatty liver disease (NAFLD), that accumulate over time. An epidemiological survey further revealed that the risk of cholecystectomy is associated with high-fat and high-cholesterol (HFHC) dietary intake. Mounting evidence suggests that cholecystectomy is associated with disrupted gut microbial homeostasis and dysregulated bile acids (BAs) metabolism. However, the effect of an HFHC diet on gastrointestinal complications after cholecystectomy has not been elucidated. Here, we aimed to investigate the effect of an HFHC diet after cholecystectomy on the gut microbiota–BA metabolic axis and elucidate the association between this alteration and the development of intestinal inflammation. In this study, a mice cholecystectomy model was established, and the levels of IL-Iβ, TNF-α, and IL-6 in the colon were increased in mice fed an HFHC diet for 6 weeks. Analysis of fecal BA metabolism showed that an HFHC diet after cholecystectomy altered the rhythm of the BA metabolism by upregulating liver CPY7A1, CYP8B1, and BSEP and ileal ASBT mRNA expression levels, resulting in increased fecal BA levels. In addition, feeding an HFHC diet after cholecystectomy caused a significant dysbiosis of the gut microbiota, which was characterized by the enrichment of the metabolic microbiota involved in BAs; the abundance of pro-inflammatory gut microbiota and related pro-inflammatory metabolite levels was also significantly higher. In contrast, the abundance of major short-chain fatty acid (SCFA)-producing bacteria significantly decreased. Overall, our study suggests that an HFHC diet after cholecystectomy promotes intestinal inflammation by exacerbating the gut microbiome and BA metabolism dysbiosis in cholecystectomy. Our study also provides useful insights into the maintenance of intestinal health after cholecystectomy through dietary or probiotic intervention strategies.

Keywords: post-cholecystectomy; gut microbiota; bile acids; diet; cholesterol; inflammation

1. Introduction

The gallbladder (GB) is primarily responsible for the storage and concentration of bile acids (BAs) secreted by the liver. Generally, GB contraction is stimulated by cholecystokinins secreted through the duodenum during the interdigestive period to expel bile [1]. Bile salts and BAs facilitate the absorption of dietary lipids [2,3]. Post-cholecystectomy (PC) can alter the dynamic balance of the BA metabolism, resulting in increased BA reabsorption and enterohepatic circulation [4]. According to epidemiological surveys, PC increases the risk of colorectal cancer (CRC) [5] and non-alcoholic fatty liver disease (NAFLD) [6], but further studies are needed to confirm the relationship, as well as to clarify the mechanism of action. Studies have shown that PC can disrupt gut microbiota homeostasis and perturb the bile acid metabolism [7], a potential risk after cholecystectomy. Moreover, the risk of cholecystectomy is often associated with the excessive intake of a high-fat, high-cholesterol (HFHC) diet [8,9] that further disrupts gut microbial homeostasis and the BA metabolism after cholecystectomy [10,11].

The gut microbiota metabolism is an important microbial pathway for the BA metabolism and is involved in the conversion of unconjugated and secondary BAs. Therefore, the composition of the gut microbiota is essential for maintaining a stable BA pool, which has a positive effect on host health [12]. Specifically, the modification of primary BAs by the gut microbiota, mainly through four metabolic pathways (ncoupling, dehydroxylation, oxidation, and exosomalization) increases the diversity of the BA pool and overall hydrophobic primary BAs [13]. In contrast, BAs, as an antimicrobial agent, can affect gut microbial homeostasis directly and through indirect effects [14]. Bacteria containing BA-metabolizing enzymes such as bile salt hydrolase (BSH) are favored because they are tolerant to the toxic effects of BAs [15]. In addition to their digestive role, BAs act as important signaling molecules that can significantly influence pathways such as metabolism and immunity in the host [16]. First, the strong hydrophobicity of BAs can exert carcinogenic effects by damaging the cells and inducing inflammation [17]. Additionally, BAs can indirectly affect the intestinal inflammatory milieu by activating or inhibiting BA receptors, such as FXR and TGR5 [16].

Dietary patterns have attracted widespread attention as a key factor affecting health. Diets rich in saturated fats and cholesterol, often associated with the Western diet [18], and malnutrition resulting from imbalanced energy or nutrient intake have been linked to the development of a variety of inflammatory diseases, such as inflammatory bowel disease, ulcerative colitis, and Crohn's disease [19]. In addition, diet is a key factor influencing gut microbial homeostasis and the BA metabolism. Primarily, fat and fiber intake can significantly alter the gut microbiota and BA metabolism [20]. Cholesterol is an important prerequisite for BA synthesis, and chronic HFHC intake can upregulate the BA synthesis pathway, thereby increasing overall host BA levels [21]. Diets rich in dietary fiber help to maintain intestinal flora diversity and normal metabolic function [22]. The gut microbiota ferments dietary fiber to produce short-chain fatty acids (SCFAs). SCFAs play an important role in maintaining intestinal barrier function; in addition, SCFAs can reduce oxygen levels in the intestinal lumen and maintain normal immunometabolic pathways [23]. In addition, an HFHC diet can affect intestinal health by increasing intestinal barrier permeability and disrupting gut microbial homeostasis [24]. Thus, diverse dietary intake can influence host health by influencing the gut microbiota–BA axis.

High-fat and high-cholesterol diets have been widely used to simulate mice models of diseases, such as obesity [25], NAFLD [26], and hypercholesterolaemia [27], caused by excessive fat and cholesterol intake. Based on these findings, we hypothesized that an HFHC diet after cholecystectomy may exacerbate the dysbiosis of gut microbial homeostasis and BA metabolic rhythms in cholecystectomy, thereby promoting intestinal inflammation. We established a cholecystectomized mice model and fed an HFHC diet for 6 weeks. Systematic investigations were conducted based on the changes in intestinal histopathology, fecal BA metabolism, BA-related gene expression, intestinal microbiota composition, and metabolic pathways to explore the effects of an HFHC diet on the BA metabolism and microbiota balance in cholecystectomy. The results of our study provide evidence that an HFHC diet after cholecystectomy promotes the development of colonic inflammation and its associated mechanisms to provide new and valuable insights into the prevention of related diseases after cholecystectomy through dietary strategies or probiotic supplementation strategies.

2. Materials and Methods

2.1. Animals and Feeding

The C57BL/6J mice PC model has been widely used in various studies [7]. Therefore, C57BL/6J mice were used in this study for experiments. C57BL/6J mice were of specific-pathogen-free (SPF) grade (6–8 weeks, male) (SPF Biotechnology, Beijing, China). Mice were housed in a 12 h diurnal cycle at a constant temperature and humidity of 22 ± 1 °C and 50 ± 10%, respectively.

In order to simulate the two dietary patterns of HFHC and low fat and low cholesterol (LFLC) after cholecystectomy, we established a higher level of cholesterol intake in the experimental group under the premise of a reasonable combination of various nutrients. HFHC group: feeding an irradiation-sterilized HFHC diet (60% of energy from fat, 26% from carbohydrate, and 14% from protein; added an extra 1.8% of cholesterol; TP 23400-180, Trophic Animal Feed High-Tech Co., Ltd., Nantong, China). LFLC group: feeding an irradiation-sterilized LFLC diet (10% energy from fat, 76% from carbohydrates, and 14% from protein; added an extra 0.2% of cholesterol; TP 23402-020, Trophic Animal Feed High-Tech Co., Ltd., Nantong, China). Refer to Table S1 for feed formulation details. This study was approved by the Experimental Animal Ethics Committee of Jiangnan University (Qualification number: JN. No20220930c0550401[403]).

In the PC group, the GB duct was ligated, and the GB was removed after bile emptying. Mice in the negative control group underwent sham surgery (NC).

After one week of acclimation, the mice were randomly divided into three treatment groups: cholecystectomy and sham surgery. As shown in Figure 1a, the experimental groups were as follows: (1) cholecystectomy and HFHC feeding (Figure 1b) (HFHC-PC) (n = 9); (2) cholecystectomy and LFLC feeding (Figure 1b) (LFLC-PC) (n = 9); and (3) sham operation and LFLC feeding (Figure 1c) (LFLC-NC) (n = 9).

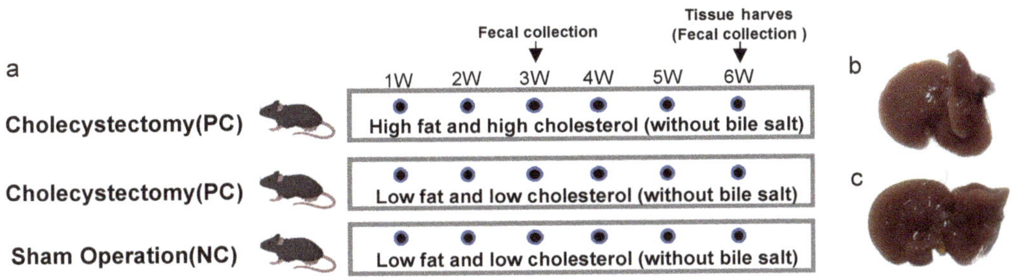

Figure 1. Animal experiments (**a**). Mice grouping instructions. (**b**,**c**). Diagram of cholecystectomy (**b**) with sham surgery (**c**).

2.2. Histological Analysis

Colon tissue specimens were end-fixed in 4% paraformaldehyde for more than 24 h, and sections were eventually stained with hematoxylin and eosin (H&E) and examined microscopically [28]. Please refer to the Supplementary Material for the detailed procedure.

2.3. Microbiome Analysis

Please refer to the Supplementary Material for the detailed sequencing procedure for fecal 16S-RNA. Briefly, Microbial Ecology Quantitative Analysis Platform 2 (QIIME2) was used to analyze the raw sequencing data [29]. First, raw sequencing data were quality filtered and demultiplexed using the DADA2 package of the QIIME2 platform. Reads were assigned using open-reference amplicon sequence variants (ASVs). Finally, the Silva Bacterial Database was used for sequence alignment. GraphPad Prism 8 and R were used for data analysis and visualization, and Python NumPy and SciPy libraries were used for ASV tracking. Microbial co-abundance analysis was performed using the Chiplot website chiplot (https://www.chiplot.online/#Bar-plot, accessed on 15 April 2023). Spearman correlation, heatmap analysis, and visualization were performed using OmicStudio tools (https://www.omicstudio.cn/tool, accessed on 7 June 2023). Kyoto Encyclopedia of Genes and Genomes (KEGG) and KEGG orthology (KO) enrichment analysis and pathway annotation were based on the Gene Denovo (https://www.genedenovo.com/, accessed on 7 June 2023) and KEGG pathway database (http://www.genome.jp/kegg/, accessed on 7 June 2023), respectively.

2.4. BA Measurements

Liquid chromatography–tandem mass spectrometry was used to determine the absolute abundance of the target BAs [30]. For sample pre-treatment, freeze-dried fecal samples were weighed (approximately 50 mg). Grinding and homogenization were performed using methanol (100%). A 0.22 μm membrane was used for filtration and stored in an injection bottle for LC-MS analysis.

UPLC-Q Exactive system (UPLC: UltiMate 3000); column: ACQUITY UPLC® HSS T3 (1.8 μm, 2.1 × 100 mm) was used for quantitative analysis of BAs. An aqueous solution of 1 mM ammonium acetate (phase A) and a methanolic solution of 1 mM ammonium acetate (phase B) were used for elution. Gradient elution conditions are listed in Table S2.

2.5. RNA Extraction and Quantitative Real-Time PCR (RT-qPCR)

Total RNA was extracted using the Total RNA Isolation Kit (Vazyme, R401-01, Nanjing, China) and reverse transcribed into cDNA using HiScript III Reverse Transcriptase (Vazyme #R333, Nanjing, China). RT-qPCR was performed to detect the corresponding gene expression. The relative level of change in target genes was calculated using $2^{-\Delta\Delta CT}$. Please refer to Table S3 for the primers used for RT-qPCR.

2.6. Analysis of Cytokines in the Colonic Tissues by Enzyme-Linked Immunosorbent Assay (ELISA)

ELISA kit (Valukine ELISA) (R&D Systems, Shanghai, China) was used for the detection of IL-1β and TNF-α levels in the colon.

Bicinchoninic Acid Assay kits (Beyotime Biotechnology, Shanghai, China) were used to determine the total protein content of all colonic tissues [31].

2.7. Untargeted Metabolomics

A UIUI3000 high-performance liquid chromatography (HPLC) system (Thermo Fisher Technologies, Waltham, MA, USA) was used in conjunction with a high-resolution Q Active Mass Spectrometer (Thermo Fisher Technologies, Waltham, MA, USA) to analyze fecal metabolites. The preparation methods of the metabolites, analytical parameters of HPLC-MS, and analytical methods for the metabolite data are described in detail in the Supplementary Material.

2.8. Determination of Plasma Biochemical Indices

The plasma was stored at −80 °C. After thawing, 80 μL of plasma was collected and diluted to 240 μL with 0.9% normal saline. Blood total cholesterol (TC), triglyceride (TG), high-density lipoprotein cholesterol (HDL-C), and glucose (Glu) levels were determined using an automatic biochemistry analyzer [32].

2.9. Determination of Fecal SCFA Contents

Analysis of SCFA levels in samples was performed using gas chromatography–mass spectrometry (GC-MS) [33]. The sample processing method was described by Wang et al. [34]. Detailed parameters for GC-MS testing are provided in the Supplementary Material.

2.10. Statistical Analysis

Statistical analysis of the data was performed using R or GraphPad Prism 8. Data are expressed as median or means ± SEM. The *t*-test, ANOVA, and Mann–Whitney test were used to test for differences in the data. Statistical significance was set at $p < 0.05$. The *p*-values in the figure represent the following: ns, $p > 0.05$ (not significant, may not be indicated); * $p < 0.05$; ** $p < 0.01$; *** $p < 0.001$; and **** $p < 0.0001$.

3. Results

3.1. Pro-Inflammatory Effects of Cholecystectomy on the Intestine Exacerbated by an HFHC Diet

We first examined whether cholecystectomy and feeding an HFHC diet after cholecystectomy resulted in changes in serum biochemistry, histology, and expression levels of inflammatory cytokines. The results showed that all three groups of mice gained weight during the experimental period (Figure 2b), with a significant difference in weight gain on day 30 in the HFHC-PC group compared to the LFLC-PC group ($p < 0.05$) (Figure 2a). However, there was no significant difference in food intake (Figure 2c). Similarly, we observed significantly increased serum TG ($p < 0.001$), HDL-C ($p < 0.01$), TC ($p < 0.05$), and Glu ($p < 0.05$) levels in the HFHC-PC group (Figure 2j–m). Compared to the LFLC-NC group, the LFLC-PC group showed a significant increase in IL-10 ($p < 0.05$) level, whereas IL-1β, IL-6, and NF-κB only showed an upward trend. In addition, compared to the LFLC-PC group, the HFHC-PC group showed increased levels in colonic cytokines IL-1β ($p < 0.01$), TNF-α ($p < 0.05$), IL-6 ($p < 0.01$), IL-10, and NF-κB (Figure 2e–i), although there was no significant tissue damage (Figure 2d). Thus, feeding an HFHC diet for 6 weeks after cholecystectomy elevated the serum levels of glycolipid metabolism in mice. It also resulted in increased expression of colonic inflammatory factors.

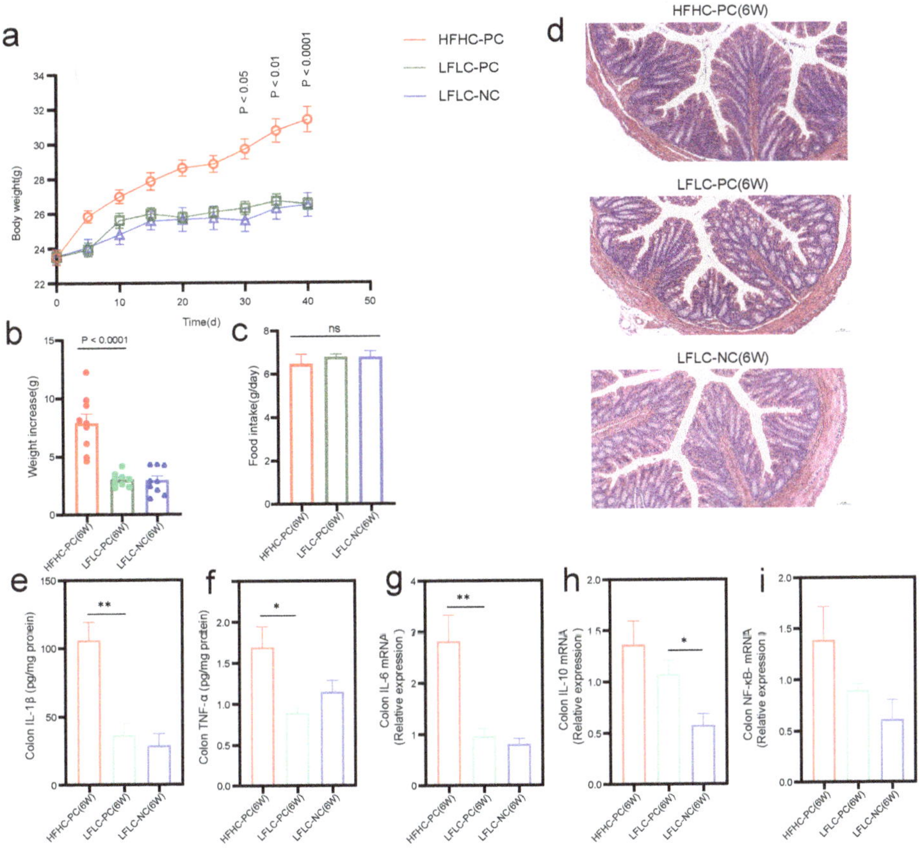

Figure 2. *Cont.*

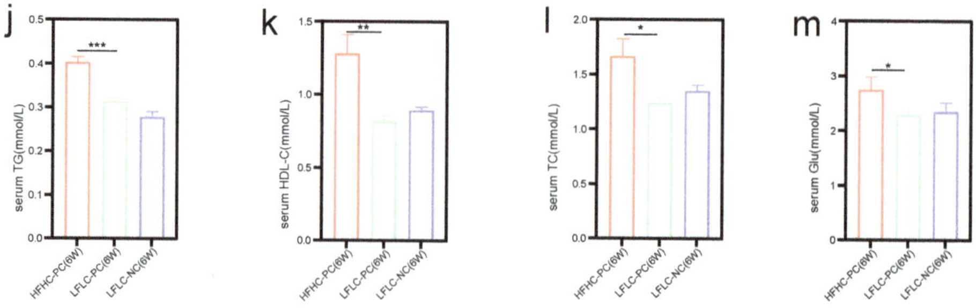

Figure 2. HFHC feeding and PC induce an inflammatory colonic environment in mice. (**a**): Changes in body weight of mice throughout surgical molding and different dietary feeding. (**b**): Weight increase in mice from week 1 to 6. (**c**): Mean food intake of mice throughout the experimental cycle. (**d**): Representative hematoxylin-and-eosin-stained sections in HFHC−PC, LFLC−PC, and LFLC−NC groups at week 6. (**e**,**f**): ELISA assay was used to detect IL-1β and TNF-α levels in the colon. (**g**–**i**): Relative mRNA expression of IL-6, IL-10, and NF-κB in the colon. (**j**–**m**): Serum TG, HDL-C, TC, and Glu levels. * $p < 0.05$, ** $p < 0.01$, *** $p < 0.001$, ns, nonsignificant.

3.2. HFHC Diet Exacerbates the Dysbiosis of Gut Microbial Homeostasis in Cholecystectomy

The gut microbial–BA axis is an important pathway for the metabolism of BAs in the colon, further modifying primary BAs to secondary BAs. The fecal microbiota was also identified. Cholecystectomy did not alter the alpha diversity of gut microbiota (Figure 3a,b). Feeding an HFHC diet for 6 weeks after cholecystectomy resulted in a significant increase in alpha diversity (Figure 3a,b). PCoA showed that the LFLFC-PC and LFLC-NC groups were significantly different at week 6 (but not at week 3) (Figure 3c,d), whereas the HFHD-PC and LFLC-PC groups were significantly different at both weeks 3 and 6 (Figure 3f,g). Mice fed an HFHC diet after cholecystectomy also transitioned along with the first principal coordinates from weeks 3 to 6, whereas mice after cholecystectomy did not follow the same gut microbiota transition (Figure 3e,h). Stacked histograms show changes in the gut microbiota at the phylum (Figure 3i), family (Figure 3j), and genus levels (Figure 3k). Notably, at weeks 3 and 6, the HFHC-PC group Firmicutes/Bacteroidetes abundance ratio showed a decreasing trend, which was negatively correlated with obesity (Figure 3l). Furthermore, we identified bacteria with significant differences at the genus level (Figure 3m,n). In the analysis of the gut microbial co-abundance network, the HFHC-PC group showed more complex relationships with increasing time than the LFLC-PC group (Figure S1a–d). Compared with the LFLC-NC group, the LFLC-PC group was significantly enriched in *Ruminococcaceae UCG 014* and *Romboutsia* at week 3, whereas *Parasutterella* and *Parabacteroides* showed a decreasing trend in abundance. At week 6, *Parasutterella*, *Odoribacter*, and *Enterococcus* were significantly enriched, whereas *Desulfovibrio*, *Acetatifactor*, and *Eubacterium coprostanoligenes groups* showed a decreasing trend (Figure 3m). Feeding an HFHC diet after cholecystectomy resulted in more complex microbiota differences. At week 3 or 6, the HFHC-PC group was highly enriched in several genera involved in BA metabolism, such as *Akkermansia*, *Parasutterella*, *Dubosiella*, *Bacteroides*, *Parabacteroides*, and *Family XIII AD3011 group*, etc. (Figure 3n). In addition, *Eubacterium nodatum group*, *Flavonifractor*, *Erysipelatoclostridium*, *Negativibacillus*, *Muribaculum*, *Clostridium innocuum group*, and *Tyzzerella* were also significantly enriched in the HFHC-PC group (Figure 3n). In contrast, *Lachnoclostridium*, *Ruminiclostridium 5*, *Fecalibaculum*, *Anaerotruncus*, *Ruminococcaceae UCG 010*, and *Ruminiclostridium* exhibited decreasing trends (Figure 3n). The results indicated that PC can affect gut microbiota homeostasis through time accumulation. In addition, feeding an HFHC diet after cholecystectomy exacerbates the disruption of gut microbiota homeostasis by cholecystectomy, resulting in alterations in the structure of gut microbiota diversity and differential bacterial profiles.

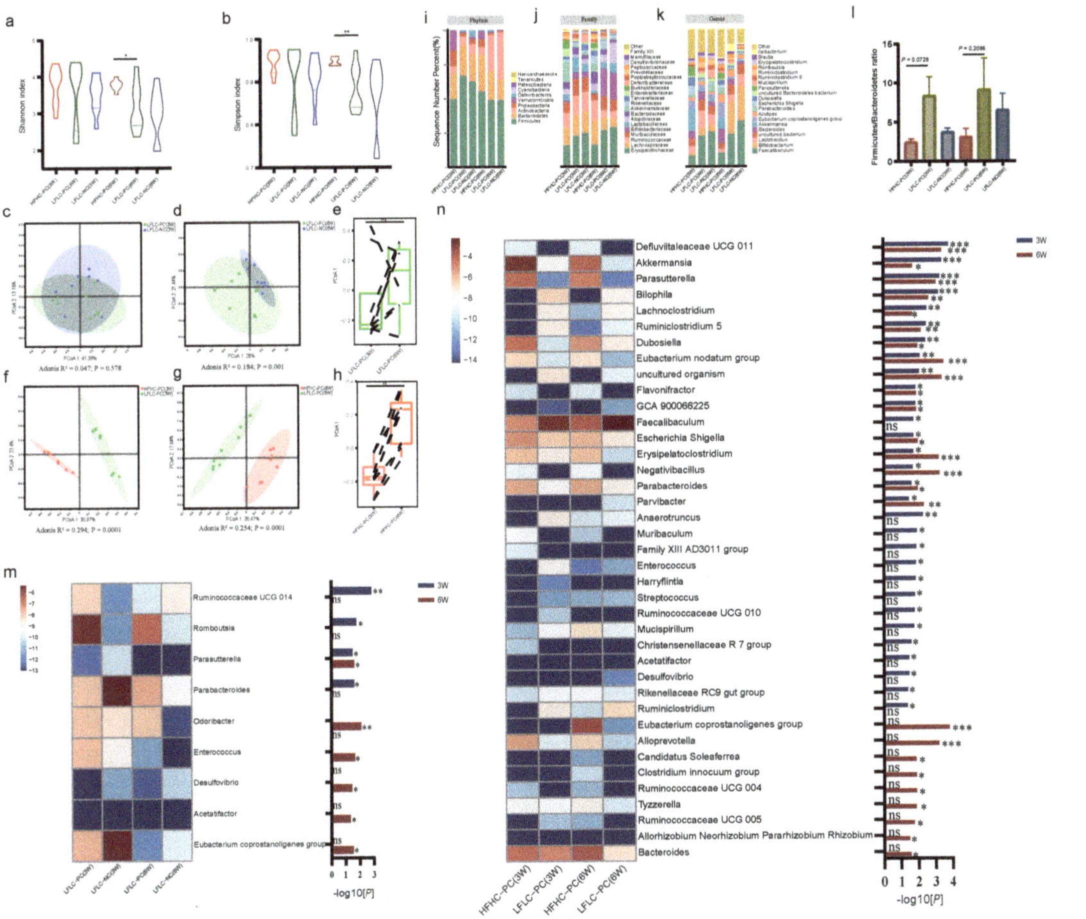

Figure 3. HFHC diet and PC altered gut microbial homeostasis. (**a**,**b**): Shannon or Simpson index of fecal microbiota (weeks 3 and 6). (**c**,**d**): Microbial clustering based on Bray Curtis distances in the LFLC−PC and LFLC−NC groups at weeks 3 (**c**) and 6 (**d**), visualized using principle coordinate analysis (PCoA). (Adonis; R2 = 0.047, p = 0.578 at week 3; R2 = 0.184, p = 0.001 at week 6; LFLC−PC vs. LFLC−NC). (**f**,**g**): Microbial clustering based on Bray Curtis distances in the HFHC−PC and LFLC−PC groups at weeks 3 (**f**) and 6 (**g**), visualized using principle coordinate analysis (PCoA) (Adonis; R2 = 0.294, p = 0.0001 at week 3; R2 = 0.254, p = 0.0001 at week 6; HFHC−PC vs. LFLC−PC). (**e**,**h**): Boxplot showing changes in microbiome from weeks 3 to 6, in the HFHC−PC (**h**) andLFLC−PC (**e**) groups. In both groups, the HFHC diet resulted in an increase along the first principal axis (** $p < 0.01$; ns, nonsignificant). (**i**–**k**): The relative abundance of gut microbiota at Phylum (**i**), Family (**j**), and Genus (**k**) levels from different groups (the HFHC−PC, LFLC−PC, and LFLC−NC groups). (**l**): Firmicutes/Bacteroidetes ratio. (**m**,**n**): Heat-map analysis of bacteria in fecal samples from cholecystectomized (**m**) and differentially diet-fed (**n**) mice at weeks 3 and 6, respectively. The color indicates the median relative abundance of bacteria in that group of samples. The significance of the difference in bacteria between the two groups is shown on the right. The bar color indicates the statistical significances (p value, values converted by −log10) of bacteria between two groups. * $p < 0.05$, ** $p < 0.01$, *** $p < 0.001$, ns, nonsignificant. The two groups were compared using Mann–Whitney test.

3.3. Disturbed BA Metabolism Attributed to Cholecystectomy Exacerbated by HFHC Diet

We examined BA levels in the colonic and fecal samples of mice. Principal coordinate analysis (PCoA) showed that the HFHC-PC group had different fecal BA clusters compared to the LFLC-PC and LFLC-NC groups at weeks 3 and 6 (Figure 4a,b). Analysis of BA levels in the colon showed increased levels of chenodeoxycholic acid (CDCA) and bile acids (CA) in the HFHC-PC group at week 6 compared to those in the LFLC-PC group, with no significant differences in other BAs (Figure 4c). Although the LFLC-PC group showed similar fecal BA profiles to the LFLC-NC group after weeks 3 and 6, we found that the levels of CDCA, β-muricholic acid (β-MCA), and DCA increased in the fecal samples (Figure 4d). However, the HFHC-PC group showed higher levels of primary and secondary BA metabolism. Specifically, CDCA, β-MCA, and DCA levels increased significantly at weeks 3 and 6. Second, glycoursodeoxycholic acid (GDCA) and taurolithocholic acid (TLCA) levels significantly increased only at week 3 and LCA levels only at week 6 (Figure 4d). Cholecystectomy significantly upregulated liver CYP7B1 and BSEP mRNA expression compared to the LFLC-NC group (Figure 4g,j). Feeding an HFHC diet after cholecystectomy significantly upregulated the liver CYP7A1, CYP8B1, FXR, and BSEP (Figure 4e,f,i,j) and ileum ASBT (Figure 4k) mRNA expression. Furthermore, we observed that neither cholecystectomy nor an HFHC diet resulted in significant differences in liver CYP27a1 mRNA expression (Figure 4h). In conclusion, feeding an HFHC diet after cholecystectomy similarly exacerbates the disturbances in the BA metabolism, resulting in elevated levels of primary and secondary BA metabolism.

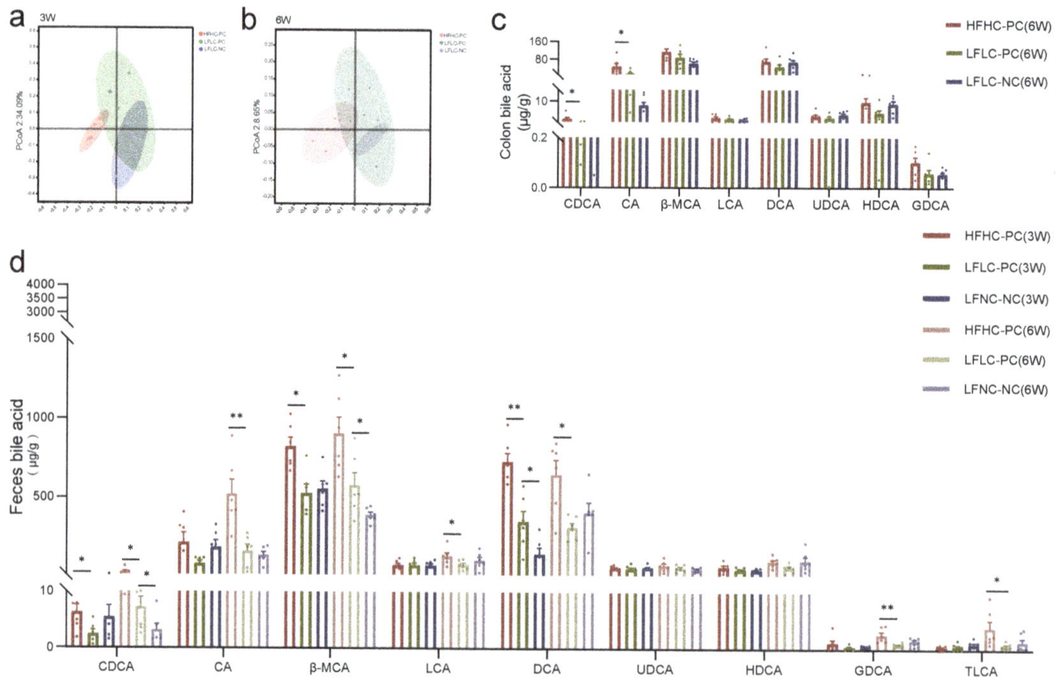

Figure 4. *Cont.*

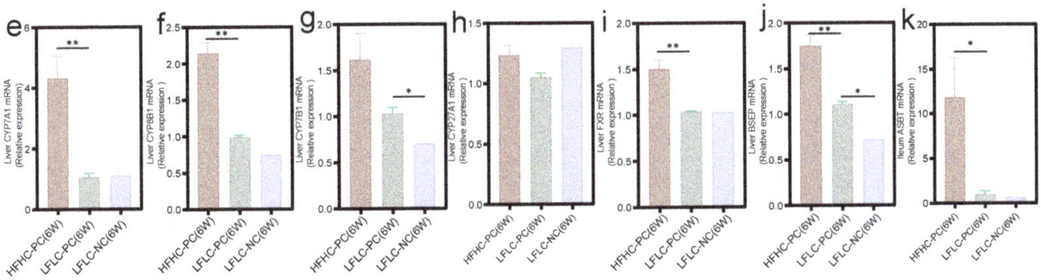

Figure 4. HFHC diet and PC altered BAs metabolic homeostasis. (**a**,**b**): PCoA analysis of fecal BAs profile at week 3 (**a**) or 6 (**b**) in the HFHC−PC, LFLC−PC, and LFLC−NC groups. (**c**): The relative concentration of colonic total CDCA, CA, β-MCA, LCA, DCA, ursodeoxycholic (UDCA), hyodeoxycholic acid (HDCA), and GDCA in the HFHC−PC, LFLC−PC, and LFLC−NC groups at week 6, respectively. (**d**): The relative concentration of feces total CDCA, CA, β-MCA, LCA, DCA, UDCA, HDCA, GDCA, and TLCA in the HFHC−PC, LFLC−PC, and LFLC−NC groups at weeks 3 and 6. (**e**–**k**): Relative mRNA expression of CYP7A1 (**e**), CYP8B1 (**f**), CYP7B1 (**g**), CYP27A1 (**h**), FXR (**i**), and BSEP (**j**) in liver, and ASBT (**k**) in the colon. * $p < 0.05$, ** $p < 0.01$.

3.4. Alterations in Gut Microbiota Associated with BA Metabolism

Spearman's correlation analysis was performed to determine the correlation between the differential gut microbiota and fecal BAs. The results showed a significant correlation between gut microbiota and BA metabolism. Specifically, *Parabacteroides* and *Parasutterella* were strongly and positively correlated with altered CA, CDCA, and TLCA in the LFLC-PC group at week 3, respectively (Figure 5a). *Parasutterella*, *Enterococcus*, and *Acetatifacor* were strongly and positively correlated with altered CDCA, β-MCA, and GDCA in the LFLC-PC group at week 6, respectively (Figure 5b). In addition, *Parasutterella, Defluviitaleaceae UCG 011, Erysipelatoclostridium, Escherichia Shigella, Family XIII AD3011 group, Eubacterium nodatum group, Parabacteroides, Akkermansia, Candidatus Soleaferrea, Flavonifractor, Alloprevotella, Negativibacillus, Ruminococcaceae UCG 004, Tyzzerella, Bacteroides*, and *Ruminococcaceae UCG 005* were strongly positively correlated with alterations in primary BA metabolism (CDCA and β-MCA) in the HFHC-PC group at week 3 or 6 (Figure 5c,d). *Parasutterella, Defluviitaleaceae UCG 011, Escherichia Shigella, Dubosiella, Akkermansia, Flavonifractor, Muribaculum, Eubacterium nodatum group, Ruminococcaceae UCG 004, Alloprevotella, Eubacterium coprostanoligenes group, Negativibacillus, Parabacteroides, Erysipelatoclostridium, Tyzzerella, Escherichia Shigella, Candidatus Soleaferrea*, and *Dubosiella* were strongly positively correlated with alterations in secondary BA metabolism (such as LCA, DCA, GDCA, and TLCA) at week 3 or 6 (Figure 5c,d). In summary, we further identified that feeding an HFHC diet after cholecystectomy can disrupt gut microbiota homeostasis and BA metabolism through the gut microbe–BA axis.

3.5. HFHC Diet Exacerbates the Effects of Cholecystectomy on the Metabolic Function of the Gut Microbiota

The gut microbiota is extensively involved in basic host metabolic activities, and this vast potential function affects whole-body metabolism and is a key factor in altering the metabolic profile of the host. Therefore, we further used PICRUSt predictions to determine the effects of cholecystectomy and feeding the HFHC diet after cholecystectomy on gut microbiota function in mice, and we further analyzed them in the context of the KEGG database (Figures S2a–f and S3a–f). Analysis of differential metabolic pathways showed that feeding an HFHC diet after either cholecystectomy or cholecystectomy significantly affected the metabolic pathways associated with the seven functional classes of the microbiota. Secondary BA biosynthesis and lipopolysaccharide biosynthesis proteins were significantly upregulated, and arachidonic acid metabolism was significantly downregulated in the LFLC-PC group compared to those in the LFLC-NC group (Figure 6a). Feeding an HFHC diet after cholecystectomy resulted in more differential metabolic pathways. Specifically, compared to the LFLC-PC group, the HFHC-PC group showed significantly upregulated arachidonic acid metabolism, biosynthesis of unsaturated fatty acids, steroid biosynthesis, primary BA biosynthesis, fatty acid biosynthesis, nitrogen metabolism, lipopolysaccharide biosynthesis, bacterial secretion system, bile secretion, pathways in cancer, and NAFLD disease metabolic pathways (Figure 6b). In addition, secondary BA biosynthesis was significantly reduced at week 3 and increased at week 6 (Figure 6b). Notably, mismatch repair, DNA repair, and recombination proteins were significantly downregulated (Figure 6b). Functional predictions further revealed that alterations in gut microbiota homeostasis were accompanied by corresponding changes in metabolic function, which may have more profound effects on the host.

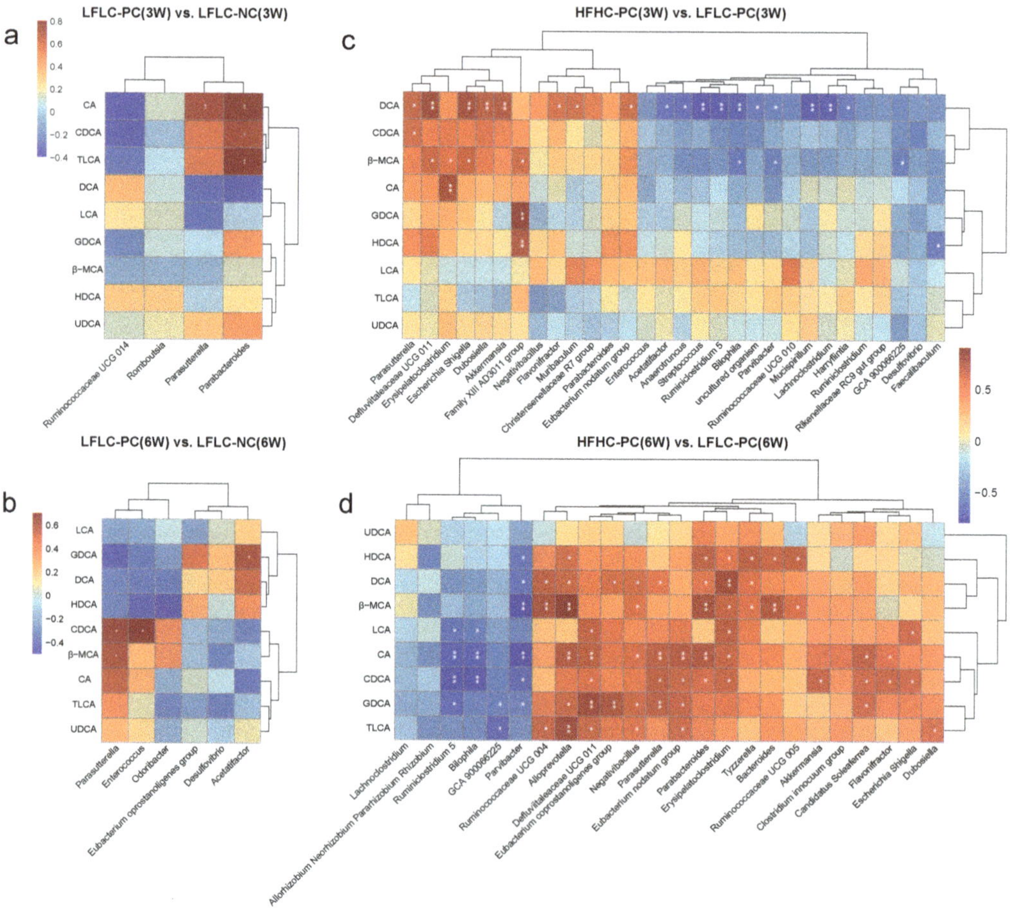

Figure 5. Effect of different diets and PC on BA metabolism in relation to gut microbiota. (**a**,**b**): Spearman's correlation between gut microbiota and fecal BAs in LFLC−PC vs. LFLC−NC groups at weeks 3 (**a**) and 6 (**b**). (**c**,**d**): Spearman's correlation between gut microbiota and BAs in HFHC−PC vs. LFLC−PC groups at weeks 3 (**c**) and 6 (**d**). Red denotes a positive correlation; blue denotes a negative correlation. The color intensity is proportional to the strength of the Spearman's correlation. * $p \leq 0.05$, ** $p \leq 0.01$.

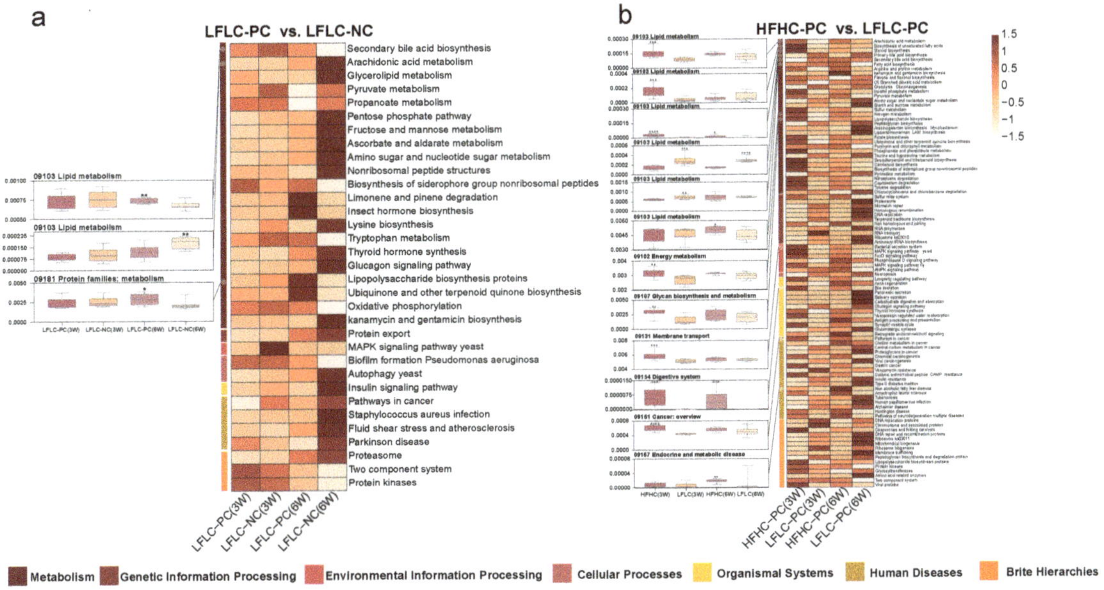

Figure 6. HFHC diets and PC altered gut microbiota metabolism in mice. PICRUSt analysis in the KEGG pathways. (**a**): HFHC−PC vs. LFLC−PC groups (at weeks 3 and 6). (**b**): LFLC−PC vs. LFLC−NC groups (at weeks 3 and 6). The boxplots (**left**) show the relative abundance of the metabolic pathway of the HFHC−PC, LFLC−PC, and LFLC−NC groups (at weeks 3 and 6). All boxplots represent the min to max of the distribution; the median is shown as a thick line in the middle of the box. Heat maps (**right**) show differential metabolic pathways between the two groups (a: top 60 pathways). The color indicates the median relative abundance of the metabolic pathway in the group. Mann–Whitney test was used for comparison between the two groups ($p < 0.05$). * $p < 0.05$, ** $p < 0.01$, *** $p < 0.001$, **** $p < 0.0001$.

3.6. HFHC Diet Exacerbates Dysbiosis of Metabolite Metabolism by Cholecystectomy

Next, we examined alterations in bacteria-derived metabolites due to microbial changes. At week 6, untargeted metabolomics analysis showed that cholecystectomy had a small effect on bacterial metabolites (Figures 7a,c and S4a,b), whereas feeding an HFHC diet after cholecystectomy significantly altered the metabolite classification levels in mice (Figures 7b,d and S4c,d). Compared to the LFLC-NC group, the differential metabolites in the LFLC-PC group were 1,5-Anhydro-D-glucitol-2 and D-(+)-Galactose at week 6 (Figure 7e). A total of 26 differential metabolites were examined in the HFHC-PC group compared to the LFLC-PC group at week 6, including 19 upregulated and 7 downregulated metabolites (Figure 7f). Importantly, arachidonic acid was significantly enriched in the HFHC-PC group (Figure 7f), and this substance is important for the cytotoxic effects of BAs. Similarly, to clarify the specific relationship between these metabolites and gut microbiota, we used Spearman's correlation analysis to correlate differential metabolites with differential microbiota. The results showed that alterations in the gut microbiota were accompanied by the upregulation or downregulation of metabolites. Among these, arachidonic acid was strongly and positively correlated with *Parasutterella*, *Negativibacillus*, *Candidatus Soleaferrea*, *Eubacterium nodatum group*, *Defluviitaleaceae UCG 011*, *Erysipelatoclostridium*, *Alloprevotella*, *Parabacteroides*, *Tyzzerella*, *Bacteroides*, and *Flavonifractor*, and it was strongly and negatively correlated with *uncultured organism* and *Parvibacter* (Figure S5). SCFAs are the main product of the breakdown of indigestible carbohydrates by the gut microbiota, and the HFHC-PC group showed a depleted content of acetate acid and butyric acid (Figure 7g,h). The results showed that feeding an HFHC diet after cholecystectomy altered fecal metabolic profiles in mice.

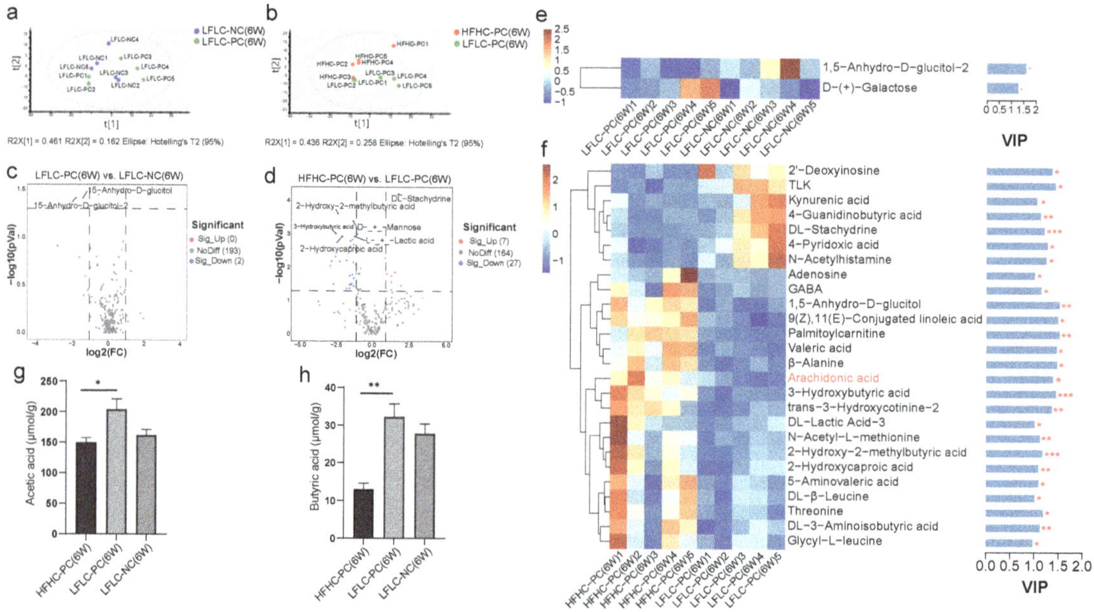

Figure 7. HFHC diet and PC altered the fecal metabolites in mice. (**a**,**b**): Principal component analysis (PCA) at week 6 (LFLC−PC vs. LFLC−NC (**a**); HFHC−PC vs. LFLC−PC (**b**)). (**c**,**d**): Volcanic map of all differential metabolites and known metabolites ($p < 0.05$) (LFLC−PC vs. LFLC−NC (**c**); HFHC−PC vs. LFLC−PC (**d**)). (**e**,**f**): Heat map analysis of fecal differential metabolites at week 6 in HFHC−PC vs. LFLC−PC groups (**e**) and LFLC−PC vs. LFLC−NC (**f**). The color indicates the median relative abundance of the metabolite in the group of samples. The metabolite clustering tree is shown on the left. The metabolite variable importance (VIP) in the projected values indicates the contribution of the metabolite to the difference between the two groups, as shown on the right. Higher VIP values indicate greater differences in the composition of that metabolite between the two groups. The differential metabolites were set as not less than 1. (**g**,**h**): Acetic acid, Butyric acid. The statistical significance (p−value) of the differential metabolites is marked on the right of the bar chart. p values were determined using a t-test. * $p \leq 0.05$, ** $p \leq 0.01$, *** $p \leq 0.001$.

4. Discussion

Cholecystectomy is often accompanied by a range of adverse gastrointestinal symptoms (diarrhea and abdominal pain), leading to the development of PC syndrome [35]. Further epidemiological investigations have suggested that cholecystectomy may increase the risk of diseases, such as CRC [5] and NAFLD [6]. However, the risk of cholecystectomy may be associated with the dysbiosis of gut microbiota and disturbances of the BA metabolism following cholecystectomy [7]. Diet is a key factor that influences BA metabolism and microbial homeostasis [36]. Previous studies have shown that an HFHC diet is positively associated with the development of PC syndrome [9,37] and NAFLD [38] and negatively associated with the consumption of whole grains, legumes, fish, and vegetables. In addition, a population-based cohort study of 1,033,955 also showed that the risk of cholecystectomy was associated with a high intake of ham, whereas adherence to a diet rich in fruits, vegetables, legumes, and olive oil was associated with a reduced risk of cholecystectomy [8]. In summary, an HFHC diet after cholecystectomy is a potential factor that increases the risk of cholecystectomy. However, whether high dietary cholesterol intake exacerbates disturbances in BA metabolism and disrupts gut microbial homeostasis after cholecystectomy remains unknown.

Based on this, we successfully constructed a cholecystectomized mice model and fed diets with different levels of fat and cholesterol. The results showed that cholecystectomy significantly increased the expression levels of colonic IL-10, whereas NF-κB showed an increasing trend. However, an HFHC diet after cholecystectomy further increased the levels of the colonic pro-inflammatory cytokines IL-1β, TNF-α, IL-6, and NF-κB, although no significant damage could be detected in histology. Our study suggests that the intake of an HFHC diet after cholecystectomy increases the risk of intestinal pro-inflammation.

Furthermore, we clarified the possible factors of an HFHC diet that promote inflammation after cholecystectomy. The gut microbiota can influence host health through its direct involvement in immune and metabolic pathways [39]. The results showed that an HFHC diet after cholecystectomy exacerbated the disruptive effects of cholecystectomy on the structural and metabolic functions of the gut microbiota. During the experimental period, we found that the effect of cholecystectomy on the structure of the gut microbiota was largely dependent on time, which altered the beta diversity at week 6. In addition, feeding the HFHC diet after cholecystectomy significantly increased the alpha diversity (week 6) and altered the beta diversity (weeks 3 and 6) of the microbiota. Although decreased microbial diversity is associated with several diseases [40], higher diversity does not necessarily imply a healthier microbial community. This may be due to the fact that the HFHC diet promoted the colonization of species that have damaging effects on the intestinal barrier [41]. Interestingly, the ratio of Firmicutes to Bacteroides (F/B), a well-known biomarker of obesity, showed an increasing trend in many HFHC studies [42]. However, in our study, the F/B ratio in the HFHC-PC group showed a decreasing trend at both weeks 3 and 6 compared to that in the LFLC-PC group. Further analysis revealed that some representative genera of the phylum Bacteroides (such as *Bacteroides* and *Parabacteroides*) were significantly enriched in the HFHC-PC group and that they all had the ability to metabolize BAs [43], thus leading to a decreasing trend in the F/B ratio.

We further analyzed how the gut microbiota was altered at the genus level. Simultaneously, the abundances of some pathogenic bacteria with pro-inflammatory effects were significantly higher in the HFHC-PC group, such as *Defluviitaleaceae UCG 011*, *Flavonifractor*, *Erysipelatoclostridium*, and *Tyzzerella*. These results were consistent with those of previous studies on HFHC diets [44,45]. It has been hypothesized that they act either directly through secreted products or through the activation of the immune system. In addition, feeding an HFHC diet after cholecystectomy further increased the ability of cholecystectomy to enrich the microbiota associated with BA metabolism. This also suggests that unlike normal mice fed an HFHC diet, PC is also a key factor in the disruption of gut microbiota homeostasis by an HFHC diet. Studies have shown that *Enterococcus*, *Bacteroides*, and *Parabacteroides* possess BSH activity [43]. BSH activity is the main condition for the involvement of the intestinal microbiota in the BA deconjugation reaction, a process that fractures the C-24 N-acyl amide in conjugated BAs and leads to the formation of unconjugated BAs [46]. Moreover, elevated BSH levels are associated with increased bile toxicity [47]. According to reports, *Parasutterella* [48], *Odoribacter* [49], *Dubosiella* [50], *Family XIII AD3011 group* [51], *Christensenellaceae R7 group* [52], *Eubacterium coprostanoligenes group* [53], and *Alloprevotella* [54] can also regulate BA metabolism through direct colonization or indirect action. In our Spearman's correlation analysis, we further confirmed that altered levels of BA metabolizing genera were the main cause of elevated fecal secondary BA levels. The abundance of *Akkermansia*, a next-generation probiotic, has been reported to be significantly reduced in high-fat diets [55]. However, in our study, *Akkermansia* was significantly enriched by feeding an HFHC diet after cholecystectomy. Studies have demonstrated that *Akkermansia* can regulate BA metabolism by acting directly or by influencing metabolite levels [56,57]. Therefore, HFHC feeding after cholecystectomy may enrich *Akkermansia* by upregulating the BA metabolism pathway. Notably, excessive intestinal *Akkermansia* counts have been reported to damage the intestinal barrier and cause elevated pro-inflammatory cytokine expression [58]. SCFAs are products of dietary fiber fermentation by the gut microbiota, are involved in host immune regulation, and have anti-inflammatory effects. We identified several major SCFA producers in the HFHC-PC group, including *Lachnoclostridium* [59], *Fecalibaculum* [60], *Anaerotruncus* [61], and *Ruminiclostridium* [62]. These results are consistent with the fecal levels of fecal SCFAs, as feeding an HFHC diet after cholecystectomy significantly reduced the fecal levels of acetate and butyric acid. This is detrimental to the intestine and may also contribute to elevated pro-inflammatory levels in the intestine.

The gut microbiota–BA axis is the main pathway of the BA metabolism, and studies have shown that microbial diversity significantly influences the BA pool size [12]. We found that cholecystectomy only upregulated liver CYP7B1 and BSEP mRNA expression levels, whereas an HFHC diet after cholecystectomy upregulated liver CYP7A1, CYP8B1, FXR, and BSEP and ileal ASBT mRNA expression levels. This leads to further accumulation of primary and secondary BAs in the feces of those consuming an HFHC diet after cholecystectomy [63]. It consists mainly of the primary BAs CDCA, CA, and β-MCA and the secondary BAs LCA, DCA, GDCA, and TLCA. This may be attributed to increased BA synthesis and an increased number of enterohepatic cycles [64]. Meanwhile, our study suggests that the classical synthesis pathway of hepatic BAs was significantly promoted in the HFHC-PC group. In conclusion, an excessive intake of cholesterol, a precursor of BA synthesis [65], can increase BA accumulation by promoting the upregulation of BA synthase following cholecystectomy.

Owing to their strong hydrophobic properties, BAs have toxic effects on cells. The hydrophobicity of the BAs decreased in the following order: LCA > DCA > CDCA > TDCA > TCDCA [66]. For example, in studies on the mechanisms on cholestatic liver injury, it has been suggested that the intrahepatic accumulation of hydrophobic BAs (such as DCA and CDCA) may be a possible cause of liver injury [67].

Previous studies have reported that high levels of secondary BAs can have adverse effects on the host, mainly by promoting inflammation, oxidative DNA damage, and activation of the NF-κB pathway [16]. First, BAs lead to activation of NF-κB, mainly through direct disruption of the plasma membrane, which, in turn, increases the pro-inflammatory response. This is because activated NF-κB transcribes genes encoding pro-inflammatory cytokines (such as IL-6, IL-1β, and TNF-α) in the cell nucleus [16]. In addition, DCA may lead to the increased production of pro-inflammatory cytokines, in part, by activating pro-inflammatory macrophages to polarize towards the M1 phenotype [16]. Studies have established that the chronic intake of high doses of DCA exacerbates intestinal inflammation and accelerates the transition from intestinal adenoma to colonic adenocarcinoma [68]. In conclusion, our study suggests that intake of an HFHC diet after cholecystectomy increases the metabolism of primary and secondary BAs in the intestine. High levels of BA metabolism can have adverse effects on the intestinal tract when exposed to it for long periods of time.

Perturbation of the gut microbiota and BA metabolism was further confirmed by predicting KEGG metabolic pathways. Cholecystectomy significantly upregulated secondary BA biosynthesis and lipopolysaccharide biosynthesis protein metabolic pathways in the microbiota, a phenomenon similar to that observed in the HFHC-PC group. LPS acts as a pro-inflammatory factor in the cell wall of Gram-negative bacteria and can significantly contribute to a sustained inflammatory response in immunocompromised hosts or when barrier integrity is compromised [69]. In addition, metabolic pathways associated with lipid metabolism, such as arachidonic acid metabolism, primary BA biosynthesis, and fatty acid biosynthesis were also significantly upregulated in the HFHC-PC group, consistent with the high levels of fecal BA metabolism. Importantly, the microbiota in the HFHC-PC group exhibited a lack of genetic information processing capacity compared to that in the LFLC-PC group. Examples include DNA replication, mismatch repair, and homologous recombination metabolic pathways. Among these, loss of function in homologous recombination has been shown to be a key factor in DNA repair failure [70]. In addition, DNA replication and mismatch repair play important roles in genomic stability and tumorigenesis [71]. These findings further confirm that an HFHC diet after cholecystectomy can adversely affect the intestines by disrupting gut microbiota homeostasis and affecting gut microbiota-related metabolic functions.

Untargeted metabolomics has also revealed possible reasons for the formation of a pro-inflammatory environment. We noted that arachidonic acid metabolism levels were significantly higher in the HFHC-PC group than that in the LFLC-PC group. Perturbation of the cell membrane by BAs has been reported to activate cytoplasmic phospholipase A2, which uses cyclooxygenase and lipoxygenase activities to release arachidonic acid from the cell membrane, ultimately increasing intracellular reactive oxygen species (ROS) levels [66]. In addition, TLK, kynurenic acid, 4-guanidinobutyric acid, and dl-stachydrine showed lower levels in the HFHC-PC group. TLK has been reported to play a central role in DNA repair and replication and is a potential target for novel cancer therapies [72]. In addition, kynurenic acid, 4-Guanidinobutyric acid, and dl-stachydrine possess anti-inflammatory activities. Kynurenic acid acts as an activator of various receptors (such as the aryl hydrocarbon receptor and G protein-coupled receptor) and is involved in the host immune response, with anti-inflammatory activity [73]. 4-Guanidinobutyric acid [74] and dl-stachydrine [75] can also maintain intestinal function and prevent inflammation through various molecular mechanisms.

In conclusion, our study showed that an HFHC diet after cholecystectomy promotes intestinal inflammation, mainly through the enrichment of microbiota associated with the BA metabolism and pro-inflammatory effects while decreasing the abundance of major SCFA producers. In addition, alterations in gut microbial homeostasis leading to further accumulation of fecal BAs and pro-inflammatory metabolites are key factors in the development of pro-inflammation.

5. Conclusions

Comprehensive multi-omics analyses showed that an HFHC diet after cholecystectomy in our study could further promote intestinal inflammation, and the mechanism of action was related to the exacerbated gut microbiota dysbiosis and BA disorders in cholecystectomy. There are several limitations of our study. We failed to observe significant histological changes during our experimental period. In addition, to clarify the effect of different dietary patterns on intestinal health after cholecystectomy, we set up only the cholecystectomy group in the HFHC dietary pattern. Thus, we were unable to confirm whether similar results were seen in an HFHC dietary model beyond the cholecystectomy model. In the future, we propose to investigate the long-term effects of an HFHC diet on histological changes after cholecystectomy and potential interventions to mitigate the pro-inflammatory effects. In addition, further clarification of whether cholecystectomy is a potential factor in HFHC diets impairing intestinal health could help us to better understand the risks after cholecystectomy. Despite these limitations, our study revealed the mechanisms involved in the promotion of intestinal inflammation by an HFHC diet after cholecystectomy. Long-term dietary patterns and probiotic interventions are key factors in the development of stable gut microbiota homeostasis and metabolic profiles. Targeting the gut microbiota by designing targeted food and probiotic interventions to modulate the gut microbiota with key metabolic functions to maintain a stable pool of BAs after cholecystectomy is key to improving intestinal health after cholecystectomy. In conclusion, our findings provide a theoretical basis for reducing PC risk in future clinical applications.

Supplementary Materials: The following supporting information can be downloaded at: https://www.mdpi.com/article/10.3390/nu15173829/s1, Figure S1: Microbial co-abundance analysis at genus level. (a,b): Microbial co-abundance analysis at genus level in the LFLC−PC group at weeks 3 (a) and 6 (b). (c,d): Microbial co-abundance analysis at genus level in the HFHC−PC group at weeks 3 (c) and 6 (d). Black line connections represent relevance. The color of the nodes is based on phylum and the size is based on edges connected to the nodes ($p \leq 0.05$, two-sided tests of 1000 permutations). Only lines corresponding to correlations whose magnitude is greater than 0.1 are drawn. Figure S2 KEGG enrichment analysis in LFLC−PC vs. LFLC−NC groups at 3 weeks (a–c) and 6 weeks (d–f).

(a,d): Rich Factor represents the ratio of the number of differentially expressed genes in the pathway to the total number of genes in the pathway. The degree of enrichment is represented by the Rich Factor, the number of genes is represented by the bubble size, and the significance level is represented by the bubble color. (b,e): Statistical histogram of KEGG pathway enrichment numbers. The vertical black font represents the KEGG A class, the color font represents the KEGG B class, and the number of genes in class B is shown on the abscissa. (c,f): The name of each KEGG pathway is shown on the left, and the corresponding *Q* value is shown on the right. Figure S3 KEGG enrichment analysis in HFHC−PC vs. LFLC−PC groups at 3 weeks (a–c) and 6 weeks (d- f). (a,d): Rich Factor represents the ratio of the number of differentially expressed genes in the pathway to the total number of genes in the pathway. The degree of enrichment is represented by the Rich Factor, the number of genes is represented by the bubble size, and the significance level is represented by the bubble color. (b,e): Statistical histogram of KEGG pathway enrichment numbers. The vertical black font represents the KEGG A class, the color font represents the KEGG B class, and the number of genes in class B is shown on the abscissa. (c,f): The name of each KEGG pathway is shown on the left, and the corresponding *Q* value is shown on the right. Figure S4 Metabolomics analysis of fecal samples from mice in LFLC−PC vs. LFLC−NC groups at 6 weeks (a-b), and HFHC-PC vs. LFLC-PC groups at 6 weeks (c-d). Partial least squares discriminant analysis (PLS-DA) and orthogonal partial least squares discriminant analysis (OPLS−DA). Figure S5 Spearman analysis of differential metabolite and genus genus correlation (HFHC−PC vs. LFLC−PC at 6 weeks). * $p \leq 0.05$, ** $p \leq 0.01$. Table S1. The feed formulation details. Table S2. The elution gradien. Table S3. Quantitative Real−Time Polymerase Chain Reaction (qRT−PCR) primer.

Author Contributions: F.X.: conceptualization, methodology, writing—original draft, software, writing—review and editing. Y.L.: investigation, writing—review and editing. T.D.: visualization, investigation. L.Y.: data curation, supervision. F.T.: supervision, writing—review and editing. Q.Z.: project administration, funding, writing—review and editing. W.C.: project administration, funding, writing—review and editing. Z.Y.: project administration, funding, writing—review and editing. All authors have read and agreed to the published version of the manuscript.

Funding: This work was supported by the National Natural Science Foundation of China [No. 32122067 and 32021005], the Natural Science Foundation of Jiangsu Province [BK20200084], and supported by the Fundamental Research Funds for the Central Universities JUSRP622013, 2023 New "Three" Strategy Project for Nurturing High-end Talents [2023XSMZL-GD-YZM-2023].

Institutional Review Board Statement: This study was approved by the Experimental Animal Ethics Committee of Jiangnan University (Qualification number: JN. No20220930c0550401[403]).

Informed Consent Statement: Not applicable.

Data Availability Statement: All data generated during and/or analyzed are available from the corresponding author on reasonable request.

Conflicts of Interest: The authors declare no conflict of interest.

References

1. Shaffer, E.A. Review article: Control of gall-bladder motor function. *Aliment. Pharmacol. Ther.* **2000**, *14*, 2–8. [CrossRef]
2. Maldonado-Valderrama, J.; Wilde, P.; Macierzanka, A.; Mackie, A. The role of bile salts in digestion. *Adv. Colloid. Interface Sci.* **2011**, *165*, 36–46. [CrossRef]
3. Bertolini, A.; Fiorotto, R.; Strazzabosco, M. Bile acids and their receptors: Modulators and therapeutic targets in liver inflammation. *Semin. Immunopathol.* **2022**, *44*, 547–564. [CrossRef]
4. Kullak-Ublick, G.A.; Paumgartner, G.; Berr, F. Long-term effects of cholecystectomy on bile acid metabolism. *Hepatology* **1995**, *21*, 41–45. [CrossRef]
5. Lagergren, J.; Ye, W.; Ekbom, A. Intestinal cancer after cholecystectomy: Is bile involved in carcinogenesis? *Gastroenterology* **2001**, *121*, 542–547. [CrossRef]
6. Ruhl, C.E.; Everhart, J.E. Relationship of non-alcoholic fatty liver disease with cholecystectomy in the US population. *Am. J. Gastroenterol.* **2013**, *108*, 952–958. [CrossRef] [PubMed]
7. Xu, Y.; Wang, J.; Wu, X.; Jing, H.; Zhang, S.; Hu, Z.; Rao, L.; Chang, Q.; Wang, L.; Zhang, Z. Gut microbiota alteration after cholecystectomy contributes to post-cholecystectomy diarrhea via bile acids stimulating colonic serotonin. *Gut Microbes* **2023**, *15*, 2168101. [CrossRef] [PubMed]
8. Barre, A.; Gusto, G.; Cadeau, C.; Carbonnel, F.; Boutron-Ruault, M.C. Diet and Risk of Cholecystectomy: A Prospective Study Based on the French E3N Cohort. *Am. J. Gastroenterol.* **2017**, *112*, 1448–1456.e1018. [CrossRef] [PubMed]

9. Yueh, T.P.; Chen, F.Y.; Lin, T.E.; Chuang, M.T. Diarrhea after laparoscopic cholecystectomy: Associated factors and predictors. *Asian J. Surg.* **2014**, *37*, 171–177. [CrossRef]
10. Liu, Y.; Xu, J.; Ren, X.; Zhang, Y.; Ke, Z.; Zhou, J.; Wang, Y.; Zhang, Y.; Liu, Y. Cholecystectomy-induced secondary bile acids accumulation ameliorates colitis through inhibiting monocyte/macrophage recruitment. *Gut Microbes* **2022**, *14*, 2107387. [CrossRef]
11. Park, S.; Zhang, T.; Yue, Y.; Wu, X. Effects of Bile Acid Modulation by Dietary Fat, Cholecystectomy, and Bile Acid Sequestrant on Energy, Glucose, and Lipid Metabolism and Gut Microbiota in Mice. *Int. J. Mol. Sci.* **2022**, *23*, 5935. [CrossRef] [PubMed]
12. Collins, S.L.; Stine, J.G.; Bisanz, J.E.; Okafor, C.D.; Patterson, A.D. Bile acids and the gut microbiota: Metabolic interactions and impacts on disease. *Nat. Rev. Microbiol.* **2023**, *21*, 236–247. [CrossRef]
13. Wahlstrom, A.; Sayin, S.I.; Marschall, H.U.; Backhed, F. Intestinal Crosstalk between Bile Acids and Microbiota and Its Impact on Host Metabolism. *Cell Metab.* **2016**, *24*, 41–50. [CrossRef] [PubMed]
14. Begley, M.; Gahan, C.G.; Hill, C. The interaction between bacteria and bile. *FEMS Microbiol. Rev.* **2005**, *29*, 625–651. [CrossRef]
15. Tian, Y.; Gui, W.; Koo, I.; Smith, P.B.; Allman, E.L.; Nichols, R.G.; Rimal, B.; Cai, J.; Liu, Q.; Patterson, A.D. The microbiome modulating activity of bile acids. *Gut Microbes* **2020**, *11*, 979–996. [CrossRef] [PubMed]
16. Cai, J.; Sun, L.; Gonzalez, F.J. Gut microbiota-derived bile acids in intestinal immunity, inflammation, and tumorigenesis. *Cell Host Microbe* **2022**, *30*, 289–300. [CrossRef]
17. Fu, T.; Coulter, S.; Yoshihara, E.; Oh, T.G.; Fang, S.; Cayabyab, F.; Zhu, Q.; Zhang, T.; Leblanc, M.; Liu, S.; et al. FXR Regulates Intestinal Cancer Stem Cell Proliferation. *Cell* **2019**, *176*, 1098–1112. [CrossRef]
18. Mayr, L.; Grabherr, F.; Schwärzler, J.; Reitmeier, I.; Sommer, F.; Gehmacher, T.; Niederreiter, L.; He, G.-W.; Ruder, B.; Kunz, K.T.R.; et al. Dietary lipids fuel GPX4-restricted enteritis resembling Crohn's disease. *Nat. Commun.* **2020**, *11*, 1775. [CrossRef]
19. Massironi, S.; Viganò, C.; Palermo, A.; Pirola, L.; Mulinacci, G.; Allocca, M.; Peyrin-Biroulet, L.; Danese, S. Inflammation and malnutrition in inflammatory bowel disease. *Lancet Gastroenterol. Hepatol.* **2023**, *8*, 579–590. [CrossRef]
20. Wan, Y.; Yuan, J.; Li, J.; Li, H.; Zhang, J.; Tang, J.; Ni, Y.; Huang, T.; Wang, F.; Zhao, F.; et al. Unconjugated and secondary bile acid profiles in response to higher-fat, lower-carbohydrate diet and associated with related gut microbiota: A 6-month randomized controlled-feeding trial. *Clin. Nutr.* **2020**, *39*, 395–404. [CrossRef]
21. Ferrell, J.M.; Boehme, S.; Li, F.; Chiang, J.Y. Cholesterol 7alpha-hydroxylase-deficient mice are protected from high-fat/high-cholesterol diet-induced metabolic disorders. *J. Lipid Res.* **2016**, *57*, 1144–1154. [CrossRef] [PubMed]
22. Makki, K.; Deehan, E.C.; Walter, J.; Backhed, F. The Impact of Dietary Fiber on Gut Microbiota in Host Health and Disease. *Cell Host Microbe* **2018**, *23*, 705–715. [CrossRef]
23. Dalile, B.; Van Oudenhove, L.; Vervliet, B.; Verbeke, K. The role of short-chain fatty acids in microbiota-gut-brain communication. *Nat. Rev. Gastroenterol. Hepatol.* **2019**, *16*, 461–478. [CrossRef] [PubMed]
24. Zhang, X.Y.; Chen, J.; Yi, K.; Peng, L.; Xie, J.; Gou, X.; Peng, T.; Tang, L. Phlorizin ameliorates obesity-associated endotoxemia and insulin resistance in high-fat diet-fed mice by targeting the gut microbiota and intestinal barrier integrity. *Gut Microbes* **2020**, *12*, 1842990. [CrossRef] [PubMed]
25. Wang, X.; Li, Y.; Qiang, G.; Wang, K.; Dai, J.; McCann, M.; Munoz, M.D.; Gil, V.; Yu, Y.; Li, S.; et al. Secreted EMC10 is upregulated in human obesity and its neutralizing antibody prevents diet-induced obesity in mice. *Nat. Commun.* **2022**, *13*, 7323. [CrossRef]
26. Hadjihambi, A.; Konstantinou, C.; Klohs, J.; Monsorno, K.; Le Guennec, A.; Donnelly, C.; Cox, I.J.; Kusumbe, A.; Hosford, P.S.; Soffientini, U.; et al. Partial MCT1 invalidation protects against diet-induced non-alcoholic fatty liver disease and the associated brain dysfunction. *J. Hepatol.* **2023**, *78*, 180–190. [CrossRef]
27. Al-Sheraji, S.H.; Ismail, A.; Manap, M.Y.; Mustafa, S.; Yusof, R.M.; Hassan, F.A. Hypocholesterolaemic effect of yoghurt containing Bifidobacterium pseudocatenulatum G4 or Bifidobacterium longum BB536. *Food Chem.* **2012**, *135*, 356–361. [CrossRef] [PubMed]
28. Liu, Y.; Sheng, Y.; Pan, Q.; Xue, Y.; Yu, L.; Tian, F.; Zhao, J.; Zhang, H.; Zhai, Q.; Chen, W. Identification of the key physiological characteristics of Lactobacillus plantarum strains for ulcerative colitis alleviation. *Food Funct.* **2020**, *11*, 1279–1291. [CrossRef]
29. Qian, W.; Li, M.; Yu, L.; Tian, F.; Zhao, J.; Zhai, Q. Effects of Taurine on Gut Microbiota Homeostasis: An Evaluation Based on Two Models of Gut Dysbiosis. *Biomedicines* **2023**, *11*, 1048. [CrossRef]
30. John, C.; Werner, P.; Worthmann, A.; Wegner, K.; Todter, K.; Scheja, L.; Rohn, S.; Heeren, J.; Fischer, M. A liquid chromatography-tandem mass spectrometry-based method for the simultaneous determination of hydroxy sterols and bile acids. *J. Chromatogr. A* **2014**, *1371*, 184–195. [CrossRef]
31. Lu, W.; Deng, Y.; Fang, Z.; Zhai, Q.; Cui, S.; Zhao, J.; Chen, W.; Zhang, H. Potential Role of Probiotics in Ameliorating Psoriasis by Modulating Gut Microbiota in Imiquimod-Induced Psoriasis-Like Mice. *Nutrients* **2021**, *13*, 2010. [CrossRef] [PubMed]
32. Liu, B.; Yu, L.; Zhai, Q.; Li, M.; Li, L.; Tian, F.; Chen, W. Effect of water-soluble polysaccharides from Morchella esculenta on high-fat diet-induced obese mice: Changes in gut microbiota and metabolic functions. *Food Funct.* **2023**, *14*, 5217–5231. [CrossRef] [PubMed]
33. Tian, P.; O'Riordan, K.J.; Lee, Y.K.; Wang, G.; Zhao, J.; Zhang, H.; Cryan, J.F.; Chen, W. Towards a psychobiotic therapy for depression: Bifidobacterium breve CCFM1025 reverses chronic stress-induced depressive symptoms and gut microbial abnormalities in mice. *Neurobiol. Stress.* **2020**, *12*, 100216. [CrossRef] [PubMed]
34. Wang, L.; Hu, L.; Xu, Q.; Jiang, T.; Fang, S.; Wang, G.; Zhao, J.; Zhang, H.; Chen, W. Bifidobacteria exert species-specific effects on constipation in BALB/c mice. *Food Funct.* **2017**, *8*, 3587–3600. [CrossRef]

35. Ruiz-Clavijo Garcia, D.; Vila Costas, J.; Prieto Martinez, C.; Elizalde Apesteguia, I.; Tarifa Castilla, A.; Mercado Gutierrez, M.; Casi Villarroya, M.; Urman Fernandez, J.M.; Herrera Cabezon, F.J. Cystic duct remnant syndrome as a cause of post-cholecystectomy syndrome. *Gastroenterol. Hepatol.* **2016**, *39*, 722–724. [CrossRef]
36. Yokota, A.; Fukiya, S.; Islam, K.B.; Ooka, T.; Ogura, Y.; Hayashi, T.; Hagio, M.; Ishizuka, S. Is bile acid a determinant of the gut microbiota on a high-fat diet? *Gut Microbes* **2012**, *3*, 455–459. [CrossRef]
37. Shin, Y.; Choi, D.; Lee, K.G.; Choi, H.S.; Park, Y. Association between dietary intake and postlaparoscopic cholecystectomic symptoms in patients with gallbladder disease. *Korean J. Intern. Med.* **2018**, *33*, 829–836. [CrossRef]
38. Shim, P.; Choi, D.; Park, Y. Association of Blood Fatty Acid Composition and Dietary Pattern with the Risk of Non-Alcoholic Fatty Liver Disease in Patients Who Underwent Cholecystectomy. *Ann. Nutr. Metab.* **2017**, *70*, 303–311. [CrossRef]
39. Peredo-Lovillo, A.; Romero-Luna, H.E.; Jimenez-Fernandez, M. Health promoting microbial metabolites produced by gut microbiota after prebiotics metabolism. *Food Res. Int.* **2020**, *136*, 109473. [CrossRef]
40. Pickard, J.M.; Zeng, M.Y.; Caruso, R.; Núñez, G. Gut microbiota: Role in pathogen colonization, immune responses, and inflammatory disease. *Immunol. Rev.* **2017**, *279*, 70–89. [CrossRef]
41. Rohr, M.W.; Narasimhulu, C.A.; Rudeski-Rohr, T.A.; Parthasarathy, S. Negative Effects of a High-Fat Diet on Intestinal Permeability: A Review. *Adv. Nutr.* **2020**, *11*, 77–91. [CrossRef] [PubMed]
42. Zhang, J.; Wei, J.; Liu, T.; Tang, J.; Zhang, X.; Feng, F.; Cai, H.; Zhao, M. Food additive glycerol monocaprylate modulated systemic inflammation and gut microbiota without stimulating metabolic dysfunction in high-fat diet fed mice. *Food Res. Int.* **2023**, *167*, 112734. [CrossRef] [PubMed]
43. Song, Z.; Cai, Y.; Lao, X.; Wang, X.; Lin, X.; Cui, Y.; Kalavagunta, P.K.; Liao, J.; Jin, L.; Shang, J.; et al. Taxonomic profiling and populational patterns of bacterial bile salt hydrolase (BSH) genes based on worldwide human gut microbiome. *Microbiome* **2019**, *7*, 9. [CrossRef] [PubMed]
44. Han, X.; Feng, Z.; Chen, Y.; Zhu, L.; Li, X.; Wang, X.; Sun, H.; Li, J. Effects of High-Fructose Corn Syrup on Bone Health and Gastrointestinal Microbiota in Growing Male Mice. *Front. Nutr.* **2022**, *9*, 829396. [CrossRef]
45. Lozano, C.P.; Wilkens, L.R.; Shvetsov, Y.B.; Maskarinec, G.; Park, S.Y.; Shepherd, J.A.; Boushey, C.J.; Hebert, J.R.; Wirth, M.D.; Ernst, T.; et al. Associations of the Dietary Inflammatory Index with total adiposity and ectopic fat through the gut microbiota, LPS, and C-reactive protein in the Multiethnic Cohort-Adiposity Phenotype Study. *Am. J. Clin. Nutr.* **2022**, *115*, 1344–1356. [CrossRef]
46. Ridlon, J.M.; Harris, S.C.; Bhowmik, S.; Kang, D.J.; Hylemon, P.B. Consequences of bile salt biotransformations by intestinal bacteria. *Gut Microbes* **2016**, *7*, 22–39. [CrossRef]
47. Foley, M.H.; O'Flaherty, S.; Allen, G.; Rivera, A.J.; Stewart, A.K.; Barrangou, R.; Theriot, C.M. Lactobacillus bile salt hydrolase substrate specificity governs bacterial fitness and host colonization. *Proc. Natl. Acad. Sci. USA* **2021**, *118*, e2017709118. [CrossRef]
48. Yu, Z.; Wang, Y.; Zhang, F.; Ma, R.; Yang, X.; Yang, K.; Mi, A.; Ran, L.; Wu, Y. Deletion of hepatic growth hormone receptor (GHR) alters the mouse gut microbiota by affecting bile acid metabolism. *Gut Microbes* **2023**, *15*, 2221098. [CrossRef]
49. Sato, Y.; Atarashi, K.; Plichta, D.R.; Arai, Y.; Sasajima, S.; Kearney, S.M.; Suda, W.; Takeshita, K.; Sasaki, T.; Okamoto, S.; et al. Novel bile acid biosynthetic pathways are enriched in the microbiome of centenarians. *Nature* **2021**, *599*, 458–464. [CrossRef]
50. Zhuge, A.; Li, S.; Lou, P.; Wu, W.; Wang, K.; Yuan, Y.; Xia, J.; Li, B.; Li, L. Longitudinal 16S rRNA Sequencing Reveals Relationships among Alterations of Gut Microbiota and Nonalcoholic Fatty Liver Disease Progression in Mice. *Microbiol. Spectr.* **2022**, *10*, e0004722. [CrossRef]
51. Sun, J.; Fan, J.; Li, T.; Yan, X.; Jiang, Y. Nuciferine Protects Against High-Fat Diet-Induced Hepatic Steatosis via Modulation of Gut Microbiota and Bile Acid Metabolism in Rats. *J. Agric. Food Chem.* **2022**, *70*, 12014–12028. [CrossRef] [PubMed]
52. Dong, Z.; Zhang, D.; Wu, X.; Yin, Y.; Wan, D. Ferrous Bisglycinate Supplementation Modulates Intestinal Antioxidant Capacity via the AMPK/FOXO Pathway and Reconstitutes Gut Microbiota and Bile Acid Profiles in Pigs. *J. Agric. Food Chem.* **2022**, *70*, 4942–4951. [CrossRef]
53. Lei, S.; He, S.; Li, X.; Zheng, B.; Zhang, Y.; Zeng, H. Effect of lotus seed resistant starch on small intestinal flora and bile acids in hyperlipidemic rats. *Food Chem.* **2023**, *404*, 134599. [CrossRef]
54. Huang, K.; Liu, C.; Peng, M.; Su, Q.; Liu, R.; Guo, Z.; Chen, S.; Li, Z.; Chang, G. Glycoursodeoxycholic Acid Ameliorates Atherosclerosis and Alters Gut Microbiota in Apolipoprotein E-Deficient Mice. *J. Am. Heart Assoc.* **2021**, *10*, e019820. [CrossRef]
55. Dai, K.; Song, Y.; Zhang, D.; Wei, Y.; Jiang, S.; Xu, F.; Wang, H.; Zhang, X.; Shao, X. Thinned peach polyphenols alleviate obesity in high fat mice by affecting gut microbiota. *Food Res. Int.* **2022**, *157*, 111255. [CrossRef] [PubMed]
56. Dong, S.; Zhu, M.; Wang, K.; Zhao, X.; Hu, L.; Jing, W.; Lu, H.; Wang, S. Dihydromyricetin improves DSS-induced colitis in mice via modulation of fecal-bacteria-related bile acid metabolism. *Pharmacol. Res.* **2021**, *171*, 105767. [CrossRef] [PubMed]
57. Xie, J.; Li, H.; Zhang, X.; Yang, T.; Yue, M.; Zhang, Y.; Chen, S.; Cui, N.; Yuan, C.; Li, J.; et al. Akkermansia muciniphila protects mice against an emerging tick-borne viral pathogen. *Nat. Microbiol.* **2023**, *8*, 91–106. [CrossRef]
58. Qu, S.; Zheng, Y.; Huang, Y.; Feng, Y.; Xu, K.; Zhang, W.; Wang, Y.; Nie, K.; Qin, M. Excessive consumption of mucin by over-colonized Akkermansia muciniphila promotes intestinal barrier damage during malignant intestinal environment. *Front. Microbiol.* **2023**, *14*, 1111911. [CrossRef]
59. Xia, W.; Khan, I.; Li, X.A.; Huang, G.; Yu, Z.; Leong, W.K.; Han, R.; Ho, L.T.; Wendy Hsiao, W.L. Adaptogenic flower buds exert cancer preventive effects by enhancing the SCFA-producers, strengthening the epithelial tight junction complex and immune responses. *Pharmacol. Res.* **2020**, *159*, 104809. [CrossRef]

60. Liang, T.; Xie, X.; Wu, L.; Li, L.; Yang, L.; Jiang, T.; Du, M.; Chen, M.; Xue, L.; Zhang, J.; et al. Metabolism of resistant starch RS3 administered in combination with Lactiplantibacillus plantarum strain 84-3 by human gut microbiota in simulated fermentation experiments in vitro and in a rat model. *Food Chem.* **2023**, *411*, 135412. [CrossRef]
61. Yan, F.; Li, N.; Shi, J.; Li, H.; Yue, Y.; Jiao, W.; Wang, N.; Song, Y.; Huo, G.; Li, B. Lactobacillus acidophilus alleviates type 2 diabetes by regulating hepatic glucose, lipid metabolism and gut microbiota in mice. *Food Funct.* **2019**, *10*, 5804–5815. [CrossRef] [PubMed]
62. Wang, S.; Tao, X.; Zhang, G.; Zhang, P.; Wang, H.; Ye, J.; Li, F.; Zhang, Q.; Nabi, M. Benefit of solid-liquid separation on volatile fatty acid production from grass clipping with ultrasound-calcium hydroxide pretreatment. *Bioresour. Technol.* **2019**, *274*, 97–104. [CrossRef] [PubMed]
63. Yu, L.; Liu, Y.; Wang, S.; Zhang, Q.; Zhao, J.; Zhang, H.; Narbad, A.; Tian, F.; Zhai, Q.; Chen, W. Cholestasis: Exploring the triangular relationship of gut microbiota-bile acid-cholestasis and the potential probiotic strategies. *Gut Microbes* **2023**, *15*, 2181930. [CrossRef] [PubMed]
64. Kullak-Ublick, G.A.; Stieger, B.; Meier, P.J. Enterohepatic bile salt transporters in normal physiology and liver disease. *Gastroenterology* **2004**, *126*, 322–342. [CrossRef] [PubMed]
65. Chiang, J.Y. Bile acid metabolism and signaling. *Compr. Physiol.* **2013**, *3*, 1191–1212. [CrossRef]
66. Jia, W.; Xie, G.; Jia, W. Bile acid-microbiota crosstalk in gastrointestinal inflammation and carcinogenesis. *Nat. Rev. Gastroenterol. Hepatol.* **2018**, *15*, 111–128. [CrossRef]
67. Woolbright, B.L.; Jaeschke, H. Novel insight into mechanisms of cholestatic liver injury. *World J. Gastroenterol.* **2012**, *18*, 4985–4993. [CrossRef]
68. Xu, M.; Shen, Y.; Cen, M.; Zhu, Y.; Cheng, F.; Tang, L.; Zheng, X.; Kim, J.J.; Dai, N.; Hu, W. Modulation of the Gut Microbiota-farnesoid X Receptor Axis Improves Deoxycholic Acid-induced Intestinal Inflammation in Mice. *J. Crohns Colitis* **2021**, *15*, 1197–1210. [CrossRef]
69. Hetemaki, I.; Jian, C.; Laakso, S.; Makitie, O.; Pajari, A.M.; de Vos, W.M.; Arstila, T.P.; Salonen, A. Fecal Bacteria Implicated in Biofilm Production Are Enriched and Associate to Gastrointestinal Symptoms in Patients With APECED—A Pilot Study. *Front. Immunol.* **2021**, *12*, 668219. [CrossRef]
70. Hoppe, M.M.; Sundar, R.; Tan, D.S.P.; Jeyasekharan, A.D. Biomarkers for Homologous Recombination Deficiency in Cancer. *J. Natl. Cancer Inst.* **2018**, *110*, 704–713. [CrossRef]
71. Baretti, M.; Le, D.T. DNA mismatch repair in cancer. *Pharmacol. Ther.* **2018**, *189*, 45–62. [CrossRef] [PubMed]
72. Segura-Bayona, S.; Villamor-Paya, M.; Attolini, C.S.; Koenig, L.M.; Sanchiz-Calvo, M.; Boulton, S.J.; Stracker, T.H. Tousled-Like Kinases Suppress Innate Immune Signaling Triggered by Alternative Lengthening of Telomeres. *Cell Rep.* **2020**, *32*, 107983. [CrossRef]
73. Li, Y.; Liu, N.; Ge, Y.; Yang, Y.; Ren, F.; Wu, Z. Tryptophan and the innate intestinal immunity: Crosstalk between metabolites, host innate immune cells, and microbiota. *Eur. J. Immunol.* **2022**, *52*, 856–868. [CrossRef] [PubMed]
74. Li, W.; Luo, L.; Zhu, J.; Yan, H.; Yang, X.; Tang, W.; Li, D.; He, D.; Wang, J.; Dai, W.; et al. Water extract of Cayratia albifolia C.L.Li root relieves zymosan A-induced inflammation by restraining M1 macrophage polarization. *Phytomedicine* **2022**, *96*, 153901. [CrossRef]
75. Cheng, F.; Zhou, Y.; Wang, M.; Guo, C.; Cao, Z.; Zhang, R.; Peng, C. A review of pharmacological and pharmacokinetic properties of stachydrine. *Pharmacol. Res.* **2020**, *155*, 104755. [CrossRef] [PubMed]

nutrients

Review

A Comprehensive Review of the Effects of Glycemic Carbohydrates on the Neurocognitive Functions Based on Gut Microenvironment Regulation and Glycemic Fluctuation Control

Jian Yin [1], Li Cheng [1,2,3,4,*], Yan Hong [1,2,3,4], Zhaofeng Li [1,2,3,4], Caiming Li [1,2,3,4], Xiaofeng Ban [1,2,3,4], Ling Zhu [1,2,3,4] and Zhengbiao Gu [1,2,3,4,*]

1 School of Food Science and Technology, Jiangnan University, Wuxi 214122, China; 7200112038@stu.jiangnan.edu.cn (J.Y.); hongyan@jiangnan.edu.cn (Y.H.); zfli@jiangnan.edu.cn (Z.L.); caimingli@jiangnan.edu.cn (C.L.); banxiaofeng@jiangnan.edu.cn (X.B.); zhuling@jiangnan.edu.cn (L.Z.)
2 State Key Laboratory of Food Science and Technology, Jiangnan University, Wuxi 214122, China
3 Collaborative Innovation Center of Food Safety and Quality Control in Jiangsu Province, Jiangnan University, Wuxi 214122, China
4 National Engineering Research Center for Functional Food, Jiangnan University, Wuxi 214122, China
* Correspondence: 8929270007@jiangnan.edu.cn (L.C.); zhengbiaogu@jiangnan.edu.cn (Z.G.)

Abstract: Improper glycemic carbohydrates (GCs) consumption can be a potential risk factor for metabolic diseases such as obesity and diabetes, which may lead to cognitive impairment. Although several potential mechanisms have been studied, the biological relationship between carbohydrate consumption and neurocognitive impairment is still uncertain. In this review, the main effects and mechanisms of GCs' digestive characteristics on cognitive functions are comprehensively elucidated. Additionally, healthier carbohydrate selection, a reliable research model, and future directions are discussed. Individuals in their early and late lives and patients with metabolic diseases are highly susceptible to dietary-induced cognitive impairment. It is well known that gut function is closely related to dietary patterns. Unhealthy carbohydrate diet-induced gut microenvironment disorders negatively impact cognitive functions through the gut–brain axis. Moreover, severe glycemic fluctuations, due to rapidly digestible carbohydrate consumption or metabolic diseases, can impair neurocognitive functions by disrupting glucose metabolism, dysregulating calcium homeostasis, oxidative stress, inflammatory responses, and accumulating advanced glycation end products. Unstable glycemic status can lead to more severe neurological impairment than persistent hyperglycemia. Slow-digested or resistant carbohydrates might contribute to better neurocognitive functions due to stable glycemic response and healthier gut functions than fully gelatinized starch and nutritive sugars.

Keywords: glycemic carbohydrates; digestive properties; glycemic fluctuation; gut microbiota; glucose metabolism; cognitive functions

1. Introduction

Glycemic carbohydrates (GCs), easily digested and absorbed by the human body and triggering glycemic response, are one of the most essential and economical sources of dietary energy for humans [1]. They mainly consist of sugars (glucose, fructose, sucrose, and maltose), oligosaccharides (malto-oligosaccharides, maltodextrins), and polysaccharides (starches) based on their degree of polymerization. Glucose is an essential fuel for the brain, and glycemic carbohydrate intake plays a crucial role in human evolution. The preference for GCs contributes to an increasing number of younger patients with metabolic diseases, such as obesity and diabetes [2], and exerts a negative impact on cognition, especially in children, the elderly, and diabetics. Therefore, understanding the effects and mechanisms of different carbohydrates on neurocognitive function is a prerequisite for a reasonable selection of diet and the search for therapeutic targets for related diseases.

Different GCs can lead to different digestion rates and products due to differences in molecular size, structure, and anti-enzymatic hydrolysis ability. Unabsorbed digestive products can be used as substrates to remodel the gut microbiota and microenvironment after entering the colon. The gut microbiota metabolites, such as short-chain fatty acids (SCFAs), neurotransmitters, and lipopolysaccharides (LPS), can be transported to the central nervous system (CNS) via the vagus nerve or blood circulation (gut–brain axis), which affect the CNS function [3]. The above-mentioned monosaccharides, disaccharides, and the widely consumed rapidly digestive starch (RDS) after gelatinization could be promptly hydrolyzed in the small intestine, while slowly digestive starch (SDS) and resistant starch (RS) might delay digestion.

GCs can induce different glycemic responses. Elevated postprandial blood glucose level, a major risk factor for prediabetes and type II diabetes (T2DM), has emerged as a global epidemic [4]. The rapidly hydrolyzed carbohydrates can cause dramatic increases and decreases in blood glucose, resulting in severe glycemic fluctuations. Conversely, delaying starch digestion helps maintain glycemic homeostasis, thereby alleviating metabolic diseases [5,6]. Frequent and severe glycemic fluctuation is the embodiment of glycometabolism disorder, which is directly related to cognitive impairment [7,8]. Experiments on children have proven that sufficient glycemic supply induced by an acute increase in glycemic levels has a short-term (throughout the morning) positive impact on memory function [9,10], while a stable glycemic level can lead to better cognitive performance in the long term [11]. However, some of the crucial issues have not been fully elucidated yet. Most in vivo studies on the mechanism of glycemic fluctuations affecting cognitive function are based on typical metabolic diseases, such as obesity [12] and diabetes [8], while there is a lack of studies on the long-term impact of food-borne glycemic fluctuations on cognitive functions.

Therefore, comprehensive studies on the association between the reported GCs' composition, gut microbiota, glycemic fluctuation patterns, glucose metabolisms, and neuron functions are highly imperative, which will help us to understand the relationship between carbohydrate consumption and cognitive functions and to conduct new studies from a more scientific perspective.

2. Glycemic Carbohydrate Digestion Rate and Glycemic Fluctuation Patterns

The monosaccharides can be absorbed directly into the small intestine, while disaccharides are converted into monosaccharides by α-glucosidases at the brush border of the small intestine mucosa. As for oligosaccharides, malto-oligosaccharides (MOS) have lower permeability than glucose, which can prolong the absorption time and energy supply, resulting in smoother glycemic fluctuations [13]. Isomaltooligosaccharides (IMO) can also be slowly hydrolyzed by α-glucosidases and induce a slight glycemic response [14]. Starches can be gradually hydrolyzed into glucose in the digestive tract by amylase and then absorbed into the blood, which is the main source of exogenous glucose causing glycemic fluctuations. According to previous studies, the digestive rates and glycemic index (GI) values of RDS, SDS, and RS were reduced sequentially, and the former induced significantly more dramatic glycemic fluctuations than the latter two [15–17]. α-Amylase first hydrolyzes starch structures to linear MOS and branched α-limit dextrins. A clear trend has been found toward incrementally slower digestion as α-limit dextrins become larger in size with more branched points [18]. As an incomplete hydrolysate of starch, maltodextrins can also be divided into rapidly, slow digestible, and resistant maltodextrins based on their anti-enzymatic ability, leading to different degrees of glycemic response [19].

Hyperglycemia, hypoglycemia, and glycemic fluctuation (the non-stable state in which blood glucose levels oscillate between peaks and valleys over a period of time) can be induced by inappropriate dietary habits and relevant diseases like obesity and diabetes. GI and glycemic load (GL = GI × amount of carbohydrate) are important indicators of the effect of food-induced glycemic response on CNS, and the effect of carbohydrates on blood glucose concentration. Researchers have found that high-GI carbohydrates are more likely to induce food addiction, suggesting that consumers may fall into a vicious circle of high-

GI carbohydrates intake, addiction, and increased consumption [20]. However, no such relation between GI and digestion rate or glycemic response has been reported. Some SDS can retard digestion and provide a stable glycemic supply, maintaining energy metabolism homeostasis in vivo [21], but have high GI values due to their complex molecular structure and low contents of digestion-resisting components [22,23]. Extended blood glucose index is a potential index to evaluate the degree of slow and sustainable release of glucose from GCs [23]. Overall, unstable glycemic status can significantly increase the pressure to control glucose homeostasis, leading to inflammation, insulin resistance (IR), glucose, and other relevant metabolism disorders, resulting in neurocognitive impairment. It is worth noting that reducing carbohydrate intake is not an ideal way to reduce glycemic fluctuation or GL. Studies have shown that a reasonable intake of carbohydrates (45% to 60% of daily energy intake) is crucial to ensuring a balanced intake of macronutrients and maintaining metabolic health [24]. Some emerging special dietary patterns such as energy-restricted/intermittent fasting diets [25] and ketogenic diets [26] have reported positive significance in assisting intervention under specialized supervision. However, they may carry risks when there is a lack of supervision or for some special populations. It has been reported that both may lead to nutrient deficiencies over a prolonged period for patients with multiple sclerosis [27]. Intermittent fasting with unreasonable timing can damage immune functions and increase inflammatory responses [28]. For most individuals, a ketogenic diet may lead to decreased appetite and insufficient nutrient intake, which exacerbates the long-term health risk of maintaining this pattern [26,29]. Additionally, a return to a regular-carb diet after a prolonged period of low-carb diet is more likely to cause acute negative consequences like disease-related carbotoxicity [6]. Therefore, the research and development of smooth glycemic response carbohydrates could be a potential approach to reducing the potential hazards of glycemic carbohydrate consumption.

3. Susceptible Population for Diet-Induced Neurocognitive Impairments

3.1. Early and Late Life of Healthy Individuals

Dietary intervention is a moderate, time-consuming process. Some populations are vulnerable to glycemic carbohydrate-induced changes in the gut microenvironment or glycemic fluctuation-induced neurocognitive functions. The CNS is immature and susceptible to the influence of external factors in early life. Generally, the human brain maintains a high glucose utilization rate at between 4 and 10 years old due to the high metabolic rate and intense learning tasks, and then the rate gradually decreases and reaches an adult value between 16 and 18 [30]. Evidence suggests that high-sugar diet (HSD)-induced gut microbiota could impair hippocampus-dependent neurocognition in rats during childhood and adolescence [31–33]. Conversely, it was reported that HSD did not significantly affect cognitive functions in adult rats [34]. A follow-up study on dietary patterns found that a sugar-rich diet during early childhood can lead to smaller cerebral white matter volume, while a whole grains-rich diet can lead to larger cerebral gray matter volume and a larger surface area of the prefrontal cortex [35]. These results confirm that dietary patterns play a critical role in neurological health development and cognitive performance during adolescence and adulthood.

Studies have also reported a decline in age-related cerebral glucose metabolism and attenuated counter-regulatory responses in middle age [30]. Additionally, aging can exacerbate high-fat diet (HFD)-induced neuroinflammation and associated cognitive impairments [36]. Aging can lead to energy metabolism disorders, mitochondrial dysfunction, and the gradual failure of defense mechanisms against abnormal proteins. Hence, the neurons in the elderly are vulnerable to injury, leading to mild cognitive impairment, a concept of cognitive impairment intervening with normal aging and early dementia [37], or Alzheimer's disease (AD) [38]. It is reported that excessive dietary sugar intake is significantly associated with AD risk in older women [39]. Aging can also induce hippocampal inflammatory responses due to a high-calorie diet and worsen cognitive phenotypes [36]. On the other hand, it is reported that the aging trajectory of the gut microbiota is associated with metabolic diseases and neurodegenerative diseases in a chronological age-dependent manner [40,41]. Evidence shows that, compared with young mice, aged mice show spatial memory deficits, accompanied by gut microbiota imbalance, increased intestinal permeability, and increased peripheral inflammatory cytokines [42]. The transplantation of fecal bacteria from aged rats to young rats can significantly damage the cognitive functions of the latter, which might be attributed to the increased levels of proinflammatory cytokines and oxidative stress (OS) related to the elderly gut microbiota, the changes in the hippocampal synaptic structure, and the decreased expression of brain-derived neurotrophic factors (BDNF) [43].

3.2. Patients with Metabolic Diseases

Neurons are susceptible to the effects of external glucose concentration due to their inability to store glycogen. Therefore, some metabolic diseases with blood glucose fluctuations as one of the main symptoms are highly susceptible to cognitive decline (Table 1). Diabetics are prone to developing diabetes-associated cognitive decline (DACD) [44]. Some typical symptoms of diabetes, such as impaired glucose tolerance, IR, chronic hyperglycemia, glycemic fluctuations, and the resulting deterioration in gut microbiota might contribute to cognitive impairments [45]. Additionally, as a metabolic disease induced by prolonged, inappropriate dietary habits and an important driving force of T2DM, obesity has been proven to be a potent risk factor for the onset and progression of several neurological disorders [46]. Studies have shown a negative correlation between obesity indicators and some cognitive indicators in the elderly, such as episodic memory, verbal learning, AD, and vascular dementia [47]. However, it is worth noting that these findings may be interfered with by different factors, such as the cause, degree, and stages of obesity development. Since obesity cannot be distinguished from complications, such as hyperglycemia and IR, studies on the correlation between obesity and cognitive decline are sometimes controversial. Typically, obesity could induce OS by disrupting the adipose microenvironment and mediating low-grade chronic inflammation and mitochondrial dysfunction, leading to cognitive decline [48]. It is reported that obesity-related cognitive decline is accompanied by a reduction in the dendritic spine density and synaptic sites associated with obesity-induced phagocytosis of synapses [49,50].

Table 1. Studies for several diet-induced metabolic diseases and their impairments of neurocognitive functions.

	Research Model	Diet-Induced Diseases	Control	Behavioral Tests	Outcomes and Conclusions	Ref.
HUMANS	Diabetics: 40–75 years old	T2DM	People with normal glucose metabolism	Tests in 3 cognitive domains: memory/attention/information processing speed	Diabetics performed worse in all cognitive domains. It can be largely explained by hyperglycemia.	[8]
	Diabetics: 70.9 years old	T2DM with sever glucose variability	T2DM with relatively stable blood glucose	Annually observational follow-up for 4.8 years	Cognitive functions can be influenced by glucose variability independently of mean blood glucose.	[7]
	Young adults: 20 years old	Obesity, prediabetes	Persons with normal glucose	Inhibitory control/sustained attention/working memory	Higher glucose levels were associated with poorer cognitive performance, especially for prediabetes.	[12]

Table 1. *Cont.*

	Research Model	Diet-Induced Diseases	Control	Behavioral Tests	Outcomes and Conclusions	Ref.
MICE	8 weeks old	T2DM induced by STZ and 20% Fr solution	Healthy mice with standard chow and water	After 38 days intervention	There is a strong association between hyperglycemia, hyperinsulinemia, neuroinflammation, and cognitive dysfunction in T2DM mice model.	[51]
	4 months of age	T2DM (db/db mice): ad libitum to standard chow	db/db mice: Intermittent fasting (IF)	After 28 days of exposure	db/db: cognitive decline; db/db-IF:cognitive improved; mitochondrial biogenesis and energy metabolism gene expression in hippocampus increased; microbial metabolites re-structured.	[44]
	Juvenile: 5 weeks old; elderly: 1 year old	Obesity induced by HFD	Healthy mice with standard chow	After 11/24 weeks of exposure	Obesity causes a dysmetabolic phenotype in both age groups. Older age exacerbates neuroinflammatory response and cognitive decline.	[36]
	8 weeks old	Obesity induced by HFD and 34% Su solution	Healthy mice with standard chow and water	After 10 weeks feeding of high-calorie diet (HFD/HSD)	HFD/HSD intervention produces obesity and cognitive decline, which is accompanied by increased microglial activation and reduced numbers of dendritic spines.	[49]
	8 weeks old	Hyperglycemia induced by chronic social defeat (CSD)	Healthy mice with normal blood glucose	3- and 5 weeks post-CSD	Hyperglycemia threatens long-term glucose homeostasis and causes spatial memory dysfunction.	[52]
RATS	5 weeks old	Hyperglycemia induced by STZ (STZ group)	Blood glucose controlled with insulin injection (STZ + insulin group)	60 days after blood glucose control	Chronic hyperglycemia can compromise cognition by reducing hippocampal ERK signaling and inducing neurotoxicity.	[53]
	Rat pups	Hyperglycemia induced by STZ /glucose injection	Treated with equal citrate buffer	After 10 days of glucose injection/5 days of STZ treatment	Hyperglycemia alters substrate transport, lactate homeostasis, dendritogenesis, and glutamate—glutamine cycling in the developing hippocampus.	[54]

Notes: T2DM, type 2 diabetes; STZ, streptozotocin; HFD, high-fat diet; ERK: extracellular regulated protein kinases.

Patients with these metabolic diseases have reduced diversity of gut microbiota due to their inappropriate dietary habits and metabolic homeostasis disorders. Similarly, patients with diabetes or hyperglycemia often have reduced diversity of gut microbiota and increased gut barrier permeability [55,56]. Compared with healthy individuals, obese patients typically have higher *Firmicutes*, lower *Bacteroidetes*, and lower SCFA production in their gut, which have been proven to be potent risk factors for cognitive decline [57,58].

4. Microbiota Remodeling and Neurocognitive Functions

4.1. Glycemic Carbohydrate Diet-Induced Microbiota Remodeling

Gut microbes can respond rapidly to changes in dietary patterns. The remodeling effect of carbohydrates on gut microbes and microenvironment is significantly related to their digestive properties (see Tables S1 and S2). RS, SDS, and IMOs are the primary carbohydrates available to bacteria in the colon. The entry of RS-containing starch into the colon provides the preferred fuel for microorganisms and helps improve the gut microenvironment. Dietary RS supplementation can attenuate hyperglycemic, hyperinsulinemic, and hyperlipidemic responses by restricting gluconeogenesis, bolstering glycogenesis, and maintaining glucose and lipid homeostasis, satiety, and colonic health [59,60]. Different types of RS can lead to different dominant bacteria and SCFAs in the gut. Recent studies have confirmed that HSD also affects gut microbial composition [33].

4.2. Microbial Metabolites and Neurocognitive Functions

Accumulating studies have reported the effects of HSD, high-sugar and fat diets (also known as Western diets), and ketogenic diets on cognitive functions through the gut–brain axis. Currently, the negative impact of excessive intake of high-sugar beverages and desserts on cognitive functions in children and adolescents warrants further exploration. Studies have shown that gut microbiota optimization could help improve DACD or mild cognitive impairment [44] and AD [61]. It was reported that five different genera, namely *Bifidobacterium, Bacteroides, Faecalibacterium, Akkermansia,* and *Roseburia,* were negatively associated with T2DM, while *Ruminococcus, Fusobacterium,* and *Blautia* were positively associated with T2DM [62]. The abundance of these microorganisms was influenced by carbohydrate intake to some extent (Tables S1 and S2). The prolonged signal communications between the gut microbiota and CNS through microbial metabolites often interfere with host metabolism and cognitive functions. RS and SDS remodel the gut microbiota and increase the production of some beneficial metabolites, such as neurotransmitters, glycerophospholipids, and SCFAs, which enhance the integrity of both IEB and BBB. These metabolites can be transported to the CNS through blood circulation or the vagus nerve to help preserve healthy neurocognitive functions.

4.2.1. SCFAs

Colonic microbiota can use complex carbohydrates such as cellobiose and starch for growth and proliferation and significantly increase the production of SCFAs, such as acetate, propionate, and butyrate. The delivery of optimal levels of SCFAs to the brain can confer neuroprotective effects through the promotion of cell proliferation, neuroblast differentiation, and BDNF expression, as well as by reducing systemic inflammation. For example, sodium butyrate (300 mg/kg/d, injected for 3 weeks) was reported to be used as an effective memory-enhancing drug for mice [63,64].

Additionally, SCFAs help maintain the integrity of the intestinal epithelial barrier (IEB), thus preventing the entry of toxic microbial metabolites from bacterial-derived LPS into the body's circulation [65]. It is reported that the gut microbiota has significant effects on gut permeability [66] and blood brain barrier (BBB) integrity [67]. Impairments to both barriers increase the chance of adverse substances entering the body's circulation and the CNS. This promotes metabolic disturbances and exacerbates systemic inflammation, disrupting the neurocognitive function. Gut function impairment, such as a diminished diversity of gut microbiota and heightened permeability of the gut barrier, is more prevalent in the obese, diabetic, hyperglycemia, and elderly populations [68,69]. Akkermansia muciniphila colonizes on the mucus layer of the gastrointestinal tract. It can degrade mucin and produce SCFAs, such as acetate and propionate, to increase mucus production and intestinal epithelial cell regeneration, maintaining the dynamic stability of the mucus layer and improving IEB function [70,71]. The abundance of this bacterium is lower in patients with obesity and T2DM [72,73], while the intake of RS can increase its abundance [74]. SCFAs, represented by butyrate produced by RS fermentation in the gut, have been reported to pose a protective effect on barrier integrity [33,71,75]. Conversely, the reduced production of SCFAs induced by high fructose feeding leads to damaged IEB and elevated serum endotoxin levels, resulting in hippocampal neuroinflammatory responses and further neuronal loss [76].

4.2.2. Neurotransmitters

Certain gut bacteria can influence the expression of BDNF and neurotransmitters (such as glutamate, GABA, 5-HT, dopamine, and acetylcholine) and associated host behavior in a vagus-dependent manner or via blood circulation by influencing the synthesis of neurotransmitters in the gut cells [77,78]. For instance, the gastrointestinal production of 5-hydroxytryptamine (5-HT) [79] is directly related to CNS functions like neurocognition and depression. Intestinal *Alistipes* levels are related to the carbohydrate digestive properties, with sugar and RDS intake increasing their abundance and SDS or RS intake decreasing their abundance (Tables S1 and S2). *Alistipes* can hydrolyze tryptophan, a precursor of serotonin, to indole, decreasing the availability of 5-HT [80], while the intervention of *Bifidobacterium* spp. or *Clostridium* spp. increases the availability of 5-HT and its precursor levels [79,81].

4.2.3. Glycerophospholipids

Neural membranes contain several classes of glycerophospholipids essential for membrane integrity and stability [82,83]. A study on bumblebees shows that the production of glycerophospholipids associated with the intestinal bacterial phosphoenolpyruvate-dependent phosphotransferase system could significantly improve long-term memory capacity [84]. These glycerophospholipids are synthesized by glycolipid metabolism in vivo or in the gut bacteria and are subsequently absorbed into the body. Glycerophospholipids can generate second messengers through further degradation, such as arachidonic acid, platelet activating factor, and diacylglycerol, which are strongly associated with synaptic plasticity and cognitive ability [83].

5. Glycemic Fluctuations and Neurocognitive Functions

The brain only accounts for 2% of the body's weight but consumes 20% of the oxygen and 25% of the glucose of the whole body. Energy metabolism disorders of neurons that exist in AD appeared earlier than β-amyloid (A-β) deposition [85]. As the primary peripheral organ of glucose metabolism, the liver undergoes similar changes to the CNS under unstable glycemic levels. Glucose fluctuation can affect neuronal functions by disturbing glucose metabolism, inducing neurotoxic substances, or interfering directly with calcium homeostasis.

5.1. Glycemic Fluctuation-Induced Glucose Metabolic Disorders

Glucose metabolism is the core of connections among glycemic levels, other metabolic pathways, and neurocognitive functions. In the CNS, a close energy and substance coupling relationship exists between astrocytes and neurons. As for energy supply, astrocytes rely mainly on glycolysis, and neurons use oxidative phosphorylation and the tricarboxylic acid (TCA) cycle [86]. Neurons are more sensitive to the perception of glucose fluctuations than astrocytes due to their high energy demand, higher affinity, and the higher turnover rate of glucose transporter-3 (GLUT3) for glucose than GLUT1 [87]. As shown in Figure 1A, when astrocytes are exposed to high glucose, the increased pyruvate might be converted to lactate. It can be shuttled into neurons to be converted into pyruvate and then into the TCA cycle [88]. Glutamate is secreted during neuronal excitation induced by elevated glucose levels, and then absorbed by astrocytes. This process activates Na^+/K^+ATPase, a key factor in promoting glucose uptake by GLUTs. In vitro studies suggest that astrocytes can detect the synaptic activity of glutamate neurons through glutamate transport activity and convert it into metabolic signals, so that the nerve cells can take up glucose as needed [89,90].

Dysregulation of glucose metabolism can lead to pathogenesis and T2DM complications, leading to IR and glycemic variability [91]. Long-term chronic hyperglycemia (>15 mmol/L) might lead to metabolic disorders and increased anaerobic metabolism [53]. Long-term stable or intermittent hyperglycemia can promote the generation of several neurotoxic substances. Correspondingly, recurrent non-severe hypoglycemia can lead to cognitive dysfunction in diabetics. Improper coordination of hypoglycemic drugs, diet, and exercise can easily lead to hypoglycemia (<3 mmol/L), an independent risk factor for DACD [92,93]. Hypoglycemia leads to insufficient energy supply, abnormal glucose metabolism, and reduced synaptic plasticity in the hippocampus [94]. Additionally, studies have shown that intermittent high glucose can lead to more severe chronic diabetes complications than sustained high glucose [95–97]. It has been reported that the repetition of hyper- and hypoglycemic cycles appears to contribute to IR, T2DM, and obesity [98]. In vitro studies have found that, compared with the cells cultured with constant high glucose, the cells cultured with fluctuating glucose are more prone to mitochondrial dysfunction and cellular DNA damage [99].

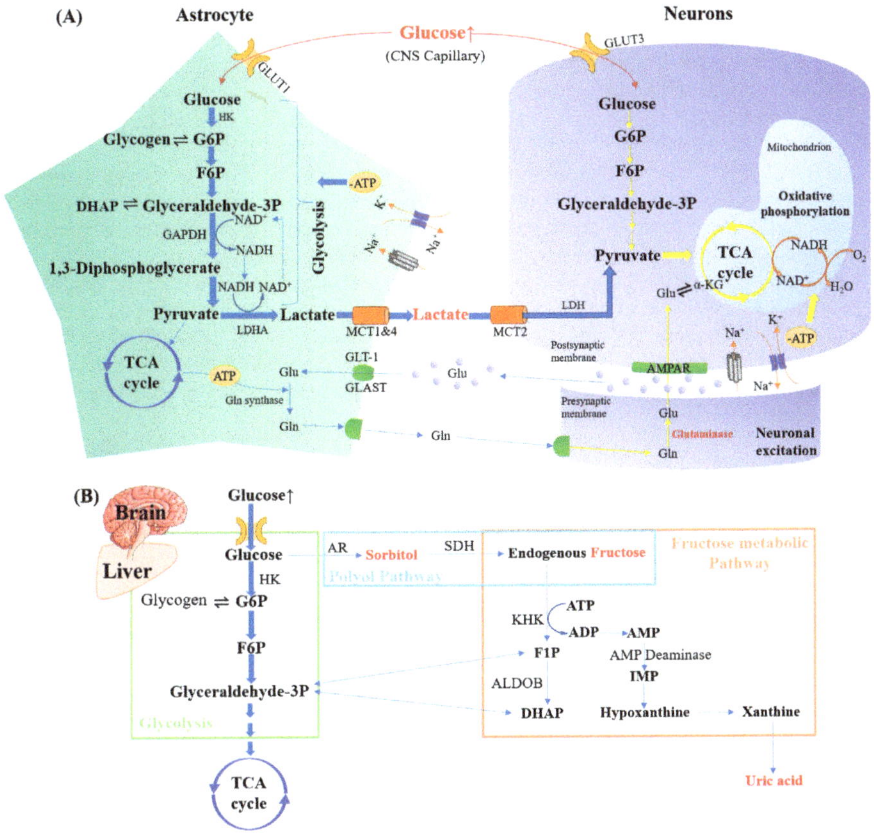

Figure 1. Glucose metabolism disorders and the production of harmful glycometabolites. (**A**) Glucose metabolism and the accumulation of lactate between astrocytes and neurons upon high glucose. Excessive glucose intake effectively activates glycolysis in astrocytes and TCA cycling and oxidative phosphorylation in neurons. Increased pyruvate produced in astrocytes might be converted to lactate, which can be then shuttled into neurons and converted into pyruvate. (**B**) The accumulation of sorbitol, fructose, and uric acid upon high glucose. When HK is saturated upon high glucose, the polyol pathway and fructose metabolism pathway can be activated so that the sorbitol, fructose, and the uric acid can be produced and accumulated. ADP, adenosine diphosphate; ALDOB, aldolase B; AMP, adenosine monophosphate; AMPAR, alpha-amino-3-hydroxy-5-methyl-4-isoxazole propionic acid receptor; ATP, adenosine triphosphate; DHAP, dihydroxyacetone phosphate; F1P, fructose-1-phosphate; G6P, glucose-6-phosphate; Gln, glutamine; Glu, glutamic acid; GLAST, glutamate aspartate transporter; GLT-1, glutamate transporter-1; GLUT, glucose transporter; IMP, inosine monophosphate; LDH, lactate dehydrogenase; LDHA, lactate dehydrogenase-A: MCT, monocarboxylate transporter; NAD^+/NADH, nicotinamide adenine dinucleotide (oxidized/reduced); PSAT1, phosphoserine aminotransferase 1; SDH, sorbitol dehydrogenase.

Although both GLUT1 and GLUT3 are non-insulin dependent, GLUT4 is highly expressed in the hippocampus in an insulin-dependent manner [100]. Disordered glucose metabolism may lead to IR and further cognitive decline. Then, the insulin-like growth factors-1 (IGF-1) can also bind and activate insulin receptors and subsequent pathways, which play an important role in brain neurogenesis, A-β clearance, and neuronal trophic support. Excessive insulin caused by IR competes with A-β for insulin-degrading enzymes, thereby reducing the degradation and consequent deposition of A-β [101]. Moreover, glycogen synthase kinase-3β (GSK-3β), one of the major tau kinases in the insulin-P13K-AKT signaling pathway, can be activated by IR [102,103]. IGF-1 resistance and enhanced GSK-3β activity can cause tau hyperphosphorylation, leading to synaptic dysfunction and neuronal apoptosis [104]. In addition, IR is also associated with OS and neuroinflammation.

5.2. *Neurotoxic Substances and Neurocognitive Functions*

Intracellular glucose fluctuation may activate several glycolysis-related pathways, such as the polyol, fructose metabolism, advanced glycation end products (AGEs), protein kinase C (PKC), and hexosamine pathways. Disordered glycolysis and some glycolytic bypass pathways can produce harmful glycometabolites and many common neurotoxic substances, such as AGEs, reactive oxygen species (ROS), and proinflammatory cytokines, thus affecting neurocognitive functions. In addition to causing direct damage to neurons, neurotoxic substances can increase the pathologic permeability of BBB by damaging the brain microvasculature and destroying the tight junction between the brain microvascular endothelial cells. As such, more toxic substances could enter the brain and induce more severe inflammatory responses and cognitive decline [105,106].

5.2.1. Glycometabolites

Excess lactic acid and other acidic metabolites will be released by enhanced anaerobic metabolism in the astrocytes under chronic hyperglycemia, which might lead to acidosis and hypoxia damage to neurons and ultimately endanger the CNS [107,108]. In the polyol pathway, the first enzyme, aldose reductase (AR), has a lower affinity for glucose than HK in glycolysis. As shown in Figure 1B, the saturation of hexokinase (HK) under high glucose concentrations can activate the polyol pathway, producing sorbitol and fructose. The activated polyol pathway induces intracellular accumulation of sorbitol, resulting in tissue swelling and direct tissue toxicity due to the poor membrane permeability of sorbitol [100].

Furthermore, excessive intake of fructose and endogenous fructose production can over-activate the fructose metabolic pathway, leading to various metabolic disorders and even dependence on sugar consumption [109–111]. The intake of GCs, such as glucose and maltodextrin [112], can also stimulate this process. Evidence suggests that excessive activation of the cerebral fructose metabolism is associated with cognition decline [113]. The activation of ketohexokinase (KHK) in this pathway leads to a significant consumption of intrahepatic phosphate and ATP levels, and an increase in uric acid levels [113,114]. Uric acid in the serum can cross BBB into the brain and induce neuronal death by stimulating mitochondrial OS and neuroinflammation, thereby resulting in cognitive decline [115,116]. Additionally, fructose promotes the production of AGEs, as discussed later.

5.2.2. AGEs

Intracellular AGEs are harmful to cells, as they induce the loss or alteration of normal cellular protein or lipid functions. Increased AGEs promote axonal atrophy and/or degeneration and reduce the innate ability of neurons to self-repair [117]. Additionally, it increases matrix metalloproteinase production, exacerbating nerve fiber damage further [118]. High glycemic levels may promote the formation of AGEs in the following ways (Figure 2).

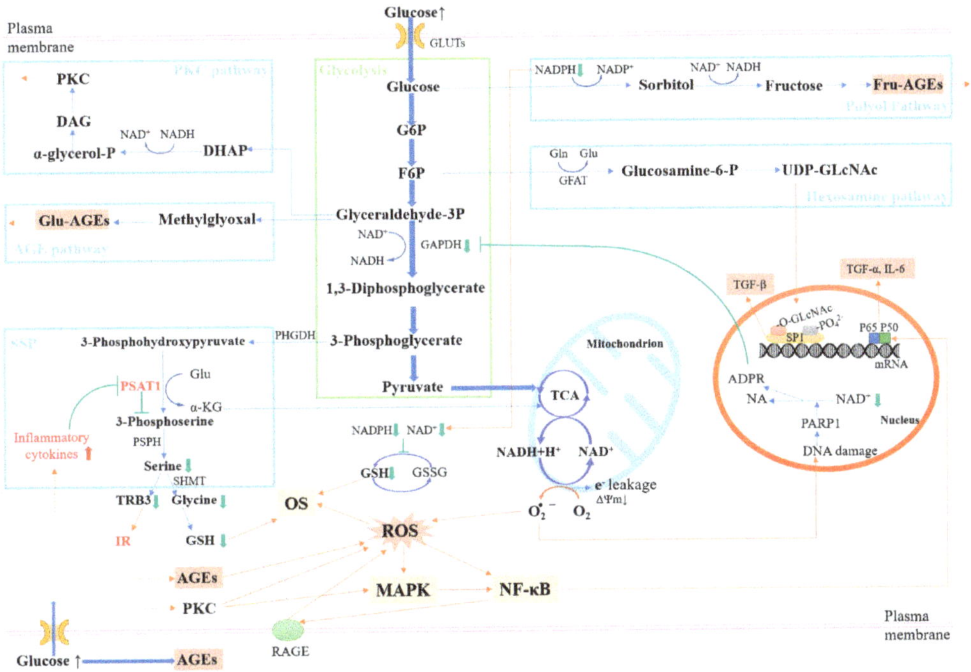

Figure 2. Neurotoxic substances triggered by a high glucose level. Fluctuating intracellular glucose may activate some glycolysis bypasses such as the polyol pathway, SSP, fructose metabolism pathway, AGE pathway, PKC pathway, and hexosamine pathway. They can produce a number of common neurotoxic substances, such as AGEs, ROS, and proinflammatory cytokines, thus affecting neurocognitive functions. α-KG, α-ketoglutarate; ADPR, adenosine diphosphate ribose; DAG, diacylglycerol; GFAT, fructose-6-phosphate amido transferase; GSH, antioxidant glutathione; GSSG, glutathione (oxidized); IL-6, interleukin 6; MAPK, mitogen-activated protein kinases; NA, nicotinic acid; NADP$^+$, nicotinamide adenine dinucleotide phosphate (oxidized); NADPH, nicotinamide adenine dinucleotide phosphate (reduced); NF-κb, kappa-light-chain enhancer of activated B cells; O-GLcNAc, O-linked-N-acetylglucosaminylation; PSAT1, phosphoserine aminotransferase1; TGF, the transforming growth factor; TRB3, tribbles homolog 3.

Firstly, hyperglycemia results in non-enzymatic glycation of excess glucose with amino acids, proteins, lipids, or nucleic acids. The Maillard reaction between the carbonyl group and amino group generates a Schiff base and then obtains the relatively stable ketoamine compounds, namely Amadori products, through Amadori rearrangement. Glucose-derived AGEs (Glu-AGEs) can be formed after further rearrangements [119]. Secondly, excess glucose activates the polyol pathway and consumes NAD$^+$ during the oxidation of sorbitol to fructose, resulting in an increase in the ratio of NADH/NAD$^+$. NAD$^+$ is the coenzyme of glyceraldehyde-3-phosphate dehydrogenase (GAPDH) in glycolysis. Hence, excessive consumption of NAD$^+$ might induce the accumulation of its upstream substrates represented by glyceraldehyde-3-phosphate (G3P). G3P can be converted into highly reactive methylglyoxal, a precursor of AGEs [100,120]. Similarly, fructose produced by the polyol pathway can also form Fru-AGEs. In addition, glucose-induced OS can activate an NAD$^+$-dependent DNA repair enzyme called poly(ADP-Ribose) polymerase (PARP) by inducing DNA damage, which inhibits the GAPDH activity by catabolizing the NAD$^+$-derived ADPR [87,121]. Thirdly, the produced fructose can be phosphorylated to fructose-3-phosphate (F3P) and converted into 3-deoxyglucosone further. Both compounds are effective glycation agents contributing to AGEs formation [120,122]. However, studies on F3P promoting AGE formation are only processed for the rat lens. There is no evidence of the occurrence of this process in hippocampal neurons.

5.2.3. ROS

The brain expends a significant amount of oxygen to sustain its normal physiological functions, yet it possesses higher lipid levels and lower concentrations of antioxidant enzymes compared to other organs [123,124]. Consequently, it is highly susceptible to oxidative stress (OS), a pivotal factor contributing to neuronal degeneration. The high sensitivity of neurons and glial cells to OS is mainly due to the excessive production of ROS in the mitochondrial respiratory chain under high glucose concentrations leading to OS, neuroinflammation, and apoptosis, as summarized in Figure 2.

In the early stages of hyperglycemia, elevated glucose level provides more fuel for the TCA cycle, thereby increasing the production of electron donors (NADH). The resulting electron transfer chain overload might lead to electron leakage and ROS formation in the mitochondria. In the cytoplasm, excessive glucose may activate the polyol pathway, depleting NADPH, a cofactor of glutathione reductase, leading to OS [87]. Then the PKC pathway can be activated by an increased synthesis of diacylglycerol, a PKC agonist [120]. PKC is known to induce cellular ROS by activating NADPH oxidases [125]. Additionally, the interaction between extracellular AGEs and their receptor RAGE can activate diverse signal transduction cascades and induce the production of downstream ROS [126]. The non-enzymatic glycation of proteins is accompanied by an oxidation reaction. Under aerobic conditions, Amadori products can generate products such as pentosidine through the oxidation pathway and release free radicals to cause OS [127]. Intracellular AGEs may aggravate OS, which itself up-regulates RAGE through NF-κB activation, thereby creating a vicious cycle [87]. Moreover, 3-phosphoglycerate generated by glycolysis can be gradually metabolized to L-serine through the serine synthesis pathway (SSP) with glutamate consumption and α-ketoglutarate production [128,129]. Serine is a synthetic precursor to glycine, which can be metabolized to produce the antioxidant glutathione to protect neurons from OS. However, higher levels of glutamate and lower levels of glycine have been reported in the plasma of diabetics, contributing to higher OS levels [130,131]. Particularly, it has been reported that the enhanced impairment of intermittent high/low glucose can activate OS through the endoplasmic reticulum (ER) stress response than stable high/low glucose [34,96,132].

5.2.4. Proinflammatory Cytokines

Persistent, chronic, and low-grade inflammation is one of the common symptoms of most neurodegenerative diseases. As shown in Figure 2, constant or oscillating high glucose may up-regulate the expression of proinflammatory cytokines and induce the inflammatory cascade reaction, leading to apoptosis of the nerve cells. In addition, it is reported that elevated levels of inflammatory factors like tumor necrosis factor-α (TNF-α) in T2DM mice lead to reduced expression of phosphoserine aminotransferase1 in SSP, inhibiting the synthesis of serine and tribbles homolog 3, thus resulting in decreased insulin sensitivity, or even IR [131].

AGEs and their binding with RAGE can induce an inflammatory cascade by activating the nuclear factor kappa B (NF-κB) pathway [126,133]. ROS can also activate the NF-κB pathway and promote the production of inflammatory cytokines. The binding of inflammatory cytokines like TNF-α and their receptors can also trigger ROS formation through various potential pathways [134]. PKC can activate the NF-κB pathway by activating the mitogen-activated protein kinase (MAPK) pathway [126]. Then, high glucose can inhibit GADPH and induce the accumulation of upstream products such as fructose-6-phosphate (F6P), which can activate another bypass of glycolysis called the hexosamine pathway. F6P can be converted into glucosamine-6-phosphate and subsequent uridine diphosphate-*N*-acetylhexosamine (UDP-GlcNAc) under glutamine F6P aminotransferase. UDP-GlcNAc can combine with serine and threonine residues of the transcription factor Sp1, resulting in an increased O-GlcNAcylation of SP1 and increased expression of Sp1-dependent genes, such as the transforming growth factor-β, which may result in neurovascular impairment [100,121]. In addition, the peroxisome proliferator-activated receptors (PPARs) play an important role in regulating energy metabolism. Several studies on peripheral tissue cells have reported that hyperglycemia down-regulates the expression of PPARs and induces inflammatory responses [135,136]. In the gut, the intake of RS has been shown to inhibit intestinal inflammation by reducing the production of pro-inflammatory mediators (such as TNF-α and NF-κB) and SCFAs and increasing the expression of the nuclear transcription factor PPARγ [137]. Additionally, research on peripheral tissues has reported that glucose fluctuations can increase the expression of inflammatory factors than hyperglycemia, providing insights into the mechanisms of the effects of glucose fluctuations on neuronal cells [138].

5.3. *Calcium Overload and Neurocognitive Functions*

Glucose level is not only an energy signal but also a status signal. Calcium is a common intracellular second messenger. With increased glucose acting as an upstream extracellular signal binding to its receptor, Ca^{2+} enters the cell and triggers a significant increase in the cytoplasmic Ca^{2+} concentration [139,140]. Severe glucose fluctuations in the circulation cause persistent hyperglycemic stimulation in the nerve cells, leading to the dysregulation of intracellular calcium homeostasis and neuropathy by affecting the expression and function of Ca^{2+} channels (for Ca^{2+} influx) or pumps (for Ca^{2+} efflux) [140,141]. An in vitro study demonstrated that a high extracellular glucose level (50 mM) significantly increased the cytoplasmic Ca^{2+} concentration and gene expression of the store-operated calcium channel (SOCE)-related protein STIM1 in rat primary hippocampal neurons, mediating more Ca^{2+} influx through the calcium release-activated calcium channel protein Orai on the plasma membrane [140,142]. In addition, the activation of PKC can promote Ca^{2+} influx by activating the voltage-gated calcium channels (VGCCs) on the plasma membrane further [143]. Disruption of Ca^{2+} homeostasis is mainly manifested by a large Ca^{2+} influx due to altered cell membrane permeability. The ER is the main storage site for Ca^{2+} in eukaryotic cells. Ca^{2+} influx triggers Ca^{2+} release from the ER, leading to intracellular Ca^{2+} overload, which can induce neuronal hypofunction or structural damage in the following ways (Figure 3).

5.3.1. Disrupt Energy Metabolisms Associated with Ca^{2+}

Mitochondrial Ca^{2+} overload, triggered by cytoplasmic Ca^{2+} overload, allows the formation and deposition of calcium phosphate in the mitochondria, thereby affecting the oxidative phosphorylation capacity and leading to reduced ATP synthesis and impaired energy production [144,145]. Normally, Ca^{2+} flowing into the cytoplasm can be partially bound to calmodulin (CaM) and activate the target enzymes such as adenosine 5′-monophosphate (AMP)-activated protein kinase (AMPK) through prior activation of CaMKII (Ca^{2+}/CaM-dependent protein kinase). Impaired mitochondrial ATP production and CaMKII overactivation due to Ca^{2+} overload can over activate AMPK, adversely affecting the regulation of energy balance, particularly in the brain [139].

5.3.2. Trigger Neuron Injury and Apoptosis

Above all, increased ER Ca^{2+} depletion due to Ca^{2+} overload can lead to ER stress. It is reported that ER stress-mediated apoptosis is involved in hyperglycemia-induced synaptic and neuronal injury of the hippocampus [146]. Continuous ER stress can activate caspase-12 and lead to apoptosis by increasing the expression of calpain, a calcium-dependent protease [147]. A higher glucose level can also increase the ratio of Bax/Bcl-2 on the membrane and activate caspase 3 [140]. Furthermore, Ca^{2+} overload leads to excessive activation of intracellular Ca^{2+}-dependent phospholipases, calpain, and nucleic acid endonucleases in the nucleus, thus destabilizing the cell membrane and cytoskeleton and causing DNA damage [145]. In addition, the increased pro-apoptotic protein Bax caused by high glucose can translocate to the outer membrane of mitochondria [148]. The loss of the mitochondrial membrane potential ($\Delta\Psi m \downarrow$) and the leakage of electrons/mitochondrial Ca^{2+} overload-induced electron donors can lead to the formation of ROS. The increased Bax, the collapse of $\Delta\Psi m$, and the resulting increase in ROS can induce the formation of the mitochondrial permeability transition pore, which can increase the release of cytochrome C from the mitochondria into the cytosol, thereby activating caspase 3 and initiating the mitochondria-dependent intrinsic apoptotic pathways [149–151].

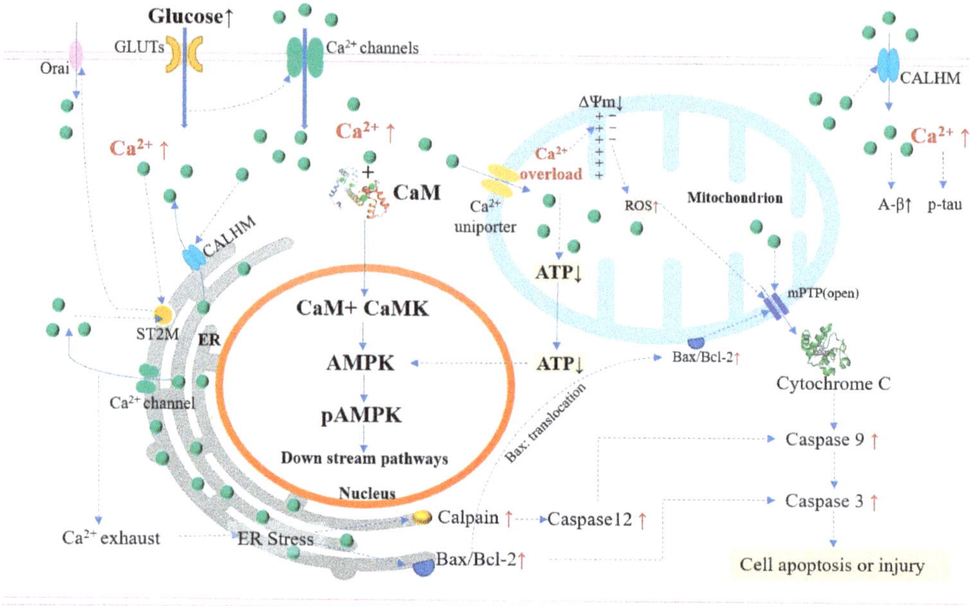

Figure 3. Calcium overload and its adverse effects on neurological function induced by high glucose stimulation. The increased extracellular glucose triggers a significant increase in the cytoplasmic Ca^{2+} concentration. Calcium overload may lead to disrupted energy metabolism, neuron injury/apoptosis, and neurotoxic protein accumulation. (AMPK, adenosine 5′-monophosphate (AMP)-activated protein kinase; Bcl-2, B-cell lymphoma-2; Bax, Bcl-2-associated x; CALHM, calcium homeostasis modulator protein; mPTP, mitochondrial permeability transition pore; Orai, calcium release-activated calcium channel protein; ST2M, stromal interaction molecule).

5.3.3. Promote Neurotoxic Protein Accumulation

Ca^{2+} overload can increase the neuroinflammation levels and A-β deposition by activating the calcium homeostasis modulator proteins [152]. A-β can also lead to mitochondrial Ca^{2+} dyshomeostasis and mitochondrial dysfunction [148]. Excessive cytosolic Ca^{2+} can induce tau hyperphosphorylation, while tau contributes to mitochondrial Ca^{2+} overload in neurons [151]. The intracellular accumulation of phosphorylated tau can trigger nuclear Ca^{2+}/CaMKIV signaling, aggravating tau hyperphosphorylation and promoting neurodegeneration [153].

5.4. Glucose Fluctuations Trigger More Severe Impairments

Accumulated studies have confirmed some credible molecular mechanisms of cellular damage induced by glycemic fluctuations, such as triggered inflammatory responses and OS. However, the reason why glucose fluctuations can trigger more severe impairment than constant high/low glucose is still unclear. It is inferred that an organism possesses a certain degree of environmental adaptability and develops homeostasis adapted to the environment in which it is located. Persistent high/low blood glucose is a relatively unhealthy but stable environment. In this new environment, the organism tends to counteract the toxic effects of glucose through many feedback regulatory mechanisms to reduce impairment. However, glycemic fluctuation is a variable or even irregular process, making it difficult to develop adaptive stabilization mechanisms and feedback regulation, leading to disrupted homeostasis and accumulated impairments.

5.5. The Interaction between Glycemic Fluctuations and Gut Microbiota

Hyperglycemia or severe glycemic fluctuations can also affect the gut microenvironment, thereby promoting the adverse effects of glycemic fluctuations and causing more serious impairment. However, this phenomenon has not received much attention. Studies have confirmed that diabetes and hyperglycemia, which are characterized by glucose variability, negatively affect the gut functions, as generally manifested by reduced gut microbial diversity, weak gut barrier integrity, and increased pathogenic bacterial diversity [55,56,58]. Brittle diabetes (BDM) is a kind of unstable diabetes characterized by severe glycemic fluctuations. As such, the difference between BDM and non-Brittle T2DM can reflect the influence of glycemic fluctuation as an independent factor on gut microbiota and cognitive ability. BDM has been associated with a lower abundance of *Akkermansia muciniphila*, *Fusobacterium*, and *Prevotella copri*, with a corresponding enrichment of *Bacteroides vulgatus* and *Veillonella denticariosi* [154,155]. As discussed earlier, a significant decrease in the abundance of *A. muciniphila* induced by glycemic fluctuations could disrupt the intestinal barrier integrity. Additionally, hyperglycemia can disrupt the integrity of tight and adherent junctions through overexpression of GLUT2 [156]. The increased intestinal barrier permeability and GLUT2 overexpression lead to the formation of a vicious cycle, which can accelerate the absorption rate of carbohydrate digestion products, thereby interfering with glycemic fluctuations and contributing to cognitive impairment.

6. Carbohydrate Dietary Strategies Beneficial for Neurocognitive Functions

Table 2 summarizes the studies for different types of GC intervention-induced changes in neurocognitive functions. To facilitate a balanced, prolonged nutritional intake and reduce the health risks associated with specific dietary patterns, it is recommended to ensure an appropriate proportion of carbohydrate daily intake [24], especially for populations with a tradition of high carbohydrate consumption such as Asians [157]. Given that cognitive decline frequently coincides with certain metabolic disorders, there has been a significant focus on exploring optimal dietary patterns as a gentle and sustained approach to either enhance cognitive development or prevent cognitive decline. SDS, RS, and many whole grains could reduce the risks of these metabolic diseases through a smooth postprandial glucose response and positive regulation of the gut microenvironment, thus hindering and delaying the related cognitive decline [158,159].

Table 2. Studies for different types of GCs intervention-induced changes in neurocognitive functions.

	Research Model	Dietary Patterns		Control	Exposure	Behavioral Tests	Outcomes and Conclusions	Ref.
HUMANS	Women: 50–79 years old	HSD	Usual diet (higher dietary sugar intake)	Behavioral modification training	8.1 years	Annually observational follow-up for 15 years	An estimated increase of 10 g/day in total sugar intake was associated with an increased AD risk by 1.3–1.4%.	[39]
	Young adults: about 23 years of age	NNS	Fr/Gl/Su solution (equal sweetness intensity)	Sucralose solution	Instant testing	After 250 mL solution drink	Gl and Su led to poorer performance on the assessed tasks as opposed to Fr and placebo, especially under the fasting condition.	[160]
	Healthy elderly (72.9 years old) participants	Whole grains	High hydrostatic pressurizing brown rice (UHHPBR)	Polished white rice (WR)	24 months	After 24 months of exposure	Long-term consumption of UHHPBR increases information processing speed in the elderly, suggesting a protective effect of UHHPBR administration against age-related cognitive decline.	[161]

Table 2. *Cont.*

	Research Model	Dietary Patterns		Control	Exposure	Behavioral Tests	Outcomes and Conclusions	Ref.
MICE	Juvenile: 4 weeks old	Fr	High Fr diet (30% calories)	Standard chow	12 weeks	—	High Fr feeding leads to damaged IEB, elevated serum endotoxin levels, hippocampal neuroinflammatory response, and neuronal loss.	[76]
	11 weeks old	Whole grains	Oat β-glucan added in HFD	HFD; Standard chow	15 weeks	After 15 weeks of exposure	β-glucan intake can improve gut barrier function, reduce endotoxemia, and enhance cognitive function via more optimized synaptic and signaling pathways in critical brain areas.	[162]
	18 weeks old		BWF	Standard chow	15 weeks	After 26 weeks of exposure	BWF intake can suppresses cognitive decline by increasing hippocampal BDNF production in SAMP8 mice.	[163]
RATS	Adolescents: PN 21; young adults: PN 56	Su	10% Su solution	0.1% sodium saccharin solution (standard chow)	4 weeks	Adolescents: PN 55; young adults: PN 91	Sucrose intervention can disrupt spatial cognition and reward-related behavior in the absence of obesity.	[164]
	Adults: age not specified		10% Su solution	Water (standard chow)	3 weeks	After 21 days of exposure	Sucrose intervention can disrupt hippocampal-dependent place recognition memory; neuroinflammation and OS play a role in this impairment.	[165]
	Adolescents: PN 28		10% Su solution	Water (standard chow)	5 weeks	PN 62	The expression of parvalbumin-immunoreactive GABAergic interneurons has decreased; both prefrontal and hippocampal functions have declined.	[166]
	8 weeks old	Fr	10% Fr solution	Water (standard chow)	8 months	After 8 months of exposure	High Fr diet induced peripheral IR and an abnormal insulin-signaling pathway in the hippocampus, which exacerbated memory deficits.	[167]
	6 weeks old		15% Fr solution	Water (standard chow)	24 weeks	7, 10, 14, 16, 18, 20, 22, and 24 weeks	IR/cognitive dysfunction appeared from 7th/20th week. Fr-induced neuroinflammation and OS impaired neuronal signaling and synaptic plasticity.	[168]
	8 weeks old		10% Fr solution	Water (standard chow)	7 months	After 7 months of exposure	The induced cognitive deficits are related to increased OS, hypertriglyceridemia, impaired insulin signaling, and altered mitochondrial dynamics.	[169]
	Mother rats: from GD0 (gestational day)		13%/40% Fr solution	Water (standard chow)	GD0-PN 21 (offspring)	Postnatal day 60 offspring	Maternal Fr exposure during gestation and lactation can impair cognition in offspring and affect brain function at the transcriptome level.	[170]
	Adolescents: PN 30 /Adults: PN 60	HFCS	11% Su solution /11% HFCS-55	Water (Low-fat chow)	4 weeks	PN 60 /PN 90	Adolescents: both learning and memory functions have declined; adults: no significant impact.	[34]
	Juvenile /Adolescent rats: PN 26		HFCS-55	Water (standard chow)	4 weeks	PN 175	HSD in early life may confer long-lasting impairments in memory function, which are not reversible by simply removing sugars from the diet.	[31]
	Juvenile/ adolescents: PN 26–28		65% Fr + 35% Gl soluton	Water (standard chow)	6 weeks	PN 67	The abundance of P. distasonis and P. johnsonii has elevated; hippocampal function has declined.	[33]
	Healthy/T2DM adult rats	NNS	Aspartame (ASP) solution	0.9% NaCl	30 days	After 30 days of oral gavage	ASP administration to healthy/diabetic rats has shown adverse effects linked to cognitive dysfunction.	[171]
	Adolescents: PN 25		Acesulfame potassium/ saccharin/ stevia (LCS) solution	Water (standard chow)	30 days	After 30 days of exposure	Habitual-life LCS consumption has long-lasting implications for hippocampal-dependent memory in rats.	[172]
	6–7 weeks old		Su/saccharin solution	Water (standard chow)	10% Su: 4 weeks; Su/water/ saccharin: 4 weeks	After 4–8 weeks of exposure	4 weeks of Su exposure results in cognitive decline. Switching from Su to water or saccharin produces similar improvements on cognitive measures.	[173]
	8–11 weeks old	Maltodex -trin	10.4% Su/ maltodextrin solution	Water (standard chow)	17 days	After 17 days of exposure	Impaired performance on a location recognition task was found in both groups.	[112]

Notes: Fr: fructose; Gl: glucose; Su: sucrose; HFCS-55: high fructose corn syrup; PN: postnatal day; HSD, high-sugar diet; IEB: intestinal epithelial barrier; IR, insulin resistance; BDNF, brain-derived neurotrophic factor; NNS: non-nutritive artificial sweeteners.

6.1. RS Selection

The RS classification method provides references for selecting and processing starch-based foods. As a fermentable dietary fiber, RS provides effective assistance in shaping a healthier gut environment and a stable blood glucose response [174]. RSI suggests that non-refined carbohydrates that remain intact in the cell wall structures, such as whole grains, often have higher dietary fiber content and lower GI values. RSII presents naturally in some plants, such as raw potatoes, green bananas, and high-amylose corn. RSIII suggests that the way food is processed and cooked is also important for RS retention. For example, starch-based foods cooled after cooking have a higher RS content due to the retrogradation of starch; baked potatoes have higher RS than boiled potatoes due to less moisture content during heat treatment [175]. Zhanggui Wang et al. reviewed the methods of yielding RSIII from different sources [176]. In food processing, the preparation of RSIV&V requires some physical and chemical modifications, usually added as additives to improve the functional characteristics of the products.

6.2. SDS Selection

Slow-digesting maltodextrin and starch have emerged as the current research hotspots. Compared to RS, SDS can maintain a stable postprandial glucose response while providing a sufficient glucose supply. It is reported that A-type raw cereal starches are slowly digested with >50% SDS by the Englyst test [177]. Currently, whole grains and legumes are recognized as the ideal dietary options with distinct health benefits, including increased cognitive functions. A study followed the dietary habits of 516 young adults (32.03 $\pm$ 5.96 y) and assessed their cognitive performance at midlife (49.03 $\pm$ 4.86 y) [178]. The findings revealed a direct correlation between increased consumption of whole grains in the diet and enhanced cognitive performance. Another investigation found that a lower dietary intake of whole grains was associated with higher inflammatory markers and decreased cognitive ability in the elderly [179]. Generally, the cognitive protective effects of whole grains are associated with smooth glycemic responses due to their slow digestive properties, beneficial gut functions, and higher abundance of functional phytochemicals.

Dietary fiber is positively associated with cognitive performance among prepubertal children [180]. The abundance of dietary fiber in whole grains and the encapsulation effect of the cell wall on starch particles are the key factors in retarding the carbohydrate digestion rate, thereby maintaining postprandial blood glucose stability and improving the gut microenvironment [181]. The abundance of β-glucan in whole grain oats and barley has been shown to prevent cognitive disorders, which may be related to its involvement in maintaining the intestinal barrier function, countering HFD-induced microglia activation and neuroinflammation, and regulating the gut microbiota [162,182]. Additionally, β-glucan can increase the viscosity of the chyme, limiting enzyme accessibility to carbohydrates, reducing the glucose absorption rate through the intestinal wall, and limiting the post-prandial glycemic response [159]. Buckwheat whole flour (BWF) intervention over the long term has been shown to successfully mitigate age-related cognitive decline in mice [163]. In a previous study, exposure to BWF significantly increased the expression of postsynaptic Arc and postsynaptic density protein-95 (PSD-95) and the mature neuronal marker NeuN in the hippocampus due to the increased abundance of *Lactococcus* and *Ruminiclostridium* in the gut. Additionally, the beneficial effect of whole grains on cognitive ability is largely related to their functional phytochemicals. The 5-heptadecylresorcinol in whole grain rye has been proven to improve cognitive functions and neuroinflammation in APP/PS1 transgenic mice [183]. Avenanthramides and avenacosides in whole grain oats have good anti-inflammatory and antioxidant properties [184]. The abundance of lipopolysaccharides in brown rice has been proven to improve cognitive functions in mice and elderly humans [161,185]. Ferulic acid in whole grains could achieve neuroprotective effects through anti-inflammatory, antioxidant, and glucose homeostasis regulating abilities [186].

It is important to highlight that individuals with limited chewing capacity and digestive functions, such as children and the elderly, need to be particularly mindful of the potential harm from the coarseness and hardness of whole grains and resistant starch (RS). Employing suitable pre-treatment methods for brown rice, such as hydrostatic treatment, is advisable to ensure its tenderness and ease of consumption [161].

6.3. Sweetener Selection

With the rapid development of society, people have gradually realized the adverse effects of excessive sugar or rapidly digested carbohydrate intake on health, including cognitive functions (Table 2). Studies have confirmed that excessive sugar intake, including glucose, sucrose, and fructose, during childhood can lead to cognitive decline compared to ungelatinized ordinary corn starch, an SDS with carbohydrates in standard chow (the study models involved are mice and rats, as shown in Table 2). Therefore, the current consensus is that reducing sugar intake can lead to better cognitive abilities under sufficient energy supply.

The invention and application of non-nutritive artificial sweeteners (NNSs) is an effective approach to reduce these risks. NNS is considered a healthier sweetener alternative due to its high sweetness, low-calorie content, and almost no involvement in body metabolism. Evidence suggests that NNSs can protect cognitive functions better than traditional sugars (Table 2). Nevertheless, there is still controversy over whether NNSs have adverse effects on cognition compared to water (control), which also generates no energy. For example, studies have found that NNS intervention leads to better cognitive abilities compared to sugar but had no significant difference compared to the water-fed group [164,173]. However, in another study, compared to the control, NNS (acesulfame, saccharin, stevia) intervention in adolescent rats induced hippocampal-dependent cognitive decline [172]. Another intervention for diabetic rats also showed that, compared with the control, the cognitive ability of rats taking aspartame solution was significantly reduced [171]. Recent reports discuss the potential negative effects of NNSs on appetite, metabolic health, and cognitive functions through various peripheral and central mechanisms [187–190]. Nevertheless, relevant evidence and conclusions are still controversial. Therefore, NNS, a traditional sugar substitute with a wide variety and insufficient evidence of long-term health effects, deserves further research.

6.4. Research Models on Diet-Induced Changes in Neuro Functions

Some research models can be drawn upon on how dietary patterns affect cognitive functions (Figure 4). Firstly, we propose studying the diet-induced changes in the gut microbiota and the correlation analysis with behavior, which could verify if these changes are the key intermediate factors between these two. The effect of highly correlated species on CNS can be further verified by subsequent animal experiments such as oral gavage of the target strain or fecal transplantation. The effect mechanisms mainly focus on the key metabolites and their signal pathways. The study approach generally involves metabolomic or transcriptomic analysis of fecal/intestinal contents/liver (place of origin), serum (transmission pathway), and target CNS regions such as the hippocampus (destination). Untargeted metabolomics allows broad-spectrum screening of differential metabolites between groups, complemented by the KEGG enrichment analysis to obtain the major metabolites affecting cognition. Targeted metabolomics is used for studies with clear targets or metabolic pathways. Forward and reverse validation based on target metabolites can increase the credibility of the study. Forward validation refers to feeding/gavaging/injecting the target metabolite to the laboratory animals based on the normal diet. Reverse validation can be performed by knocking out or silencing of genes for key enzymes or receptors for the metabolites and comparing the cognitive differences with control. Selection of study models is also important. Contrasting with the rapid and pronounced therapeutic effects typically expected from medical treatments, dietary interventions are generally appropriate for most healthy individuals or as a supplement to medical treatment in patients with specific diseases, marked by gentler effects and extended duration. Therefore, the effectiveness is generally demonstrated in populations with weaker or vulnerable cognitive functions, such as children and adolescents with immature brains in early life, diabetics, and the elderly prone to cognitive impairment.

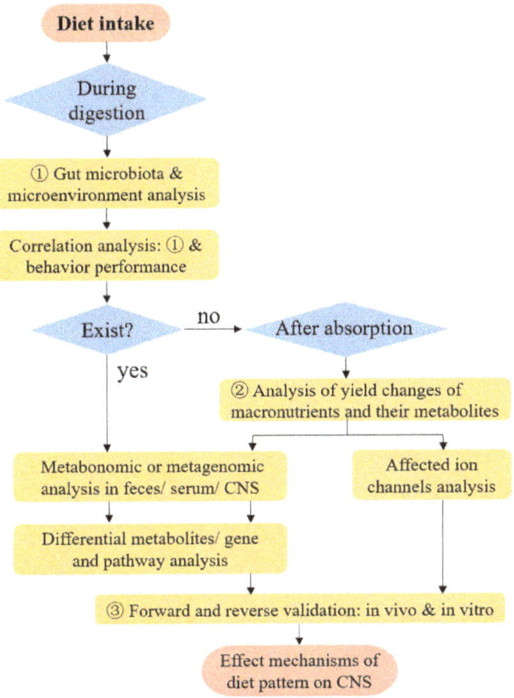

Figure 4. Referable research models of how dietary patterns affect CNS functions.

7. Conclusions

Glycemic carbohydrate is a major and economical energy source for humans, but its inappropriate consumption can lead to various metabolic and neurodegenerative diseases, including cognitive impairment. In modern society, the rapid increase in mental labor and stress and the pursuit of immediate happiness feedback have led to a sharp increase in the demand for rapidly digestible carbohydrates, such as sugar and pregelatinized starch-based foods [191–193]. However, there is substantial evidence to suggest that GCs with different digestive characteristics can lead to differences in gut microbiota diversity and glucose fluctuation patterns, which have been demonstrated have an association with neurological impairment (Figure 5), especially for those susceptible populations, including those in early and late life and those suffering from metabolic diseases such as obesity and diabetes. Unhealthy glycemic fluctuations can negatively impact brain functions in various ways by disrupting the gut microbiota structure, causing metabolic disturbances and calcium overload, and producing neurotoxic substances. Therefore, it is imperative to adjust the dietary strategies to promote the development of neurocognitive functions better, including increasing the intake of RS and SDS as appropriate, choosing whole grains as a staple instead of refined carbohydrates, and reducing sugar intake while ensuring sufficient energy intake. Additionally, as discussed in this review, there is a lack of research on how long-term intake of starch with different digestive properties affects neurocognitive function. Moreover, the existing targeted research and mechanism studies remain inadequate, with some controversial conclusions arising from the wide variety of GCs. As such, achieving a more judicious selection of carbohydrates or mitigating health risks through scientific processing while considering sensory enjoyment is still worth further study.

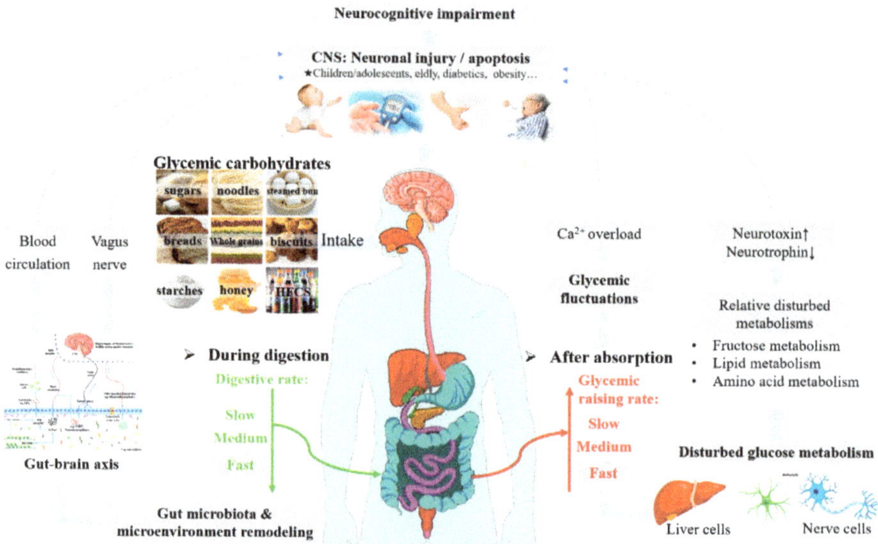

Figure 5. A summary of the effect mechanisms of glycemic carbohydrate diet on neurocognitive.

Supplementary Materials: The following supporting information can be downloaded at: https://www.mdpi.com/article/10.3390/nu15245080/s1, Table S1: Effects of monosaccharide and disaccharide intake on gut microbiota; Table S2: Effects of starch with different digestive properties intake on gut microbiota. References [31,76,194–219] are cited in the supplementary materials.

Author Contributions: J.Y. developed the original draft of the manuscript, L.C., Y.H. and Z.G. proofread and edited the final manuscript, Z.L., C.L., X.B. and L.Z. supervised and revised the literature. All authors have read and agreed to the published version of the manuscript.

Funding: This work was financially supported by National Natural Science Foundation of China (No. 22278182), the Agricultural Science and Technology Innovation Program of CAAS "Evaluation and Regulation of Nutritional Quality of Major Agricultural Products" (CAAS-XTCX20190025), the Jiangsu Province "Collaborative Innovation Center of Food Safety and Quality Control" industry development program, and the Postgraduate Research & Practice Innovation Program of Jiangsu Province (KYCX22_2399).

Conflicts of Interest: The authors declare no conflict of interest.

References

1. Lim, J.; Pullicin, A.J. Oral carbohydrate sensing: Beyond sweet taste. *Physiol. Behav.* **2019**, *202*, 14–25. [CrossRef] [PubMed]
2. Popkin, B.M. Nutrition Transition and the Global Diabetes Epidemic. *Curr. Diabetes Rep.* **2015**, *15*, 64. [CrossRef] [PubMed]
3. Cryan, J.F.; O'Riordan, K.J.; Sandhu, K.; Peterson, V.; Dinan, T.G. The gut microbiome in neurological disorders. *Lancet Neurol.* **2020**, *19*, 179–194. [CrossRef] [PubMed]
4. Zeevi, D.; Korem, T.; Zmora, N.; Israeli, D.; Rothschild, D.; Weinberger, A.; Ben-Yacov, O.; Lador, D.; Avnit-Sagi, T.; Lotan-Pompan, M. Personalized nutrition by prediction of glycemic responses. *Cell* **2015**, *163*, 1079–1094. [CrossRef]
5. Hasek, L.Y.; Phillips, R.J.; Zhang, G.; Kinzig, K.P.; Kim, C.Y.; Powley, T.L.; Hamaker, B.R. Dietary slowly digestible starch triggers the gut–brain axis in obese rats with accompanied reduced food intake. *Mol. Nutr. Food Res.* **2018**, *62*, 1700117. [CrossRef]
6. Kroemer, G.; López-Otín, C.; Madeo, F.; de Cabo, R. Carbotoxicity-noxious effects of carbohydrates. *Cell* **2018**, *175*, 605–614. [CrossRef]
7. Kim, C.; Sohn, J.-H.; Jang, M.U.; Kim, S.-H.; Choi, M.-G.; Ryu, O.-H.; Lee, S.; Choi, H.-C. Association between visit-to-visit glucose variability and cognitive function in aged type 2 diabetic patients: A cross-sectional study. *PLoS ONE* **2015**, *10*, e0132118. [CrossRef]
8. Geijselaers, S.L.; Sep, S.J.; Claessens, D.; Schram, M.T.; Van Boxtel, M.P.; Henry, R.M.; Verhey, F.R.; Kroon, A.A.; Dagnelie, P.C.; Schalkwijk, C.G. The role of hyperglycemia, insulin resistance, and blood pressure in diabetes-associated differences in cognitive performance—The Maastricht Study. *Diabetes Care* **2017**, *40*, 1537–1547. [CrossRef]

9. Ingwersen, J.; Defeyter, M.A.; Kennedy, D.O.; Wesnes, K.A.; Scholey, A.B. A low glycaemic index breakfast cereal preferentially prevents children's cognitive performance from declining throughout the morning. *Appetite* **2007**, *49*, 240–244. [CrossRef]
10. Smith, M.A.; Foster, J.K. The impact of a high versus a low glycaemic index breakfast cereal meal on verbal episodic memory in healthy adolescents. *Nutr. Neurosci.* **2008**, *11*, 219–227. [CrossRef]
11. Mahoney, C.R.; Taylor, H.A.; Kanarek, R.B.; Samuel, P. Effect of breakfast composition on cognitive processes in elementary school children. *Physiol. Behav.* **2005**, *85*, 635–645. [CrossRef] [PubMed]
12. Hawkins, M.A.; Gunstad, J.; Calvo, D.; Spitznagel, M.B. Higher fasting glucose is associated with poorer cognition among healthy young adults. *Health Psychol.* **2016**, *35*, 199. [CrossRef] [PubMed]
13. Pan, S.; Ding, N.; Ren, J.; Gu, Z.; Li, C.; Hong, Y.; Cheng, L.; Holler, T.P.; Li, Z. Maltooligosaccharide-forming amylase: Characteristics, preparation, and application. *Biotechnol. Adv.* **2017**, *35*, 619–632. [CrossRef] [PubMed]
14. Song, Y.-B.; Lamothe, L.M.; Rodriguez, N.E.N.; Rose, D.R.; Lee, B.-H. New insights suggest isomaltooligosaccharides are slowly digestible carbohydrates, rather than dietary fibers, at constitutive mammalian α-glucosidase levels. *Food Chem.* **2022**, *383*, 132456. [CrossRef] [PubMed]
15. Englyst, H.N.; Kingman, S.; Cummings, J. Classification and measurement of nutritionally important starch fractions. *Eur. J. Clin. Nutr.* **1992**, *46*, S33–S50. [PubMed]
16. Englyst, K.N.; Englyst, H.N.; Hudson, G.J.; Cole, T.J.; Cummings, J.H. Rapidly available glucose in foods: An in vitro measurement that reflects the glycemic response. *Am. J. Clin. Nutr.* **1999**, *69*, 448–454. [CrossRef] [PubMed]
17. Miao, M.; Jiang, B.; Cui, S.W.; Zhang, T.; Jin, Z. Slowly digestible starch—A review. *Crit. Rev. Food Sci. Nutr.* **2015**, *55*, 1642–1657. [CrossRef]
18. Lee, B.-H.; Hamaker, B.R. Number of branch points in α-limit dextrins impact glucose generation rates by mammalian mucosal α-glucosidases. *Carbohydr. Polym.* **2017**, *157*, 207–213. [CrossRef]
19. Kong, H.; Yu, L.; Li, C.; Ban, X.; Gu, Z.; Li, Z. Short-Clustered Maltodextrin Activates Ileal Glucose-Sensing and Induces Glucagon-like Peptide 1 Secretion to Ameliorate Glucose Homeostasis in Type 2 Diabetic Mice. *J. Agric. Food Chem.* **2022**, *70*, 12604–12619. [CrossRef]
20. Lennerz, B.; Lennerz, J.K. Food addiction, high-glycemic-index carbohydrates, and obesity. *Clin. Chem.* **2018**, *64*, 64–71. [CrossRef]
21. Della Pepa, G.; Vetrani, C.; Lupoli, R.; Massimino, E.; Lembo, E.; Riccardi, G.; Capaldo, B. Uncooked cornstarch for the prevention of hypoglycemic events. *Crit. Rev. Food Sci. Nutr.* **2022**, *62*, 3250–3263. [CrossRef] [PubMed]
22. Nadia, J.; Bronlund, J.; Singh, R.P.; Singh, H.; Bornhorst, G.M. Structural breakdown of starch-based foods during gastric digestion and its link to glycemic response: In vivo and in vitro considerations. *Compr. Rev. Food Sci. Food Saf.* **2021**, *20*, 2660–2698. [CrossRef] [PubMed]
23. Dupuis, J.H.; Liu, Q.; Yada, R.Y. Methodologies for increasing the resistant starch content of food starches: A review. *Compr. Rev. Food Sci. Food Saf.* **2014**, *13*, 1219–1234. [CrossRef]
24. Seidelmann, S.B.; Brian, C.; Cheng, S.; Mir, H.; Amil, S.; Steffen, L.M.; Folsom, A.R.; Rimm, E.B.; Willett, W.C.; Solomon, S.D. Dietary carbohydrate intake and mortality: A prospective cohort study and meta-analysis. *Lancet Public Health* **2018**, *3*, e419–e428. [CrossRef]
25. Zhang, H.; Zhang, W.; Yun, D.; Li, L.; Zhao, W.; Li, Y.; Liu, X.; Liu, Z. Alternate-day fasting alleviates diabetes-induced glycolipid metabolism disorders: Roles of FGF21 and bile acids. *J. Nutr. Biochem.* **2020**, *83*, 108403. [CrossRef]
26. Włodarek, D. Role of ketogenic diets in neurodegenerative diseases (Alzheimer's disease and Parkinson's disease). *Nutrients* **2019**, *11*, 169. [CrossRef]
27. Atabilen, B.; Akdevelioğlu, Y. Effects of different dietary interventions in multiple sclerosis: A systematic review of evidence from 2018 to 2022. *Nutr. Neurosci.* **2022**, *26*, 1279–1291. [CrossRef]
28. Janssen, H.; Kahles, F.; Liu, D.; Downey, J.; Koekkoek, L.L.; Roudko, V.; D'Souza, D.; McAlpine, C.S.; Halle, L.; Poller, W.C. Monocytes re-enter the bone marrow during fasting and alter the host response to infection. *Immunity* **2023**, *56*, 783–796. [CrossRef]
29. Crosby, L.; Davis, B.; Joshi, S.; Jardine, M.; Paul, J.; Neola, M.; Barnard, N.D. Ketogenic diets and chronic disease: Weighing the benefits against the risks. *Front. Nutr.* **2021**, *8*, 702802. [CrossRef]
30. Sünram-Lea, S.I.; Owen, L. The impact of diet-based glycaemic response and glucose regulation on cognition: Evidence across the lifespan. *Proc. Nutr. Soc.* **2017**, *76*, 466–477. [CrossRef]
31. Noble, E.E.; Hsu, T.M.; Liang, J.; Kanoski, S.E. Early life sugar consumption has long-term negative effects on memory function in male rats. *Nutr. Neurosci.* **2019**, *22*, 273–283. [CrossRef] [PubMed]
32. Noble, E.E.; Kanoski, S.E. Early life exposure to obesogenic diets and learning and memory dysfunction. *Curr. Opin. Behav. Sci.* **2016**, *9*, 7–14. [CrossRef] [PubMed]
33. Noble, E.E.; Olson, C.A.; Davis, E.; Tsan, L.; Chen, Y.-W.; Schade, R.; Liu, C.; Suarez, A.; Jones, R.B.; de La Serre, C. Gut microbial taxa elevated by dietary sugar disrupt memory function. *Transl. Psychiatry* **2021**, *11*, 194. [CrossRef] [PubMed]
34. Hsu, T.M.; Konanur, V.R.; Taing, L.; Usui, R.; Kayser, B.D.; Goran, M.I.; Kanoski, S.E. Effects of sucrose and high fructose corn syrup consumption on spatial memory function and hippocampal neuroinflammation in adolescent rats. *Hippocampus* **2015**, *25*, 227–239. [CrossRef] [PubMed]
35. Mou, Y.; Blok, E.; Barroso, M.; Jansen, P.W.; White, T.; Voortman, T. Dietary patterns, brain morphology and cognitive performance in children: Results from a prospective population-based study. *Eur. J. Epidemiol.* **2023**, *38*, 669–687. [CrossRef] [PubMed]

36. Henn, R.E.; Elzinga, S.E.; Glass, E.; Parent, R.; Guo, K.; Allouch, A.A.; Mendelson, F.E.; Hayes, J.; Webber-Davis, I.; Murphy, G.G. Obesity-induced neuroinflammation and cognitive impairment in young adult versus middle-aged mice. *Immun. Ageing* **2022**, *19*, 67. [CrossRef] [PubMed]
37. Petersen, R.C. Mild cognitive impairment as a diagnostic entity. *J. Intern. Med.* **2004**, *256*, 183–194. [CrossRef]
38. Mattson, M.P.; Arumugam, T.V. Hallmarks of brain aging: Adaptive and pathological modification by metabolic states. *Cell Metab.* **2018**, *27*, 1176–1199. [CrossRef]
39. Liu, L.; Volpe, S.L.; Ross, J.A.; Grimm, J.A.; Van Bockstaele, E.J.; Eisen, H.J. Dietary sugar intake and risk of Alzheimer's disease in older women. *Nutr. Neurosci.* **2022**, *25*, 2302–2313. [CrossRef]
40. Fu, J.; Qiu, W.; Zheng, H.; Qi, C.; Hu, S.; Wu, W.; Wang, H.; Wu, G.; Cao, P.; Ma, Z. Ageing trajectory of the gut microbiota is associated with metabolic diseases in a chronological age-dependent manner. *Gut* **2023**, *72*, 1431–1433. [CrossRef]
41. Zhou, R.; Qian, S.; Cho, W.C.; Zhou, J.; Jin, C.; Zhong, Y.; Wang, J.; Zhang, X.; Xu, Z.; Tian, M. Microbiota-microglia connections in age-related cognition decline. *Aging Cell* **2022**, *21*, e13599. [CrossRef] [PubMed]
42. Scott, K.A.; Ida, M.; Peterson, V.L.; Prenderville, J.A.; Moloney, G.M.; Izumo, T.; Murphy, K.; Murphy, A.; Ross, R.P.; Stanton, C. Revisiting Metchnikoff: Age-related alterations in microbiota-gut-brain axis in the mouse. *Brain Behav. Immun.* **2017**, *65*, 20–32. [CrossRef] [PubMed]
43. Li, Y.; Ning, L.; Yin, Y.; Wang, R.; Zhang, Z.; Hao, L.; Wang, B.; Zhao, X.; Yang, X.; Yin, L. Age-related shifts in gut microbiota contribute to cognitive decline in aged rats. *Aging* **2020**, *12*, 7801. [CrossRef]
44. Liu, Z.; Dai, X.; Zhang, H.; Shi, R.; Hui, Y.; Jin, X.; Zhang, W.; Wang, L.; Wang, Q.; Wang, D. Gut microbiota mediates intermittent-fasting alleviation of diabetes-induced cognitive impairment. *Nat. Commun.* **2020**, *11*, 855. [CrossRef] [PubMed]
45. Zheng, H.; Xu, P.; Jiang, Q.; Xu, Q.; Zheng, Y.; Yan, J.; Ji, H.; Ning, J.; Zhang, X.; Li, C. Depletion of acetate-producing bacteria from the gut microbiota facilitates cognitive impairment through the gut-brain neural mechanism in diabetic mice. *Microbiome* **2021**, *9*, 145. [CrossRef]
46. Bhat, Z.F.; Morton, J.D.; Mason, S.; Bekhit, A.E.-D.A.; Bhat, H.F. Obesity and neurological disorders: Dietary perspective of a global menace. *Crit. Rev. Food Sci. Nutr.* **2019**, *59*, 1294–1310. [CrossRef]
47. Dye, L.; Boyle, N.B.; Champ, C.; Lawton, C. The relationship between obesity and cognitive health and decline. *Proc. Nutr. Soc.* **2017**, *76*, 443–454. [CrossRef]
48. Li, H.; Ren, J.; Li, Y.; Wu, Q.; Wei, J. Oxidative stress: The nexus of obesity and cognitive dysfunction in diabetes. *Front. Endocrinol.* **2023**, *14*, 1134025. [CrossRef]
49. Cope, E.C.; LaMarca, E.A.; Monari, P.K.; Olson, L.B.; Martinez, S.; Zych, A.D.; Katchur, N.J.; Gould, E. Microglia play an active role in obesity-associated cognitive decline. *J. Neurosci.* **2018**, *38*, 8889–8904. [CrossRef]
50. Bocarsly, M.E.; Fasolino, M.; Kane, G.A.; LaMarca, E.A.; Kirschen, G.W.; Karatsoreos, I.N.; McEwen, B.S.; Gould, E. Obesity diminishes synaptic markers, alters microglial morphology, and impairs cognitive function. *Proc. Natl. Acad. Sci. USA* **2015**, *112*, 15731–15736. [CrossRef]
51. Piatkowska-Chmiel, I.; Herbet, M.; Gawronska-Grzywacz, M.; Ostrowska-Lesko, M.; Dudka, J. The role of molecular and inflammatory indicators in the assessment of cognitive dysfunction in a mouse model of diabetes. *Int. J. Mol. Sci.* **2021**, *22*, 3878. [CrossRef] [PubMed]
52. van der Kooij, M.A.; Jene, T.; Treccani, G.; Miederer, I.; Hasch, A.; Voelxen, N.; Walenta, S.; Müller, M.B. Chronic social stress-induced hyperglycemia in mice couples individual stress susceptibility to impaired spatial memory. *Proc. Natl. Acad. Sci. USA* **2018**, *115*, E10187–E10196. [CrossRef] [PubMed]
53. Remor, A.P.; Da Silva, R.A.; de Matos, F.J.; Glaser, V.; de Paula Martins, R.; Ghisoni, K.; da Luz Scheffer, D.; Andia, D.C.; Portinho, D.; de Souza, A.P. Chronic metabolic derangement-induced cognitive deficits and neurotoxicity are associated with REST inactivation. *Mol. Neurobiol.* **2019**, *56*, 1539–1557. [CrossRef] [PubMed]
54. Rao, R.; Nashawaty, M.; Fatima, S.; Ennis, K.; Tkac, I. Neonatal hyperglycemia alters the neurochemical profile, dendritic arborization and gene expression in the developing rat hippocampus. *NMR Biomed.* **2018**, *31*, e3910. [CrossRef] [PubMed]
55. Zhou, W.; Chen, G.; Chen, D.; Ye, H.; Zeng, X. The antidiabetic effect and potential mechanisms of natural polysaccharides based on the regulation of gut microbiota. *J. Funct. Foods* **2020**, *75*, 104222. [CrossRef]
56. Zhang, L.; Zhang, T.; Sun, J.; Huang, Y.; Liu, T.; Ye, Z.; Hu, J.; Zhang, G.; Chen, H.; Ye, Z. Calorie restriction ameliorates hyperglycemia, modulates the disordered gut microbiota, and mitigates metabolic endotoxemia and inflammation in type 2 diabetic rats. *J. Endocrinol. Investig.* **2023**, *46*, 699–711. [CrossRef]
57. Tai, N.; Wong, F.S.; Wen, L. The role of gut microbiota in the development of type 1, type 2 diabetes mellitus and obesity. *Rev. Endocr. Metab. Disord.* **2015**, *16*, 55–65. [CrossRef]
58. Erejuwa, O.O.; Sulaiman, S.A.; Ab Wahab, M.S. Modulation of gut microbiota in the management of metabolic disorders: The prospects and challenges. *Int. J. Mol. Sci.* **2014**, *15*, 4158–4188. [CrossRef]
59. Walsh, S.K.; Lucey, A.; Walter, J.; Zannini, E.; Arendt, E.K. Resistant starch—An accessible fiber ingredient acceptable to the Western palate. *Compr. Rev. Food Sci. Food Saf.* **2022**, *21*, 2930–2955. [CrossRef]
60. Meenu, M.; Xu, B. A critical review on anti-diabetic and anti-obesity effects of dietary resistant starch. *Crit. Rev. Food Sci. Nutr.* **2019**, *59*, 3019–3031. [CrossRef]

61. Kim, M.-S.; Kim, Y.; Choi, H.; Kim, W.; Park, S.; Lee, D.; Kim, D.K.; Kim, H.J.; Choi, H.; Hyun, D.-W.; et al. Transfer of a healthy microbiota reduces amyloid and tau pathology in an Alzheimer's disease animal model. *Gut* **2019**, *69*, 283–294. [CrossRef] [PubMed]
62. Gurung, M.; Li, Z.; You, H.; Rodrigues, R.; Jump, D.B.; Morgun, A.; Shulzhenko, N. Role of gut microbiota in type 2 diabetes pathophysiology. *EBioMedicine* **2020**, *51*, 102590. [CrossRef] [PubMed]
63. Yoo, D.Y.; Kim, D.W.; Kim, M.J.; Choi, J.H.; Jung, H.Y.; Nam, S.M.; Kim, J.W.; Yoon, Y.S.; Choi, S.Y.; Hwang, I.K. Sodium butyrate, a histone deacetylase Inhibitor, ameliorates SIRT2-induced memory impairment, reduction of cell proliferation, and neuroblast differentiation in the dentate gyrus. *Neurol. Res.* **2015**, *37*, 69–76. [CrossRef] [PubMed]
64. Intlekofer, K.A.; Berchtold, N.C.; Malvaez, M.; Carlos, A.J.; McQuown, S.C.; Cunningham, M.J.; Wood, M.A.; Cotman, C.W. Exercise and sodium butyrate transform a subthreshold learning event into long-term memory via a brain-derived neurotrophic factor-dependent mechanism. *Neuropsychopharmacology* **2013**, *38*, 2027–2034. [CrossRef] [PubMed]
65. Laukoetter, M.G.; Bruewer, M.; Nusrat, A. Regulation of the intestinal epithelial barrier by the apical junctional complex. *Curr. Opin. Gastroenterol.* **2006**, *22*, 85–89. [CrossRef] [PubMed]
66. De la Cuesta-Zuluaga, J.; Mueller, N.T.; Álvarez-Quintero, R.; Velásquez-Mejía, E.P.; Sierra, J.A.; Corrales-Agudelo, V.; Carmona, J.A.; Abad, J.M.; Escobar, J.S. Higher fecal short-chain fatty acid levels are associated with gut microbiome dysbiosis, obesity, hypertension and cardiometabolic disease risk factors. *Nutrients* **2018**, *11*, 51. [CrossRef]
67. Braniste, V.; Al-Asmakh, M.; Kowal, C.; Anuar, F.; Abbaspour, A.; Tóth, M.; Korecka, A.; Bakocevic, N.; Ng, L.G.; Kundu, P. The gut microbiota influences blood-brain barrier permeability in mice. *Sci. Transl. Med.* **2014**, *6*, 263ra158. [CrossRef]
68. Thaiss, C.A.; Levy, M.; Grosheva, I.; Zheng, D.; Soffer, E.; Blacher, E.; Braverman, S.; Tengeler, A.C.; Barak, O.; Elazar, M. Hyperglycemia drives intestinal barrier dysfunction and risk for enteric infection. *Science* **2018**, *359*, 1376–1383. [CrossRef]
69. Milenkovic, D.; Capel, F.; Combaret, L.; Comte, B.; Dardevet, D.; Evrard, B.; Guillet, C.; Monfoulet, L.-E.; Pinel, A.; Polakof, S. Targeting the gut to prevent and counteract metabolic disorders and pathologies during aging. *Crit. Rev. Food Sci. Nutr.* **2023**, *63*, 11185–11210. [CrossRef]
70. Caesar, R.; Tremaroli, V.; Kovatcheva-Datchary, P.; Cani, P.D.; Bäckhed, F. Crosstalk between gut microbiota and dietary lipids aggravates WAT inflammation through TLR signaling. *Cell Metab.* **2015**, *22*, 658–668. [CrossRef]
71. Shin, N.-R.; Lee, J.-C.; Lee, H.-Y.; Kim, M.-S.; Whon, T.W.; Lee, M.-S.; Bae, J.-W. An increase in the Akkermansia spp. population induced by metformin treatment improves glucose homeostasis in diet-induced obese mice. *Gut* **2014**, *63*, 727–735. [CrossRef] [PubMed]
72. Macchione, I.; Lopetuso, L.; Ianiro, G.; Napoli, M.; Gibiino, G.; Rizzatti, G.; Petito, V.; Gasbarrini, A.; Scaldaferri, F. Akkermansia muciniphila: Key player in metabolic and gastrointestinal disorders. *Eur. Rev. Med. Pharmacol. Sci.* **2019**, *23*, 8075–8083. [CrossRef] [PubMed]
73. Ghaffari, S.; Abbasi, A.; Somi, M.H.; Moaddab, S.Y.; Nikniaz, L.; Kafil, H.S.; Ebrahimzadeh Leylabadlo, H. Akkermansia muciniphila: From its critical role in human health to strategies for promoting its abundance in human gut microbiome. *Crit. Rev. Food Sci. Nutr.* **2022**, *63*, 7357–7377. [CrossRef] [PubMed]
74. McCarty, M.F.; Lerner, A. Perspective: Prospects for nutraceutical support of intestinal barrier function. *Adv. Nutr.* **2021**, *12*, 316–324. [CrossRef] [PubMed]
75. Liu, H.; Wang, J.; He, T.; Becker, S.; Zhang, G.; Li, D.; Ma, X. Butyrate: A double-edged sword for health? *Adv. Nutr.* **2018**, *9*, 21–29. [CrossRef] [PubMed]
76. Li, J.-M.; Yu, R.; Zhang, L.-P.; Wen, S.-Y.; Wang, S.-J.; Zhang, X.-Y.; Xu, Q.; Kong, L.-D. Dietary fructose-induced gut dysbiosis promotes mouse hippocampal neuroinflammation: A benefit of short-chain fatty acids. *Microbiome* **2019**, *7*, 98. [CrossRef]
77. O'Leary, O.F.; Ogbonnaya, E.S.; Felice, D.; Levone, B.R.; Conroy, L.C.; Fitzgerald, P.; Bravo, J.A.; Forsythe, P.; Bienenstock, J.; Dinan, T.G. The vagus nerve modulates BDNF expression and neurogenesis in the hippocampus. *Eur. Neuropsychopharmacol.* **2018**, *28*, 307–316. [CrossRef]
78. Chen, Y.; Xu, J.; Chen, Y. Regulation of neurotransmitters by the gut microbiota and effects on cognition in neurological disorders. *Nutrients* **2021**, *13*, 2099. [CrossRef]
79. Yano, J.M.; Yu, K.; Donaldson, G.P.; Shastri, G.G.; Ann, P.; Ma, L.; Nagler, C.R.; Ismagilov, R.F.; Mazmanian, S.K.; Hsiao, E.Y. Indigenous bacteria from the gut microbiota regulate host serotonin biosynthesis. *Cell* **2015**, *161*, 264–276. [CrossRef]
80. Jiang, H.; Ling, Z.; Zhang, Y.; Mao, H.; Ma, Z.; Yin, Y.; Wang, W.; Tang, W.; Tan, Z.; Shi, J. Altered fecal microbiota composition in patients with major depressive disorder. *Brain Behav. Immun.* **2015**, *48*, 186–194. [CrossRef]
81. Tian, P.; Wang, G.; Zhao, J.; Zhang, H.; Chen, W. Bifidobacterium with the role of 5-hydroxytryptophan synthesis regulation alleviates the symptom of depression and related microbiota dysbiosis. *J. Nutr. Biochem.* **2019**, *66*, 43–51. [CrossRef] [PubMed]
82. Mapstone, M.; Cheema, A.K.; Fiandaca, M.S.; Zhong, X.; Mhyre, T.R.; MacArthur, L.H.; Hall, W.J.; Fisher, S.G.; Peterson, D.R.; Haley, J.M. Plasma phospholipids identify antecedent memory impairment in older adults. *Nat. Med.* **2014**, *20*, 415–418. [CrossRef] [PubMed]
83. Farooqui, A.A.; Horrocks, L.A.; Farooqui, T. Glycerophospholipids in brain: Their metabolism, incorporation into membranes, functions, and involvement in neurological disorders. *Chem. Phys. Lipids* **2000**, *106*, 1–29. [CrossRef] [PubMed]
84. Li, L.; Solvi, C.; Zhang, F.; Qi, Z.; Chittka, L.; Zhao, W. Gut microbiome drives individual memory variation in bumblebees. *Nat. Commun.* **2021**, *12*, 6588. [CrossRef] [PubMed]

85. Butterfield, D.A.; Halliwell, B. Oxidative stress, dysfunctional glucose metabolism and Alzheimer disease. *Nat. Rev. Neurosci.* **2019**, *20*, 148–160. [CrossRef]
86. Alberini, C.M.; Cruz, E.; Descalzi, G.; Bessières, B.; Gao, V. Astrocyte glycogen and lactate: New insights into learning and memory mechanisms. *Glia* **2017**, *66*, 1244–1262. [CrossRef]
87. Sergi, D.; Renaud, J.; Simola, N.; Martinoli, M.-G. Diabetes, a contemporary risk for Parkinson's disease: Epidemiological and cellular evidences. *Front. Aging Neurosci.* **2019**, *11*, 302. [CrossRef]
88. Hubbard, J.; Binder, D. Glutamate metabolism. In *Astrocytes and Epilepsy*; Academic Press: San Diego, CA, USA, 2016; pp. 197–224. [CrossRef]
89. Voutsinos-Porche, B.; Bonvento, G.; Tanaka, K.; Steiner, P.; Welker, E.; Chatton, J.-Y.; Magistretti, P.J.; Pellerin, L. Glial glutamate transporters mediate a functional metabolic crosstalk between neurons and astrocytes in the mouse developing cortex. *Neuron* **2003**, *37*, 275–286. [CrossRef]
90. Rodriguez-Rodriguez, P.; Almeida, A.; Bolaños, J.P. Brain energy metabolism in glutamate-receptor activation and excitotoxicity: Role for APC/C-Cdh1 in the balance glycolysis/pentose phosphate pathway. *Neurochem. Int.* **2013**, *62*, 750–756. [CrossRef]
91. Wang, Y.; Fan, M.; Qian, H.; Ying, H.; Li, Y.; Wang, L. Whole grains-derived functional ingredients against hyperglycemia: Targeting hepatic glucose metabolism. *Crit. Rev. Food Sci. Nutr.* **2023**, 1–22. [CrossRef]
92. Whitmer, R.A.; Gilsanz, P.; Quesenberry, C.P.; Karter, A.J.; Lacy, M.E. Association of Type 1 Diabetes and Hypoglycemic and Hyperglycemic Events and Risk of Dementia. *Neurology* **2021**, *97*, e275–e283. [CrossRef]
93. Bourdel-Marchasson, I.; Schweizer, A.; Dejager, S. Incretin therapies in the management of elderly patients with type 2 diabetes mellitus. *Hosp. Pract.* **2011**, *39*, 7–21. [CrossRef]
94. Mushtaq, G.; Greig, N.H.; Khan, J.A.; Kamal, M.A. Status of acetylcholinesterase and butyrylcholinesterase in Alzheimer's disease and type 2 diabetes mellitus. *CNS Neurol. Disord.-Drug Targets* **2014**, *13*, 1432–1439. [CrossRef]
95. Ceriello, A.; Esposito, K.; Piconi, L.; Ihnat, M.A.; Thorpe, J.E.; Testa, R.; Boemi, M.; Giugliano, D. Oscillating glucose is more deleterious to endothelial function and oxidative stress than mean glucose in normal and type 2 diabetic patients. *Diabetes* **2008**, *57*, 1349–1354. [CrossRef]
96. Shi, X.-l.; Ren, Y.-z.; Wu, J. Intermittent high glucose enhances apoptosis in INS-1 cells. *Exp. Diabetes Res.* **2011**, *2011*, 754673. [CrossRef]
97. Zhang, Z.-Y.; Miao, L.-F.; Qian, L.-L.; Wang, N.; Qi, M.-M.; Zhang, Y.-M.; Dang, S.-P.; Wu, Y.; Wang, R.-X. Molecular mechanisms of glucose fluctuations on diabetic complications. *Front. Endocrinol.* **2019**, *10*, 640. [CrossRef]
98. Birt, D.F.; Boylston, T.; Hendrich, S.; Jane, J.-L.; Hollis, J.; Li, L.; McClelland, J.; Moore, S.; Phillips, G.J.; Rowling, M. Resistant starch: Promise for improving human health. *Adv. Nutr.* **2013**, *4*, 587–601. [CrossRef]
99. Owens, D.R.; Monnier, L.; Hanefeld, M. A review of glucagon-like peptide-1 receptor agonists and their effects on lowering postprandial plasma glucose and cardiovascular outcomes in the treatment of type 2 diabetes mellitus. *Diabetes Obes. Metab.* **2017**, *19*, 1645–1654. [CrossRef] [PubMed]
100. Tomlinson, D.R.; Gardiner, N.J. Glucose neurotoxicity. *Nat. Rev. Neurosci.* **2008**, *9*, 36–45. [CrossRef] [PubMed]
101. Bosco, D.; Fa Va, A.; Plastino, M.; Montalcini, T.; Pujia, A. Possible implications of insulin resistance and glucose metabolism in Alzheimer's disease pathogenesis. *J. Cell. Mol. Med.* **2011**, *15*, 1807–1821. [CrossRef]
102. Ying, L.; Fei, L.; Grundke-Iqbal, I.; Iqbal, K.; Gong, C.X. Deficient brain insulin signalling pathway in Alzheimer's disease and diabetes. *J. Pathol.* **2011**, *225*, 54–62. [CrossRef]
103. Zhang, Y.; Huang, N.Q.; Yan, F.; Jin, H.; Zhou, S.Y.; Shi, J.S.; Jin, F. Diabetes mellitus and Alzheimer's disease: GSK-3β as a potential link. *Behav. Brain Res.* **2017**, *339*, 57–65. [CrossRef] [PubMed]
104. Infante-Garcia, C.; Ramos-Rodriguez, J.J.; Galindo-Gonzalez, L.; Garcia-Alloza, M. Long-term central pathology and cognitive impairment are exacerbated in a mixed model of Alzheimer's disease and type 2 diabetes. *Psychoneuroendocrinology* **2016**, *65*, 15–25. [CrossRef] [PubMed]
105. Bogush, M.; Heldt, N.A.; Persidsky, Y. Blood brain barrier injury in diabetes: Unrecognized effects on brain and cognition. *J. Neuroimmune Pharmacol.* **2017**, *12*, 593–601. [CrossRef] [PubMed]
106. Geng, J.; Wang, L.; Zhang, L.; Qin, C.; Song, Y.; Ma, Y.; Chen, Y.; Chen, S.; Wang, Y.; Zhang, Z. Blood-brain barrier disruption induced cognitive impairment is associated with increase of inflammatory cytokine. *Front. Aging Neurosci.* **2018**, *10*, 129. [CrossRef] [PubMed]
107. Miranda, H.V.; El-Agnaf, O.; Outeiro, T.F. Glycation in Parkinson's disease and Alzheimer's disease. *Mov. Disord. Off. J. Mov. Disord. Soc.* **2016**, *31*, 782–790. [CrossRef] [PubMed]
108. Zhao, L.; Dong, M.; Wang, D.; Ren, M.; Zheng, Y.; Zheng, H.; Li, C.; Gao, H. Characteristic metabolic alterations identified in primary neurons under high glucose exposure. *Front. Cell. Neurosci.* **2018**, *12*, 207. [CrossRef] [PubMed]
109. Lanaspa, M.A.; Ishimoto, T.; Li, N.; Cicerchi, C.; Orlicky, D.J.; Ruzycki, P.; Rivard, C.; Inaba, S.; Roncal-Jimenez, C.A.; Bales, E.S. Endogenous fructose production and metabolism in the liver contributes to the development of metabolic syndrome. *Nat. Commun.* **2013**, *4*, 2434. [CrossRef] [PubMed]
110. Hwang, J.J.; Jiang, L.; Hamza, M.; Dai, F.; Belfort-DeAguiar, R.; Cline, G.; Rothman, D.L.; Mason, G.; Sherwin, R.S. The human brain produces fructose from glucose. *JCI Insight* **2017**, *2*, e90508. [CrossRef]
111. Lustig, R.H. Fructose: It's "alcohol without the buzz". *Adv. Nutr.* **2013**, *4*, 226–235. [CrossRef]

112. Kendig, M.D.; Lin, C.S.; Beilharz, J.E.; Rooney, K.B.; Boakes, R.A. Maltodextrin can produce similar metabolic and cognitive effects to those of sucrose in the rat. *Appetite* **2014**, *77*, 1–12. [CrossRef] [PubMed]
113. Johnson, R.J.; Gomez-Pinilla, F.; Nagel, M.; Nakagawa, T.; Rodriguez-Iturbe, B.; Sanchez-Lozada, L.G.; Tolan, D.R.; Lanaspa, M.A. Cerebral fructose metabolism as a potential mechanism driving Alzheimer's disease. *Front. Aging Neurosci.* **2020**, *12*, 560865. [CrossRef] [PubMed]
114. Herman, M.A.; Birnbaum, M.J. Molecular aspects of fructose metabolism and metabolic disease. *Cell Metab.* **2021**, *33*, 2329–2354. [CrossRef] [PubMed]
115. Shao, X.; Lu, W.; Gao, F.; Li, D.; Hu, J.; Li, Y.; Zuo, Z.; Jie, H.; Zhao, Y.; Cen, X. Uric acid induces cognitive dysfunction through hippocampal inflammation in rodents and humans. *J. Neurosci.* **2016**, *36*, 10990–11005. [CrossRef] [PubMed]
116. Desideri, G.; Gentile, R.; Antonosante, A.; Benedetti, E.; Grassi, D.; Cristiano, L.; Manocchio, A.; Selli, S.; Ippoliti, R.; Ferri, C. Uric acid amplifies Aβ amyloid effects involved in the cognitive dysfunction/dementia: Evidences from an experimental model in vitro. *J. Cell. Physiol.* **2017**, *232*, 1069–1078. [CrossRef] [PubMed]
117. Sugimoto, K.; Yasujima, M.; Yagihashi, S. Role of advanced glycation end products in diabetic neuropathy. *Curr. Pharm. Des.* **2008**, *14*, 953–961. [CrossRef]
118. Rajchgot, T.; Thomas, S.C.; Wang, J.-C.; Ahmadi, M.; Balood, M.; Crosson, T.; Dias, J.P.; Couture, R.; Claing, A.; Talbot, S. Neurons and Microglia; A Sickly-Sweet Duo in Diabetic Pain Neuropathy. *Front. Neuroence* **2019**, *13*, 25. [CrossRef]
119. Twarda-Clapa, A.; Olczak, A.; Białkowska, A.M.; Koziołkiewicz, M. Advanced glycation end-products (AGEs): Formation, chemistry, classification, receptors, and diseases related to AGEs. *Cells* **2022**, *11*, 1312. [CrossRef]
120. Tups, A.; Benzler, J.; Sergi, D.; Ladyman, S.R.; Williams, L.M. Central regulation of glucose homeostasis. *Compr. Physiol.* **2017**, *7*, 741–764. [CrossRef]
121. Du, X.-L.; Edelstein, D.; Rossetti, L.; Fantus, I.G.; Goldberg, H.; Ziyadeh, F.; Wu, J.; Brownlee, M. Hyperglycemia-induced mitochondrial superoxide overproduction activates the hexosamine pathway and induces plasminogen activator inhibitor-1 expression by increasing Sp1 glycosylation. *Proc. Natl. Acad. Sci. USA* **2000**, *97*, 12222–12226. [CrossRef]
122. Lal, S.; Szwergold, B.S.; Taylor, A.H.; Randall, W.C.; Kappler, F.; Wellsknecht, K.; Baynes, J.W.; Brown, T.R. Metabolism of fructose-3-phosphate in the diabetic rat lens. *Arch. Biochem. Biophys.* **1995**, *318*, 191–199. [CrossRef]
123. Sandhir, R.; Yadav, A.; Sunkaria, A.; Singhal, N. Nano-antioxidants: An emerging strategy for intervention against neurodegenerative conditions. *Neurochem. Int.* **2015**, *89*, 209–226. [CrossRef] [PubMed]
124. Lin, X.-m.; Sun, W.-y.; Duan, W.-j.; Gong, H.-b.; Tu, L.-f.; Li, Y.-f.; Kurihara, H.; He, R.-r. Phospholipid peroxidation: A key factor in" susceptibility" to neurodegenerative diseases. *Acta Pharm. Sin.* **2021**, *56*, 2154–2163. [CrossRef]
125. Inoguchi, T.; Li, P.; Umeda, F.; Yu, H.Y.; Kakimoto, M.; Imamura, M.; Aoki, T.; Etoh, T.; Hashimoto, T.; Naruse, M. High glucose level and free fatty acid stimulate reactive oxygen species production through protein kinase C--dependent activation of NAD (P) H oxidase in cultured vascular cells. *Diabetes* **2000**, *49*, 1939–1945. [CrossRef] [PubMed]
126. Sandireddy, R.; Yerra, V.G.; Areti, A.; Komirishetty, P.; Kumar, A. Neuroinflammation and oxidative stress in diabetic neuropathy: Futuristic strategies based on these targets. *Int. J. Endocrinol.* **2014**, *2014*, 674987. [CrossRef] [PubMed]
127. Tan, A.L.; Forbes, J.M.; Cooper, M.E. AGE, RAGE, and ROS in diabetic nephropathy. *Semin. Nephrol.* **2007**, *27*, 130–143. [CrossRef] [PubMed]
128. Snell, K. Enzymes of serine metabolism in normal, developing and neoplastic rat tissues. *Adv. Enzym. Regul.* **1984**, *22*, 325–400. [CrossRef] [PubMed]
129. Ly, C.H.; Lynch, G.S.; Ryall, J.G. A metabolic roadmap for somatic stem cell fate. *Cell Metab.* **2020**, *31*, 1052–1067. [CrossRef]
130. Lin, W.; Wang, M.; Chen, M.; Zheng, X.; Wu, Y.; Gao, D.; Yang, Z.; Tian, Z. Metabolomics and correlation network analyses of core biomarkers in type 2 diabetes. *Amino Acids* **2020**, *52*, 1307–1317. [CrossRef]
131. Yu, J.; Xiao, F.; Guo, Y.; Deng, J.; Liu, B.; Zhang, Q.; Li, K.; Wang, C.; Chen, S.; Guo, F. Hepatic phosphoserine aminotransferase 1 regulates insulin sensitivity in mice via tribbles homolog 3. *Diabetes* **2015**, *64*, 1591–1602. [CrossRef]
132. Zhang, J.; An, H.; Ni, K.; Chen, B.; Li, H.; Li, Y.; Sheng, G.; Zhou, C.; Xie, M.; Chen, S. Glutathione prevents chronic oscillating glucose intake-induced β-cell dedifferentiation and failure. *Cell Death Dis.* **2019**, *10*, 321. [CrossRef] [PubMed]
133. Singh, R.; Kishore, L.; Kaur, N. Diabetic peripheral neuropathy: Current perspective and future directions. *Pharmacol. Res.* **2014**, *80*, 21–35. [CrossRef] [PubMed]
134. Flohé, L.; Brigelius-Flohé, R.; Saliou, C.; Traber, M.G.; Packer, L. Redox regulation of NF-kappa B activation. *Free Radic. Biol. Med.* **1997**, *22*, 1115–1126. [CrossRef] [PubMed]
135. Chen, Y.J.; Chan, D.C.; Lan, K.C.; Wang, C.C.; Chen, C.M.; Chao, S.C.; Tsai, K.S.; Yang, R.S.; Liu, S.H. PPARγ is involved in the hyperglycemia-induced inflammatory responses and collagen degradation in human chondrocytes and diabetic mouse cartilages. *J. Orthop. Res.* **2015**, *33*, 373–381. [CrossRef] [PubMed]
136. Hu, Y.; Chen, Y.; Ding, L.; He, X.; Takahashi, Y.; Gao, Y.; Shen, W.; Cheng, R.; Chen, Q.; Qi, X. Pathogenic role of diabetes-induced PPAR-α down-regulation in microvascular dysfunction. *Proc. Natl. Acad. Sci. USA* **2013**, *110*, 15401–15406. [CrossRef] [PubMed]
137. Zhang, Y.; Capanoglu, E.; Jiao, L.; Yin, L.; Liu, X.; Wang, R.; Xiao, J.; Lu, B. Coarse cereals modulating chronic low-grade inflammation. *Crit. Rev. Food Sci. Nutr.* **2022**, *63*, 9694–9715. [CrossRef]
138. Li, H.; Wang, Y.; Zhang, D.; Chen, T.; Hu, A.; Han, X. Glycemic fluctuation exacerbates inflammation and bone loss and alters microbiota profile around implants in diabetic mice with experimental peri-implantitis. *Int. J. Implant Dent.* **2021**, *7*, 79. [CrossRef]

139. Marcelo, K.L.; Means, A.R.; York, B. The Ca2+/calmodulin/CaMKK2 axis: Nature's metabolic CaMshaft. *Trends Endocrinol. Metab.* **2016**, *27*, 706–718. [CrossRef]
140. Xu, Z.; Xu, W.; Song, Y.; Zhang, B.; Li, F.; Liu, Y. Blockade of store-operated calcium entry alleviates high glucose-induced neurotoxicity via inhibiting apoptosis in rat neurons. *Chem.-Biol. Interact.* **2016**, *254*, 63–72. [CrossRef]
141. Khomula, E.V.; Viatchenko-Karpinski, V.Y.; Borisyuk, A.L.; Duzhyy, D.E.; Belan, P.V.; Voitenko, N.V. Specific functioning of Cav3. 2 T-type calcium and TRPV1 channels under different types of STZ-diabetic neuropathy. *Biochim. Et Biophys. Acta (BBA)-Mol. Basis Dis.* **2013**, *1832*, 636–649. [CrossRef]
142. Hou, X.; Pedi, L.; Diver, M.M.; Long, S.B. Crystal structure of the calcium release–activated calcium channel Orai. *Science* **2012**, *338*, 1308–1313. [CrossRef] [PubMed]
143. Wu, W.-N.; Wu, P.-F.; Zhou, J.; Guan, X.-L.; Zhang, Z.; Yang, Y.-J.; Long, L.-H.; Xie, N.; Chen, J.-G.; Wang, F. Orexin-A activates hypothalamic AMP-activated protein kinase signaling through a Ca^{2+}-dependent mechanism involving voltage-gated L-type calcium channel. *Mol. Pharmacol.* **2013**, *84*, 876–887. [CrossRef]
144. Walkon, L.L.; Strubbe-Rivera, J.O.; Bazil, J.N. Calcium Overload and Mitochondrial Metabolism. *Biomolecules* **2022**, *12*, 1891. [CrossRef] [PubMed]
145. Dong, Z.; Saikumar, P.; Weinberg, J.M.; Venkatachalam, M.A. Calcium in cell injury and death. *Annu. Rev. Pathol. Mech. Dis.* **2006**, *1*, 405–434. [CrossRef] [PubMed]
146. Zhang, X.; Xu, L.; He, D.; Ling, S. Endoplasmic reticulum stress-mediated hippocampal neuron apoptosis involved in diabetic cognitive impairment. *BioMed Res. Int.* **2013**, *2013*, 924327. [CrossRef] [PubMed]
147. Liu, D.; Zhang, M.; Yin, H. Signaling pathways involved in endoplasmic reticulum stress-induced neuronal apoptosis. *Int. J. Neurosci.* **2013**, *123*, 155–162. [CrossRef] [PubMed]
148. Ferreiro, E.; Oliveira, C.R.; Pereira, C.M. The release of calcium from the endoplasmic reticulum induced by amyloid-beta and prion peptides activates the mitochondrial apoptotic pathway. *Neurobiol. Dis.* **2008**, *30*, 331–342. [CrossRef]
149. Qi, H.; Xu, G.; Peng, X.-L.; Li, X.; Shuai, J.; Xu, R. Roles of four feedback loops in mitochondrial permeability transition pore opening induced by Ca^{2+} and reactive oxygen species. *Phys. Rev. E* **2020**, *102*, 62422. [CrossRef]
150. Zhu, J.; Jin, M.; Wang, J.; Zhang, H.; Wu, Y.; Li, D.; Ji, X.; Yang, H.; Yin, C.; Ren, T. TNFα induces Ca2+ influx to accelerate extrinsic apoptosis in hepatocellular carcinoma cells. *J. Exp. Clin. Cancer Res.* **2018**, *37*, 43. [CrossRef]
151. Calvo-Rodriguez, M.; Bacskai, B.J. Mitochondria and calcium in Alzheimer's disease: From cell signaling to neuronal cell death. *Trends Neurosci.* **2021**, *44*, 136–151. [CrossRef]
152. Cheng, J.; Dong, Y.; Ma, J.; Pan, R.; Liao, Y.; Kong, X.; Li, X.; Li, S.; Chen, P.; Wang, L. Microglial Calhm2 regulates neuroinflammation and contributes to Alzheimer's disease pathology. *Sci. Adv.* **2021**, *7*, eabe3600. [CrossRef] [PubMed]
153. Wei, Y.-P.; Ye, J.-W.; Wang, X.; Zhu, L.-P.; Hu, Q.-H.; Wang, Q.; Ke, D.; Tian, Q.; Wang, J.-Z. Tau-induced Ca2+/calmodulin-dependent protein kinase-IV activation aggravates nuclear tau hyperphosphorylation. *Neurosci. Bull.* **2018**, *34*, 261–269. [CrossRef] [PubMed]
154. Shih, C.-T.; Yeh, Y.-T.; Lin, C.-C.; Yang, L.-Y.; Chiang, C.-P. Akkermansia muciniphila is negatively correlated with hemoglobin A1c in refractory diabetes. *Microorganisms* **2020**, *8*, 1360. [CrossRef] [PubMed]
155. Liu, J.; Zhou, L.; Sun, L.; Ye, X.; Ma, M.; Dou, M.; Shi, L. Association Between Intestinal Prevotella copri Abundance and Glycemic Fluctuation in Patients with Brittle Diabetes. *Diabetes Metab. Syndr. Obes.* **2023**, *16*, 1613–1621. [CrossRef] [PubMed]
156. Zhou, Z.; Sun, B.; Yu, D.; Zhu, C. Gut microbiota: An important player in type 2 diabetes mellitus. *Front. Cell. Infect. Microbiol.* **2022**, *12*, 112. [CrossRef]
157. Pajic, P.; Pavlidis, P.; Dean, K.; Neznanova, L.; Romano, R.-A.; Garneau, D.; Daugherity, E.; Globig, A.; Ruhl, S.; Gokcumen, O. Independent amylase gene copy number bursts correlate with dietary preferences in mammals. *Elife* **2019**, *8*, e44628. [CrossRef]
158. Ross, A.B.; Shertukde, S.P.; Staffier, K.L.; Chung, M.; Jacques, P.F.; McKeown, N.M. The relationship between whole-grain intake and measures of cognitive decline, mood, and anxiety—A systematic review. *Adv. Nutr.* **2023**, *14*, 652–670. [CrossRef]
159. Sanders, L.M.; Zhu, Y.; Wilcox, M.L.; Koecher, K.; Maki, K.C. Whole grain intake, compared to refined grain, improves postprandial glycemia and insulinemia: A systematic review and meta-analysis of randomized controlled trials. *Crit. Rev. Food Sci. Nutr.* **2021**, *63*, 5339–5357. [CrossRef]
160. Ginieis, R.; Franz, E.A.; Oey, I.; Peng, M. The "sweet" effect: Comparative assessments of dietary sugars on cognitive performance. *Physiol. Behav.* **2018**, *184*, 242–247. [CrossRef]
161. Kuroda, Y.; MATSUZAkI, K.; WAkATSUkI, H.; Shido, O.; Harauma, A.; Moriguchi, T.; Sugimoto, H.; Yamaguchi, S.; Yoshino, K.; Hashimoto, M. Influence of ultra-high hydrostatic pressurizing brown rice on cognitive functions and mental health of elderly Japanese individuals: A 2-year randomized and controlled trial. *J. Nutr. Sci. Vitaminol.* **2019**, *65*, S80–S87. [CrossRef]
162. Shi, H.; Yu, Y.; Lin, D.; Zheng, P.; Zhang, P.; Hu, M.; Wang, Q.; Pan, W.; Yang, X.; Hu, T. β-glucan attenuates cognitive impairment via the gut-brain axis in diet-induced obese mice. *Microbiome* **2020**, *8*, 143. [CrossRef] [PubMed]
163. Katayama, S.; Okahata, C.; Onozato, M.; Minami, T.; Maeshima, M.; Ogihara, K.; Yamazaki, S.; Takahashi, Y.; Nakamura, S. Buckwheat Flour and Its Starch Prevent Age-Related Cognitive Decline by Increasing Hippocampal BDNF Production in Senescence-Accelerated Mouse Prone 8 Mice. *Nutrients* **2022**, *14*, 2708. [CrossRef] [PubMed]
164. Kendig, M.D.; Boakes, R.A.; Rooney, K.B.; Corbit, L.H. Chronic restricted access to 10% sucrose solution in adolescent and young adult rats impairs spatial memory and alters sensitivity to outcome devaluation. *Physiol. Behav.* **2013**, *120*, 164–172. [CrossRef] [PubMed]

165. Beilharz, J.E.; Maniam, J.; Morris, M.J. Short exposure to a diet rich in both fat and sugar or sugar alone impairs place, but not object recognition memory in rats. *Brain Behav. Immun.* **2014**, *37*, 134–141. [CrossRef]
166. Reichelt, A.C.; Killcross, S.; Hambly, L.D.; Morris, M.J.; Westbrook, R.F. Impact of adolescent sucrose access on cognitive control, recognition memory, and parvalbumin immunoreactivity. *Learn. Mem.* **2015**, *22*, 215–224. [CrossRef]
167. Wu, H.-W.; Ren, L.-F.; Zhou, X.; Han, D.-W. A high-fructose diet induces hippocampal insulin resistance and exacerbates memory deficits in male Sprague-Dawley rats. *Nutr. Neurosci.* **2015**, *18*, 323–328. [CrossRef]
168. Sachdeva, A.K.; Dharavath, R.N.; Chopra, K. Time-response studies on development of cognitive deficits in an experimental model of insulin resistance. *Clin. Nutr.* **2019**, *38*, 1447–1456. [CrossRef]
169. Sangüesa, G.; Cascales, M.; Griñán, C.; Sánchez, R.M.; Roglans, N.; Pallàs, M.; Laguna, J.C.; Alegret, M. Impairment of novel object recognition memory and brain insulin signaling in fructose-but not glucose-drinking female rats. *Mol. Neurobiol.* **2018**, *55*, 6984–6999. [CrossRef]
170. Zou, Y.; Guo, Q.; Chang, Y.; Jia, L.; Zhai, L.; Bai, Y.; Sun, Q.; Wei, W. Learning and memory impairment and transcriptomic profile in hippocampus of offspring after maternal fructose exposure during gestation and lactation. *Food Chem. Toxicol.* **2022**, *169*, 113394. [CrossRef]
171. Ediga, M.G.; Annapureddy, S.; Salikineedy, K.; Nimgampalle, M. Aspartame consumption causes cognitive impairment in streptozotocin-induced diabetic Wistar rats. *Biologia* **2023**, *78*, 2393–2407. [CrossRef]
172. Tsan, L.; Chometton, S.; Hayes, A.M.; Klug, M.E.; Zuo, Y.; Sun, S.; Bridi, L.; Lan, R.; Fodor, A.A.; Noble, E.E. Early-life low-calorie sweetener consumption disrupts glucose regulation, sugar-motivated behavior, and memory function in rats. *JCI Insight* **2022**, *7*, e157714. [CrossRef] [PubMed]
173. Kendig, M.D.; Fu, M.X.; Rehn, S.; Martire, S.I.; Boakes, R.A.; Rooney, K.B. Metabolic and cognitive improvement from switching to saccharin or water following chronic consumption by female rats of 10% sucrose solution. *Physiol. Behav.* **2018**, *188*, 162–172. [CrossRef] [PubMed]
174. Keenan, M.J.; Zhou, J.; Hegsted, M.; Pelkman, C.; Durham, H.A.; Coulon, D.B.; Martin, R.J. Role of resistant starch in improving gut health, adiposity, and insulin resistance. *Adv. Nutr.* **2015**, *6*, 198–205. [CrossRef] [PubMed]
175. Raatz, S.K.; Idso, L.; Johnson, L.K.; Jackson, M.I.; Combs, G.F., Jr. Resistant starch analysis of commonly consumed potatoes: Content varies by cooking method and service temperature but not by variety. *Food Chem.* **2016**, *208*, 297–300. [CrossRef] [PubMed]
176. Wang, Z.; Wang, S.; Xu, Q.; Kong, Q.; Li, F.; Lu, L.; Xu, Y.; Wei, Y. Synthesis and Functions of Resistant Starch. *Adv. Nutr.* **2023**, *14*, 1131–1144. [CrossRef] [PubMed]
177. Zhang, G.; Hamaker, B.R. Slowly digestible starch: Concept, mechanism, and proposed extended glycemic index. *Crit. Rev. Food Sci. Nutr.* **2009**, *49*, 852–867. [CrossRef] [PubMed]
178. Fortune, N.C.; Harville, E.W.; Guralnik, J.M.; Gustat, J.; Chen, W.; Qi, L.; Bazzano, L.A. Dietary intake and cognitive function: Evidence from the Bogalusa Heart Study. *Am. J. Clin. Nutr.* **2019**, *109*, 1656–1663. [CrossRef]
179. Ozawa, M.; Shipley, M.; Kivimaki, M.; Singh-Manoux, A.; Brunner, E.J. Dietary pattern, inflammation and cognitive decline: The Whitehall II prospective cohort study. *Clin. Nutr.* **2017**, *36*, 506–512. [CrossRef]
180. Khan, N.A.; Raine, L.B.; Drollette, E.S.; Scudder, M.R.; Kramer, A.F.; Hillman, C.H. Dietary fiber is positively associated with cognitive control among prepubertal children. *J. Nutr.* **2015**, *145*, 143–149. [CrossRef]
181. Bach Knudsen, K.E. Microbial degradation of whole-grain complex carbohydrates and impact on short-chain fatty acids and health. *Adv. Nutr.* **2015**, *6*, 206–213. [CrossRef]
182. Yu, L.; Gao, Y.; Ye, Z.; Duan, H.; Zhao, J.; Zhang, H.; Narbad, A.; Tian, F.; Zhai, Q.; Chen, W. Interaction of beta-glucans with gut microbiota: Dietary origins, structures, degradation, metabolism, and beneficial function. *Crit. Rev. Food Sci. Nutr.* **2023**. [CrossRef]
183. Liu, J.; Wang, Y.; Wang, Z.; Hao, Y.; Bai, W.; Wang, Z.; Wang, J. 5-Heptadecylresorcinol, a Biomarker for Whole Grain Rye Consumption, Ameliorates Cognitive Impairments and Neuroinflammation in APP/PS1 Transgenic Mice. *Mol. Nutr. Food Res.* **2020**, *64*, 1901218. [CrossRef] [PubMed]
184. Sang, S.; Chu, Y. Whole grain oats, more than just a fiber: Role of unique phytochemicals. *Mol. Nutr. Food Res.* **2017**, *61*, 1600715. [CrossRef] [PubMed]
185. Uenobe, M.; Saika, T.; Waku, N.; Ohno, M.; Inagawa, H. Effect of continuous dewaxed brown rice ingestion on the cognitive function of elderly individuals. *J. Nutr. Sci. Vitaminol.* **2019**, *65*, S122–S124. [CrossRef] [PubMed]
186. Di Giacomo, S.; Percaccio, E.; Gullì, M.; Romano, A.; Vitalone, A.; Mazzanti, G.; Gaetani, S.; Di Sotto, A. Recent Advances in the Neuroprotective Properties of Ferulic Acid in Alzheimer's Disease: A Narrative Review. *Nutrients* **2022**, *14*, 3709. [CrossRef] [PubMed]
187. Burke, M.V.; Small, D.M. Physiological mechanisms by which non-nutritive sweeteners may impact body weight and metabolism. *Physiol. Behav.* **2015**, *152*, 381–388. [CrossRef]
188. Hamelin, H.; Poizat, G.; Florian, C.; Kursa, M.B.; Pittaras, E.; Callebert, J.; Rampon, C.; Taouis, M.; Hamed, A.; Granon, S. Prolonged consumption of sweetened beverages lastingly deteriorates cognitive functions and reward processing in mice. *Cereb. Cortex* **2022**, *32*, 1365–1378. [CrossRef]

189. Crézé, C.; Candal, L.; Cros, J.; Knebel, J.-F.; Seyssel, K.; Stefanoni, N.; Schneiter, P.; Murray, M.M.; Tappy, L.; Toepel, U. The impact of caloric and non-caloric sweeteners on food intake and brain responses to food: A randomized crossover controlled trial in healthy humans. *Nutrients* **2018**, *10*, 615. [CrossRef]
190. Lohner, S.; Toews, I.; Meerpohl, J.J. Health outcomes of non-nutritive sweeteners: Analysis of the research landscape. *Nutr. J.* **2017**, *16*, 55. [CrossRef]
191. Rutters, F.; Nieuwenhuizen, A.G.; Lemmens, S.G.; Born, J.M.; Westerterp-Plantenga, M.S. Acute stress-related changes in eating in the absence of hunger. *Obesity* **2009**, *17*, 72–77. [CrossRef]
192. Zuker; Charles, S. Food for the brain. *Cell* **2015**, *161*, 9–11. [CrossRef] [PubMed]
193. Roberts, C.J.; Campbell, I.C.; Troop, N. Increases in Weight during Chronic Stress are Partially Associated with a Switch in Food Choice towards Increased Carbohydrate and Saturated Fat Intake. *Eur. Eat. Disord. Rev.* **2013**, *22*, 77–82. [CrossRef] [PubMed]
194. Silva, J.C.P.; Mota, M.; Martins, F.O.; Nogueira, C.; Gonçalves, T.; Carneiro, T.; Pinto, J.; Duarte, D.; Barros, A.S.; Jones, J.G.; et al. Intestinal Microbial and Metabolic Profiling of Mice Fed with High-Glucose and High-Fructose Diets. *J. Proteome Res.* **2018**, *17*, 2880–2891. [CrossRef] [PubMed]
195. Do, M.H.; Lee, E.; Oh, M.-J.; Kim, Y.; Park, H.-Y. High-Glucose or -Fructose Diet Cause Changes of the Gut Microbiota and Metabolic Disorders in Mice without Body Weight Change. *Nutrients* **2018**, *10*, 761. [CrossRef] [PubMed]
196. Sun, S.; Araki, Y.; Hanzawa, F.; Umeki, M.; Kojima, T.; Nishimura, N.; Ikeda, S.; Mochizuki, S.; Oda, H. High sucrose diet-induced dysbiosis of gut microbiota promotes fatty liver and hyperlipidemia in rats. *J. Nutr. Biochem.* **2021**, *93*, 108621. [CrossRef] [PubMed]
197. Kong, C.; Gao, R.; Yan, X.; Huang, L.; Qin, H. Probiotics improve gut microbiota dysbiosis in obese mice fed a high-fat or high-sucrose diet. *Nutrition* **2019**, *60*, 175–184. [CrossRef] [PubMed]
198. Magnusson, K.; Hauck, L.; Jeffrey, B.; Elias, V.; Humphrey, A.; Nath, R.; Perrone, A.; Bermudez, L. Relationships between diet-related changes in the gut microbiome and cognitive flexibility. *Neuroscience* **2015**, *300*, 128–140. [CrossRef] [PubMed]
199. Laffin, M.; Fedorak, R.; Zalasky, A.; Park, H.; Gill, A.; Agrawal, A.; Keshteli, A.; Hotte, N.; Madsen, K.L. A high-sugar diet rapidly enhances susceptibility to colitis via depletion of luminal short-chain fatty acids in mice. *Sci. Rep.* **2019**, *9*, 1–11. [CrossRef]
200. E Noble, E.; Hsu, T.M.; Jones, R.B.; A Fodor, A.; I Goran, M.; E Kanoski, S. Early-Life Sugar Consumption Affects the Rat Microbiome Independently of Obesity. *J. Nutr.* **2017**, *147*, 20–28. [CrossRef]
201. Nickerson, K.P.; Homer, C.R.; Kessler, S.P.; Dixon, L.J.; Kabi, A.; Gordon, I.O.; Johnson, E.E.; de la Motte, C.A.; McDonald, C. The Dietary Polysaccharide Maltodextrin Promotes Salmonella Survival and Mucosal Colonization in Mice. *PLoS ONE* **2014**, *9*, e101789. [CrossRef]
202. Nickerson, K.P.; McDonald, C. Crohn's Disease-Associated Adherent-Invasive Escherichia coli Adhesion Is Enhanced by Exposure to the Ubiquitous Dietary Polysaccharide Maltodextrin. *PLoS ONE* **2012**, *7*, e52132. [CrossRef] [PubMed]
203. Kong, H.; Yu, L.; Gu, Z.; Li, C.; Ban, X.; Cheng, L.; Hong, Y.; Li, Z. Novel Short-Clustered Maltodextrin as a Dietary Starch Substitute Attenuates Metabolic Dysregulation and Restructures Gut Microbiota in *db/db* Mice. *J. Agric. Food Chem.* **2020**, *68*, 12400–12412. [CrossRef] [PubMed]
204. Kaur, A.; Chen, T.; Green, S.J.; Mutlu, E.; Martin, B.R.; Rumpagaporn, P.; Patterson, J.A.; Keshavarzian, A.; Hamaker, B.R. Physical Inaccessibility of a Resistant Starch Shifts Mouse Gut Microbiota to Butyrogenic Firmicutes. *Mol. Nutr. Food Res.* **2019**, *63*, e1801012. [CrossRef] [PubMed]
205. Sorndech, W.; Rodtong, S.; Blennow, A.; Tongta, S. Impact of Resistant Maltodextrins and Resistant Starch on Human Gut Microbiota and Organic Acids Production. *Starch* **2018**, *71*, 1800231. [CrossRef]
206. He, B.; Nohara, K.; Ajami, N.J.; Michalek, R.D.; Tian, X.; Wong, M.; Losee-Olson, S.H.; Petrosino, J.F.; Yoo, S.-H.; Shimomura, K.; et al. Transmissible microbial and metabolomic remodeling by soluble dietary fiber improves metabolic homeostasis. *Sci. Rep.* **2015**, *5*, srep10604. [CrossRef] [PubMed]
207. Guan, N.; He, X.; Wang, S.; Liu, F.; Huang, Q.; Fu, X.; Chen, T.; Zhang, B. Cell Wall Integrity of Pulse Modulates the in Vitro Fecal Fermentation Rate and Microbiota Composition. *J. Agric. Food Chem.* **2020**, *68*, 1091–1100. [CrossRef] [PubMed]
208. Rovalino-Córdova, A.M.; Fogliano, V.; Capuano, E. Effect of bean structure on microbiota utilization of plant nutrients: An in-vitro study using the simulator of the human intestinal microbial ecosystem (SHIME®). *J. Funct. Foods* **2020**, *73*, 104087. [CrossRef]
209. Tachon, S.; Zhou, J.; Keenan, M.; Martin, R.; Marco, M.L. The intestinal microbiota in aged mice is modulated by dietary resistant starch and correlated with improvements in host responses. *FEMS Microbiol. Ecol.* **2012**, *83*, 299–309. [CrossRef]
210. Li, Z.-T.; Hu, G.-A.; Zhu, L.; Zhao, Z.-C.; Jiang, Y.; Gao, M.-J.; Zhan, X.-B. In vitro digestion and fecal fermentation of highly resistant starch rice and its effect on the gut microbiota. *Food Chem.* **2021**, *361*, 130095. [CrossRef]
211. Martínez, I.; Kim, J.; Duffy, P.R.; Schlegel, V.L.; Walter, J. Resistant Starches Types 2 and 4 Have Differential Effects on the Composition of the Fecal Microbiota in Human Subjects. *PLoS ONE* **2010**, *5*, e15046. [CrossRef]
212. Zhou, Y.; Wei, Y.; Yan, B.; Zhao, S.; Zhou, X. Regulation of tartary buckwheat-resistant starch on intestinal microflora in mice fed with high-fat diet. *Food Sci. Nutr.* **2020**, *8*, 3243–3251. [CrossRef] [PubMed]
213. Zeng, H.; Huang, C.; Lin, S.; Zheng, M.; Chen, C.; Zheng, B.; Zhang, Y. Lotus Seed Resistant Starch Regulates Gut Microbiota and Increases Short-Chain Fatty Acids Production and Mineral Absorption in Mice. *J. Agric. Food Chem.* **2017**, *65*, 9217–9225. [CrossRef] [PubMed]

214. Zhou, Y.; Zhao, S.; Jiang, Y.; Wei, Y.; Zhou, X. Regulatory Function of Buckwheat-Resistant Starch Supplementation on Lipid Profile and Gut Microbiota in Mice Fed with a High-Fat Diet. *J. Food Sci.* **2019**, *84*, 2674–2681. [CrossRef]
215. Umu, Ö.C.; A Frank, J.; Fangel, J.U.; Oostindjer, M.; da Silva, C.S.; Bolhuis, E.J.; Bosch, G.; Willats, W.G.T.; Pope, P.B.; Diep, D.B. Resistant starch diet induces change in the swine microbiome and a predominance of beneficial bacterial populations. *Microbiome* **2015**, *3*, 1–15. [CrossRef] [PubMed]
216. Wang, S.; Zhang, B.; Chen, T.; Li, C.; Fu, X.; Huang, Q. Chemical Cross-Linking Controls in Vitro Fecal Fermentation Rate of High-Amylose Maize Starches and Regulates Gut Microbiota Composition. *J. Agric. Food Chem.* **2019**, *67*, 13728–13736. [CrossRef]
217. Upadhyaya, B.; McCormack, L.; Fardin-Kia, A.R.; Juenemann, R.; Nichenametla, S.; Clapper, J.; Specker, B.; Dey, M. Impact of dietary resistant starch type 4 on human gut microbiota and immunometabolic functions. *Sci. Rep.* **2016**, *6*, 28797. [CrossRef]
218. Qin, R.; Wang, J.; Chao, C.; Yu, J.; Copeland, L.; Wang, S.; Wang, S. RS5 Produced More Butyric Acid through Regulating the Microbial Community of Human Gut Microbiota. *J. Agric. Food Chem.* **2021**, *69*, 3209–3218. [CrossRef]
219. Zhou, Q.; Fu, X.; Dhital, S.; Zhai, H.; Huang, Q.; Zhang, B. In vitro fecal fermentation outcomes of starch-lipid complexes depend on starch assembles more than lipid type. *Food Hydrocoll.* **2021**, *120*, 106941. [CrossRef]

nutrients

MDPI

Article

Lactobacillus helveticus-Derived Whey-Calcium Chelate Promotes Calcium Absorption and Bone Health of Rats Fed a Low-Calcium Diet

Wei Hu [1,2], Zhiwen Pei [1,2], Aonan Xia [1,2], Yang Jiang [1,2], Bo Yang [1,2], Xiaoming Liu [1,2,*], Jianxin Zhao [1,2], Hao Zhang [1,2] and Wei Chen [1,2,3]

1 State Key Laboratory of Food Science and Technology, Jiangnan University, Wuxi 214122, China; 6210112027@stu.jiangnan.edu.cn (W.H.); 6210113068@stu.jiangnan.edu.cn (Z.P.); 7210112107@stu.jiangnan.edu.cn (A.X.); 7160112009@vip.jiangnan.edu.cn (Y.J.); bo.yang@jiangnan.edu.cn (B.Y.); jxzhao@jiangnan.edu.cn (J.Z.); zhanghao@jiangnan.edu.cn (H.Z.); chenwei66@jiangnan.edu.cn (W.C.)
2 School of Food Science and Technology, Jiangnan University, Wuxi 214122, China
3 National Engineering Research Center for Functional Food, Jiangnan University, Wuxi 214122, China
* Correspondence: liuxm@jiangnan.edu.cn; Tel.: +86-13812501690

Abstract: This study investigated the characteristics of *Lactobacillus helveticus*-derived whey-calcium chelate (LHWCC) and its effect on the calcium absorption and bone health of rats. Fourier-transform infrared spectroscopy showed that carboxyl oxygen atoms, amino nitrogen atoms, and phosphate ions were the major binding sites with calcium in LHWCC, which has a sustained release effect in simulated in vitro digestion. LHWCC had beneficial effects on serum biochemical parameters, bone biomechanics, and the morphological indexes of the bones of calcium-deficient rats when fed at a dose of 40 mg Ca/kg BW for 7 weeks. In contrast to the inorganic calcium supplement, LHWCC significantly upregulated the gene expression of transient receptor potential cation V5 (TRPV5), TRPV6, PepT1, calcium-binding protein-D9k (Calbindin-D9k), and a calcium pump (plasma membrane Ca-ATPase, PMCA1b), leading to promotion of the calcium absorption rate, whereas $Ca_3(PO_4)_2$ only upregulated the TRPV6 channel in vivo. These findings illustrate the potential of LHWCC as an organic calcium supplement.

Keywords: whey-calcium chelate; low-calcium diet; calcium absorption; bone health

1. Introduction

Calcium mainly exists in the form of phosphates in bones and teeth, accounting for approximately 1.5% to 2% of the normal human body [1]. Calcium plays multiple physiological functions in the body and plays a crucial role in maintaining bone health. There is a greater demand for calcium in children and adolescents during their rapid growth period and the accumulation of calcium can achieve optimal peak bone mass in the early stages of life [2]. Although serum calcium can be maintained within the normal range through bone resorption, dietary intake of calcium is the only source of calcium supplementation in the body's bones, and low calcium intake and bioavailability may lead to calcium deficiency. Long-term calcium deficiency in the body can lead to spasms, osteoporosis, and chondropathy. At present, calcium deficiency is a common global problem, and calcium intake in China is below the WHO's daily recommended intake (1000 mg/d) [3], which calls for the attention of academia and the food industry in China.

In response to the current situation of calcium deficiency, calcium supplements such as inorganic calcium salts and organic calcium salts have been developed. Among them, organic calcium chelates such as amino acid-calcium chelates and protein hydrolysate-calcium chelates are known for their fast absorption rate and low energy consumption [4], with diversified sources such as soy protein hydrolysates [5], cucumber seed [6], casein hydrolysates [7], egg yolk hydrolysates [8], et al. The function of protein hydrolysate-calcium chelates has also been validated in vivo and in vitro [9]. Hua et al. [10] reported that after supplementation with *Chlorella pyrenoidosa* protein hydrolysate-calcium chelate (CPPH-Ca) to the male SD rats (3 weeks old), fed with the low-calcium diet, the physical and biomechanical properties of femurs and the gene expressions of transient receptor potential cation V5 (TRPV5), TRPV6, calcium-binding protein-D9k (Calbinding-D9k), and a calcium pump (plasma membrane Ca-ATPase, PMCA1b) in calcium-deficient rats were significantly improved by CPPH-Ca [10].

Lactobacillus helveticus is one of the commonly used lactic acid bacteria in the production of fermented dairy products such as yogurt and cheese [11]. It has a strong protein hydrolytic ability, which endows its fermented dairy products with rich and diverse bioactive peptide profiles with functions in the regulation of blood pressure [12], the immune system [13], cognition [14], et al. *L. helveticus* CCFM1263 has been shown to be highly efficient in casein hydrolysis and the generation of bioactive peptides [15]. The dairy protein hydrolysates of *L. helveticus* CCFM1263 would be a desirable agent for the development of functional calcium chelates. Therefore, in the present study, we aimed to investigate the characteristics of *Lactobacillus helveticus*-derived whey-calcium chelate (LHWCC) and its effect on the calcium absorption and bone health of rats fed with low-calcium diets.

2. Materials and Methods

2.1. Materials

Skim milk powder (lactose > 51.8%, protein > 35.8%) was provided by Bright Dairy Co., Ltd. (Shanghai, China). Chemicals, enzymes, and bile were purchased from Sigma Aldrich (Shanghai, China). Pepsin (Sigma P6887) and pancreatin (Sigma, P7545 8 USP) were of porcine origin, whereas bile (Sigma B8631) was of bovine origin. *Lactobacillus helveticus* CCFM1263 was isolated from naturally fermented dairy products in China and was deposited in the Culture Collection of Food Microorganisms (CCFM) of Jiangnan University (Wuxi, China). The AIN-93G rodent diet was purchased from Jiangsu Xietong Biology Co., Ltd. (Nanjing, Jiangsu, China). Nuclease-free water, FastPure cell/tissue total RNA isolation kit V2, HiScript III RT SuperMix for qPCR (+gDNA wiper), and ChamQ Universal SYBR qPCR Master Mix were purchased from Vazyme Biotech Co., Ltd. (Nanjing, Jiangsu, China). The primers for TRPV5, TRPV6, PepT1, Calbindin-D9k, Na^+/Ca^{2+} exchange mechanism (NCX), PMCA1b and β-actin were compounded by the Genewiz Biotechnology Co., Ltd. (Suzhou, Jiangsu, China).

2.2. Preparation of Whey-Calcium Chelate

The preparation method described by Wang et al. [16] was used with moderate modifications. The strains were sub-cultured three times in MRS medium and then twice in sterile reconstituted skim milk (11% *w*/*w*) at 37 °C prior to use. After two washes in Tris-HCl (pH 6.5), 2% cultures with an initial concentration of 1–5 × 10^8 CFU/mL were inoculated with sterile reconstituted skim milk (11% *w*/*w*) and incubated for 48 h at 37 °C. Then, 1 mol/L NaOH was added to adjust the sample to pH 4.6, heated at 95 °C for 10 min, and centrifuged. After centrifugation, the supernatant was filtered with 0.45 μM organic filter membrane and freeze-dried as lyophilized *Lactobacillus helveticus* whey (LHW). Then, LHW was dissolved in deionized water at a concentration of 3 mg/mL and mixed with $CaCl_2$ at a Ca^{2+} concentration of 1 mg/mL. The solution was stirred at pH 7.6, 40 °C for 120 min [17]. Then, ethanol was added to remove free calcium from the samples. After centrifugation, the precipitate was freeze-dried to obtain LHWCC (125.85 ± 4.31 mg Ca/g).

2.3. Fourier-Transform Infrared Spectroscopy (FT-IR)

The FT-IR spectrum of LHW and LHWCC was recorded from 4000 to 400 cm^{-1} using a Nicolet Summit FT-IR spectrometer iS50 (Thermo Fisher Scientific Inc., Waltham, MA, USA).

2.4. *In Vitro Digestion*

In vitro digestion was based on the standardized COST INFOGEST protocol [18]. In the digestion test, samples were taken at the beginning and end of the oral phase, at 0, 15, and 120 min of simulated gastric juice digestion, and at 0, 15, 30, 60, and 120 min of simulated intestinal juice digestion. Then, the samples were centrifuged at 8000 r/min for 10 min at 4 °C, and the calcium concentration of the supernatant was measured.

2.5. *Animal Experiments*

Male SD rats (n = 48, 3 weeks old, 55 ± 10 g) were purchased from the Vital River Laboratory Animal Technology Co., Ltd. (Beijing, China). The animal experimental protocol was approved by the Animal Ethics and Welfare Committee of Jiangnan University (Wuxi, China), and the IACUC Issue No. was JN.No 20230530S1200730[247]. Animal feeding conditions met SPF level requirements, and during the entire experimental period, rats were free to eat commercial food, which was prepared according to the AIN-93 [19] (normal diet: 5000 mg Ca/kg; low-calcium diet: 1000 mg Ca/kg) [10], and drink freely. At the beginning of the experiment, the initial body length, body weight, and tail length were measured. During a 7-week experiment, the length and weight of rats were measured every week. The rats in the control group were fed the normal diet and the remaining rats were fed a low-Ca diet. The rats were randomly assigned into six groups, and the details of the experimental design are shown in Figure 1.

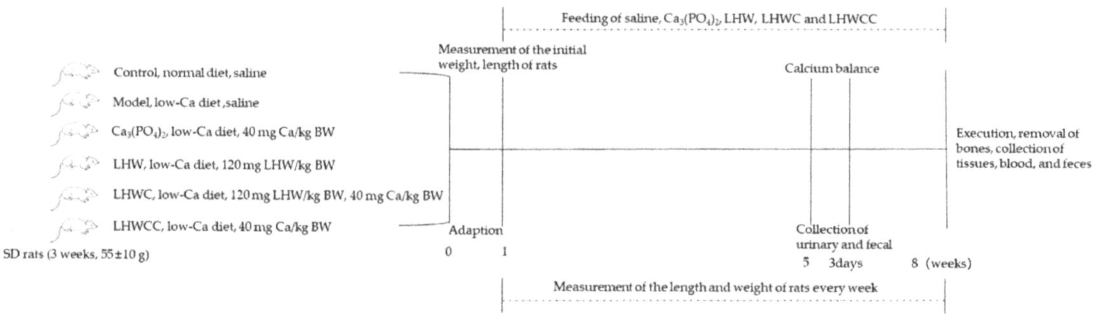

Figure 1. The flowchart of animal experiment. Note: the rats in the control group were fed the normal diet (5000 mg Ca/kg), and the remaining rats were fed a low-Ca diet (1000 mg Ca/kg).

2.6. *Analysis of Serum Biochemical Indexes*

The serum levels of calcium and ALP in different groups of rats were analyzed with analytical reagent kits (Nanjing Jiancheng Bioengineering Institute, Nanjing, China).

2.7. *Analysis of Femur Length, Diameter, and Weight*

The femurs that were cleaned of soft tissue were placed in a constant weight box and dried thoroughly in the drying oven for 10 h until reaching constant weight (under the condition that the lid is opened at 80 °C for 6 h and then closed at 115 °C for 4 h). Then, the dry weight of the femur was weighed and the length of the femur was measured. The diameter from the descending third rotor to the junction of the femoral shaft was determined as the femoral diameter.

2.8. *Analysis of Calcium Content in Femur*

After being dried, a 100 mg femur was dissolved in 7 mL of 16 mol/L HNO_3 to determine calcium content by flame atomic absorption spectrometry (AA-240, Varian Medical Systems, Palo Alto, CA, USA). The atomic absorbance was monitored at 422.7 nm, and the Ca content in the femur was expressed on a mg/g dry basis [20].

2.9. BMD and Bone Mass Measurements

The BMD of the femur was measured using a micro-CT (PerkinElmer Quantum GX, Waltham, MA, USA). Bone and trabecular-related indexes of the proximal femoral were obtained using the built-in software of the micro-CT. The operation parameters were as follows: 90 kV tube potential, 88 μA tube current, 86 mm FOV, high-resolution scan mode, 4 min scanning time, and 0.1 mm Cu X-ray filter according to the method of Chen et al. [21]. Calculations included bone volume (BV), bone surface (BS), bone volume/tissue volume (BV/TV), bone surface/tissue volume (BS/TV), trabecular separation (Tb.Sp), trabecular thickness (Tb·Th), and connectivity density (Conn.D).

2.10. Bone Biomechanical Strength Measurements

A three-point bending mechanical test was performed on the left femur diaphysis using a TA-XT plus texture analyzer (Stable Micro Systems, Godalming, Surrey, UK). The maximum fracture force, i.e., the maximum bone load, was measured using a three-point bending test at a test speed of 1 mm/s. The test was performed with a fulcrum span of 16 mm according to the method of Ye et al. [22] with slight modification.

2.11. Analysis of Calcium-Apparent Absorption and Retention Rate

The calcium intake and fecal and urinary calcium content were determined by AAS during the last 3 days of treatment. The calcium metabolism was calculated according to Wang et al. [23] with the following formula:

$$\text{Apparent calcium absorption rate (ACAR) (\%)} = (\text{Calcium Intake} - \text{Fecal Calcium})/\text{Calcium Intake} \times 100\%. \tag{1}$$

$$\text{Calcium accumulation rate (CAR) (\%)} = (\text{Calcium Intake} - \text{Fecal Calcium} - \text{Urinary Calcium})/\text{Calcium Intake} \times 100\%. \tag{2}$$

2.12. RNA Extraction and Real-Time RT-PCR

The intestinal tissue was ground and the RNA was obtained according to the instructions of the total RNA extraction kit. The nucleic acid purity (OD260/280 = 1.8–2.2, OD260/230 $\geq$ 2.0) and concentration were tested. The samples were reverse transcribed into cDNA according to the instructions of the reverse transcription kit. The primer reference was Li et al. [6], and the gene primer sequence was shown in Table 1. β-Actin was selected as the housekeeping gene. Relative gene expressions were calculated by the comparative $2^{-\Delta\Delta Ct}$ method.

Table 1. Primers used in the measurement of mRNA expression.

Gene	Primer Sequence
TRPV6	forward 5′-CACCCAGTGGACGTATGGAC-3′ reverse 5′-CTCGTGCGGTTATTGGTCCT-3′
TRPV5	forward 5′-ACGTATGGACCCCTGACCTC-3′ reverse 5′-GAATTTGGCGAGCCTCTCGT-3′
Calbindin-D9K	forward 5′-GGCAACCAGACACCAGAATGA-3′ reverse 5′-TGACAACTGGTCTGGATCACC-3′
NCX-1	forward 5′-TTGAGATTGGAGAACCCCGT-3′ reverse 5′-ATGTGAAGCCACCAAGCTCA-3′
PMCA1b	forward 5′-AGTGATTGTTGCTTTTACGGGC-3′ reverse 5′-AGAGACTCAGTGGGTGGTTCCG-3′
PepT1	forward 5′-ATCTACCATACGTTTGTTGC-3′ reverse 5′-CTGGGGCTGAAACTTCTT-3′
β-Actin	forward 5′-CACCCAGCACAATGAAGATCAAGAT-3′ reverse 5′-CCAGTTTTTAAATCCTGAGTCAAGC-3′

2.13. Statistical Analysis

Data for each group were expressed as mean ± SD (n = 8). For data analysis, one-way analysis of variance (ANOVA) was conducted using IBM SPSS Statistics 26 software (SPSS Inc, Chicago, IL, USA). Graphing and data processing were performed using GraphPad Prism 9.0.

3. Results

3.1. Fourier Transform-Infrared Spectroscopy of LHWCC

The infrared spectra of LHW and LHWCC in the wavelength range of 400–4000 cm^{-1} are shown in Figure 2, and the infrared spectrum of the calcium chelate showed significant changes. LHWCC had obvious fluctuations at 3410 cm^{-1}, 2104 cm^{-1}, 1591 cm^{-1}, 1422 cm^{-1}, and 1072 cm^{-1}. The characteristic peaks of amide A and amide B bands in the sample at 3388 cm^{-1} are significantly weakened and shifted, which was caused by the inductive effect or the dipole field effect, indicating the binding of calcium ions with N-H [24]. The absorption peak of LHW at 2170 cm^{-1} corresponding to the phosphate group O=P-O-H disappeared after chelation, indicating that H in the phosphate group was replaced by calcium ions. The absorption peak of LHWCC weakened at 1600 cm^{-1} and 1400 cm^{-1}, indicating that -COOH participated in the formation of chelates in the form of covalent bonds [25] with calcium ions to form -COO-Ca. The absorption peak of LHWCC shifted at 1072 cm^{-1}, which might be due to the formation of C-O-Ca by the combination of -CO bond and calcium [26]. The changes in absorption peaks in the range of 800–500 cm^{-1} could be attributed to the effect of chelation on the vibration of C-H and N-H bonds in carboxyl oxygen atoms, amino nitrogen atoms, and phosphate ions in compounds such as peptides in LHWCC.

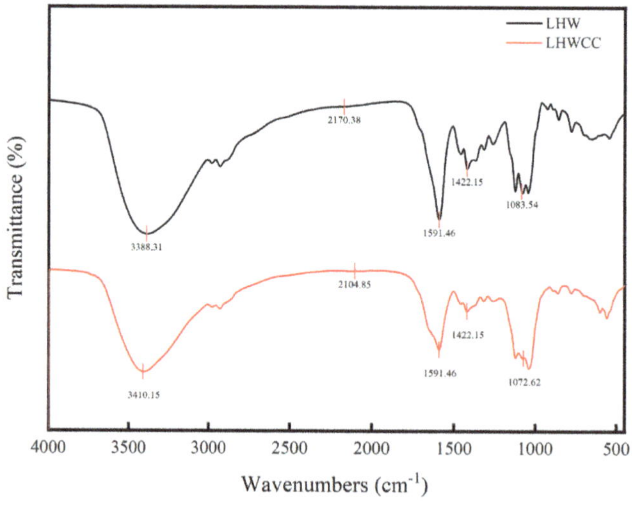

Figure 2. Fourier transform-infrared spectra of LHW and LHWCC in the regions of 4000 to 400 cm^{-1}.

3.2. Soluble Calcium Content of LHWCC In Vitro Digestion

As shown in Figure 3, there were significant differences in the dissolution characteristics of different calcium agents during the simulated oral digestion stage. $Ca_3(PO_4)_2$ was almost insoluble in the simulated saliva, and the solubility of LHWCC was around 30%. In the simulated gastric digestion stage, the solubility of both calcium agents significantly increased as an acidic environment (pH 3.0) increased calcium solubility [9]. $Ca_3(PO_4)_2$ was almost completely dissolved when entering the simulated gastric juice and subsequently maintained a solubility of over 90%. The solubility of LHWCC during gastric digestion increased with time, from the initial 70% to 100%, which was consistent with grape seed polypeptide calcium chelate [27]. This indicated that LHWCC has a certain sustained-release effect, which can reduce the rapid release of calcium ions in the stomach.

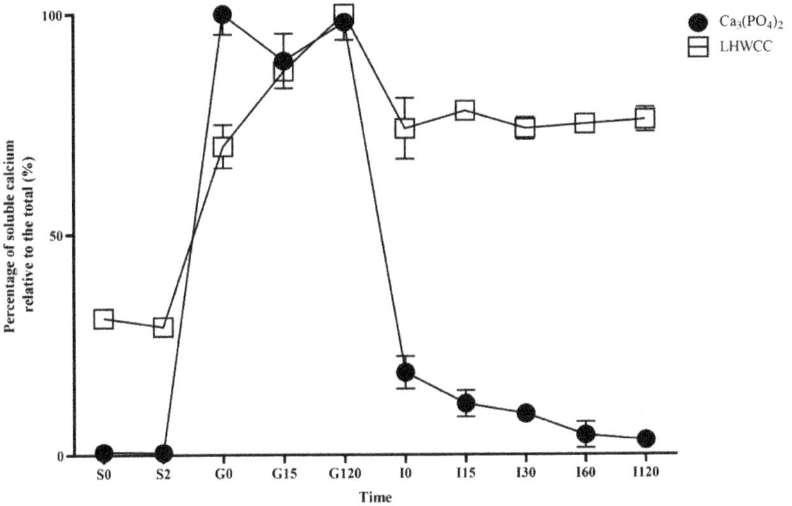

Figure 3. Changes in percentage of soluble calcium (relative to the total of calcium) for $Ca_3(PO_4)_2$ and LHWCC during in vitro digestion.

After entering the intestinal buffer, the solubility of $Ca_3(PO_4)_2$ rapidly decreased to 20% and gradually decreased to 3% with time. On the other hand, the solubility of LHWCC slightly decreased to 70% when entering the alkaline environment of the intestine and remained stable afterward.

3.3. *Effect of LHWCC on Weight, Body Length, and Tail Length Gain*

Figure S1 shows the weight changes in rats during the experiment. The weight of rats in different treatment groups showed steady growth, and there was no significant difference among the groups in body weight and length ($p > 0.05$). The low calcium treatment resulted in slow tail growth. The treatments with LHW, co-administration of $Ca_3(PO_4)_2$ with LHW (LHWC), and LHWCC significantly increased the tail length of rats, whereas $Ca_3(PO_4)_2$ had no significant effect on tail length compared to the model group.

3.4. *Effect of LHWCC on Femoral and Serum Indicators*

Figure 4A–F summarizes the changes in femoral and serum biochemical parameters. A low-calcium diet led to a significant decrease in bone length ($p < 0.001$), bone diameter ($p < 0.01$), bone weight ($p < 0.005$), and bone and serum calcium content ($p < 0.005$), with a significant increase in ALP activity ($p < 0.005$). Treatments with $Ca_3(PO_4)_2$ and LHWCC significantly increased bone length, as well as bone and serum calcium content, with no significant difference in most indicators among the groups fed with $Ca_3(PO_4)_2$, LHWC, and LHWCC ($p > 0.05$). $Ca_3(PO_4)_2$, LHWC, and LHWCC treatment resulted in significantly lower ALP activity compared to the model group ($p < 0.001$), with a stronger effect of LHWC and LHWCC on ALP activity than that of the $Ca_3(PO_4)_2$ ($p < 0.001$). LHW had no effect on serum ALP activity in rats and the weight of the femur ($p < 0.05$), whereas the intake of LHW had an impact on both femur and serum calcium content. These results indicated that supplementation of LHW was beneficial for restoring femoral morphology and calcification in the state of low calcium, whereas LHWCC was as effective in the improvement of the serum and femoral indicators as $Ca_3(PO_4)_2$, and even more effective in the improvement of ALP activity in calcium-deficient rats.

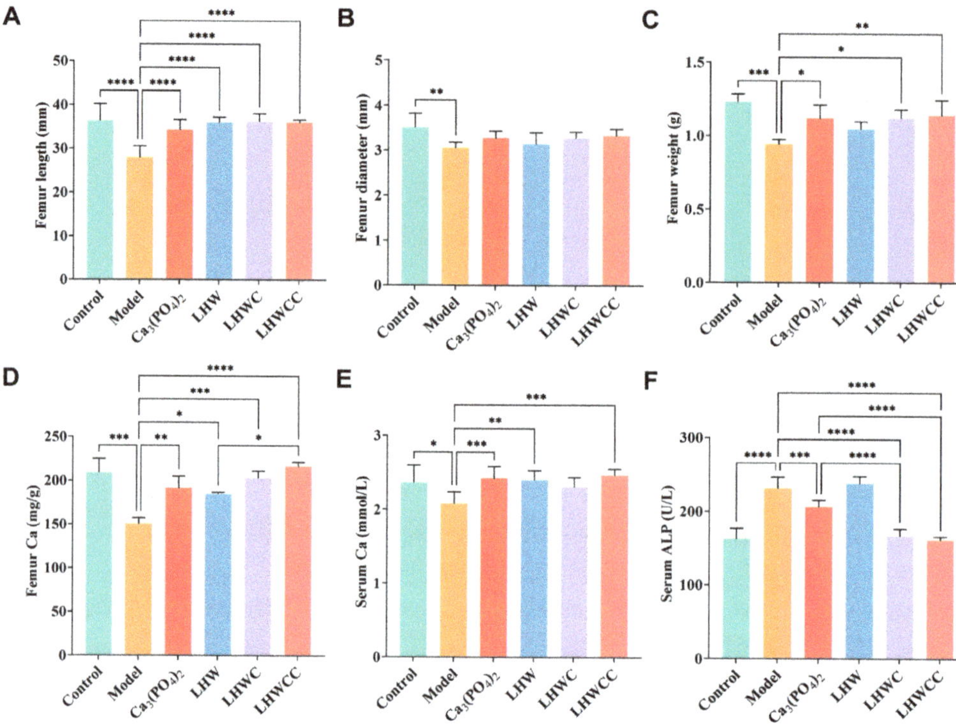

Figure 4. Changes in the bone morphology and calcium content and serum biochemical parameters of rats (**A**), femur length (**B**), femur diameter (**C**), femur weight (**D**), femur calcium (**E**), serum calcium (**F**), serum ALP. Data are expressed as the mean ± SD ($n = 8$). * $p < 0.05$; ** $p < 0.01$; *** $p < 0.005$; **** $p < 0.001$.

3.5. Bone Biomechanical Parameters and Histomorphometry

The three-dimensional (3D) reconstruction of micro-CT images of the left femoral trabecular bone is shown in Figure 5. Compared with the control group, the bone trabeculae of low-calcium rats were sparse, with large gaps and obvious damage in their morphology and network connectivity structure. Supplementation with $Ca_3(PO_4)_2$, LHWC, and LHWCC all resulted in a significant effect on the bone trabeculae and an increase in thickness and connectivity, with LHWCC as the improvement of the microstructure of bone trabeculae and enhancing bone quality. On the other hand, LHW only showed a weak influence on the morphology of bone trabeculae.

The results of bone mass are shown in Figure 6. Low calcium treatment resulted in a significant decrease in femoral bone density ($p < 0.001$), BS/TV ($p < 0.001$), and BV/TV ($p < 0.005$) in rats (Figure 6A–C). After treatment, femoral BMD improved significantly in all groups, and the BMD of rats in LHWCC group was the highest. Bone mass was remarkably recovered with the intervention of $Ca_3(PO_4)_2$, LHW and LHWC, and LHWCC, with LHWCC showing a stronger regulating effect on bone loss than $Ca_3(PO_4)_2$ ($p < 0.05$).

Low calcium treatment significantly reduced the thickness and the connectivity density ($p < 0.001$) and increased the separation of bone trabeculae ($p < 0.05$) (Figure 6D–F) as indicated by indexes such as Th.Tb (an indicator of the thickness of the trabecular bone), Th.Sp (an indicator of the bone trabecular separation), and Conn.D (an indicator of the degree of trabecular bone separation). Both $Ca_3(PO_4)_2$ and LHWCC showed significant effects on promoting bone trabeculae. The coadministration of LHW and $Ca_3(PO_4)_2$ had a significant effect on restoring Th.Tb ($p < 0.05$) and Conn.D ($p < 0.005$), with no effect on Th.Sp, whereas no influence on bone trabeculae was recorded by LHW treatment.

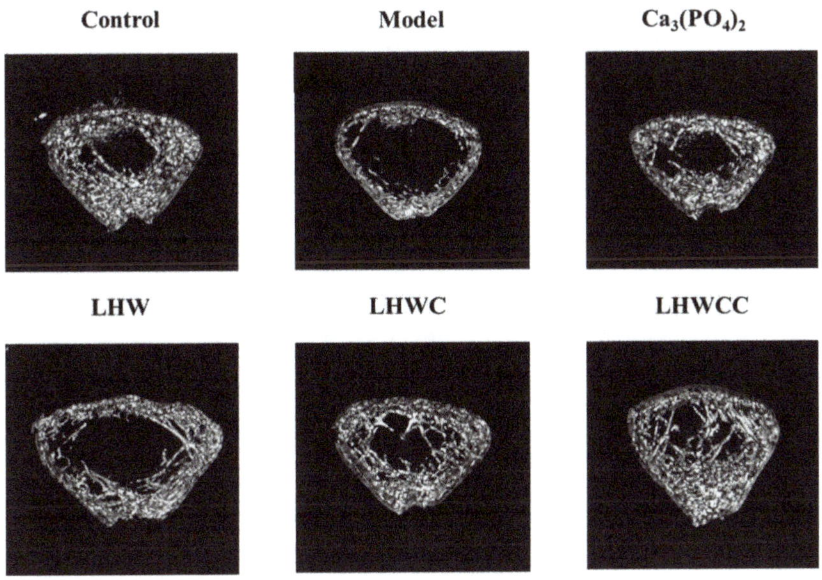

Figure 5. Three-dimensional micro-CT images of the distal femur of rats.

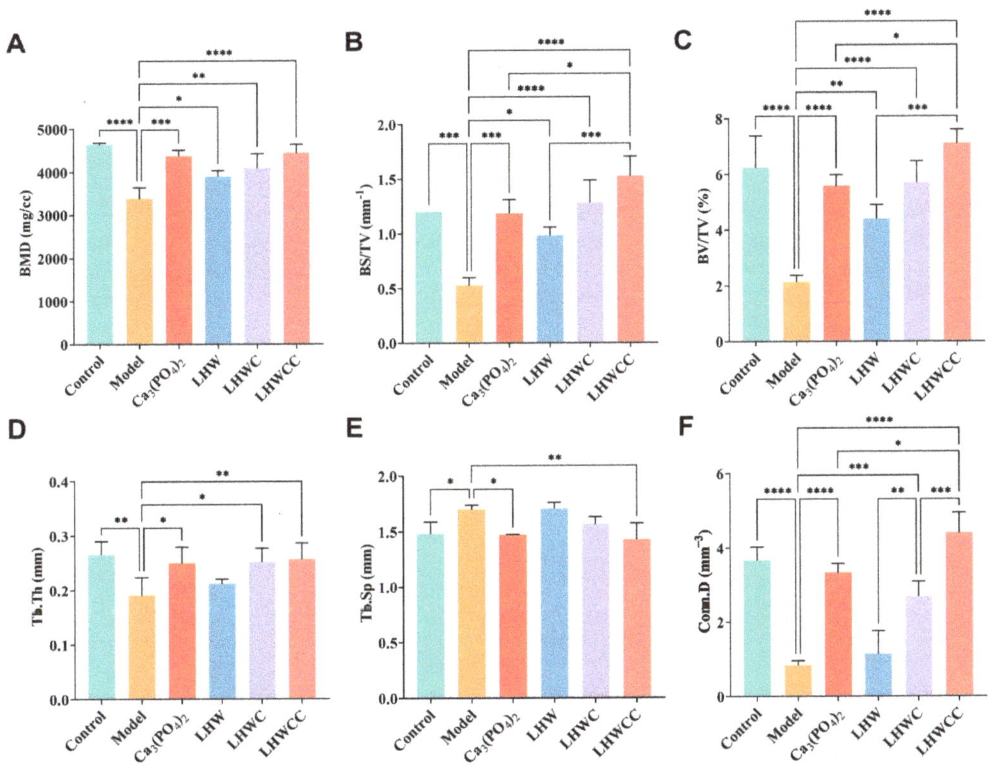

Figure 6. Changes in BMD and bone mass of rats (**A**), BMD (**B**), BS/TV (**C**), BV/TV (**D**), Tb.Th. (E), Tb.Sp (**F**), Conn.D. Data are expressed as the mean ± SD (n = 8). * $p < 0.05$; ** $p < 0.01$; *** $p < 0.005$; **** $p < 0.001$.

3.6. *Effects on Bone Biomechanical Strength*

From Figure 7, it can be seen that low calcium intake resulted in significant decreases in the maximum bone load ($p < 0.005$) and maximum deflection. Supplementation with $Ca_3(PO_4)_2$, LHWC, and LHWCC significantly improved bone biomechanics ($p < 0.001$) in rats, whereas LHW showed no effect. There was no significant difference between the regulating effect of $Ca_3(PO_4)_2$ and LHWCC on hardness, whereas LHWCC performed better than $Ca_3(PO_4)_2$ in fracturability.

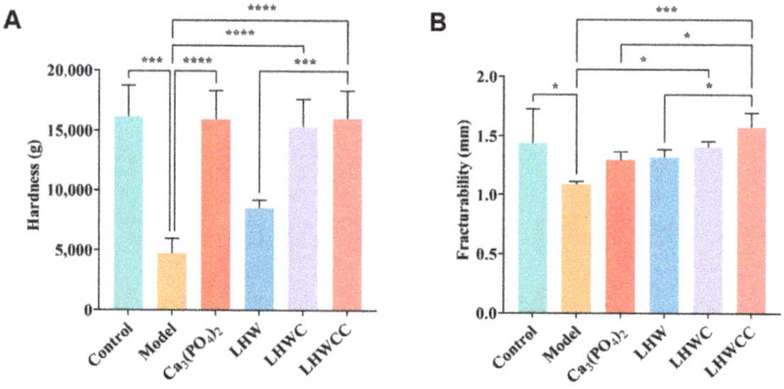

Figure 7. Changes in bone biomechanical property of rats (**A**), hardness (**B**), fracturability. Data are expressed as the mean ± SD ($n = 8$). * $p < 0.05$; *** $p < 0.005$; **** $p < 0.001$.

3.7. *Effect of LHWCC on Calcium Balance*

From Figure 8, it can be seen that the apparent calcium absorption rate (ACAR) and calcium accumulation rate (CAR) of the model group were significantly increased compared to the control group ($p < 0.001$), which might be due to pathological compensation formed to maintain calcium concentration in the body in a calcium-deficient state [5]. $Ca_3(PO_4)_2$ treatment significantly decreased both ACAR and CAR. Although LHW treatment did not result in changes in calcium balance, the combination of $Ca_3(PO_4)_2$ with LHW showed higher calcium absorption rates than that of $Ca_3(PO_4)_2$ alone ($p < 0.001$), indicating that LHW could promote the absorption and accumulation of inorganic calcium in rats. When LHW was chelated with calcium, its apparent absorption rate increased to 80%, indicating that the chelation had a beneficial effect on calcium absorption and retention in calcium-deficient rats compared to inorganic calcium in the body [28], which is consistent with the pattern of calcium release of $Ca_3(PO_4)_2$ and LHWCC during in vitro digestion.

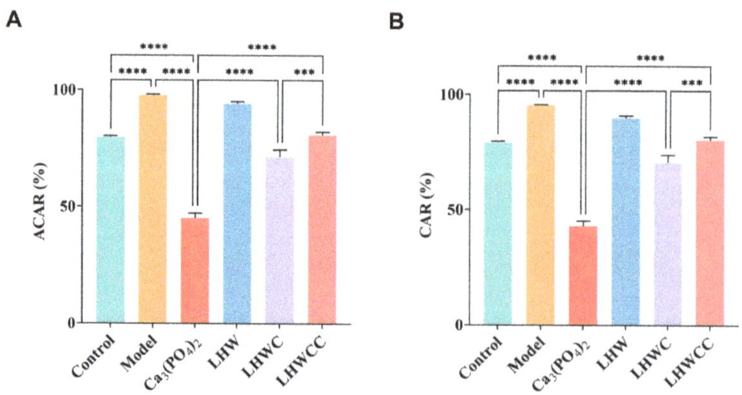

Figure 8. Changes in calcium metabolism of rats (**A**), apparent calcium absorption rate (ACAR) (**B**), calcium accumulation rate (CAR). Data are expressed as the mean ± SD ($n = 8$). *** $p < 0.005$; **** $p < 0.001$.

3.8. Gene Expression of Corresponding Receptors in the Intestines of Rats

The expression of calcium absorption-related genes in the small intestine of rats is shown in Figure 9, and the inorganic calcium salt and organic chelates varied in the regulation of the related gene expression. The expression levels of TRPV5, TRPV6, PepT1, and Calbindin-D9k significantly increased by LHWC and LHWCC treatments, whereas $Ca_3(PO_4)_2$ showed notable elevation of the expression of TRPV6 and PMCA1b. In addition, compared to the control, LHWCC showed increased expression levels of TRPV5/6, PepT1, and Calbindin D9k. Among all the treatments, LHWCC showed the strongest regulating effect. On the other hand, LHW only significantly increased the expression of PepT1. However, none of the treatments had an impact on the expression of NCX-1.

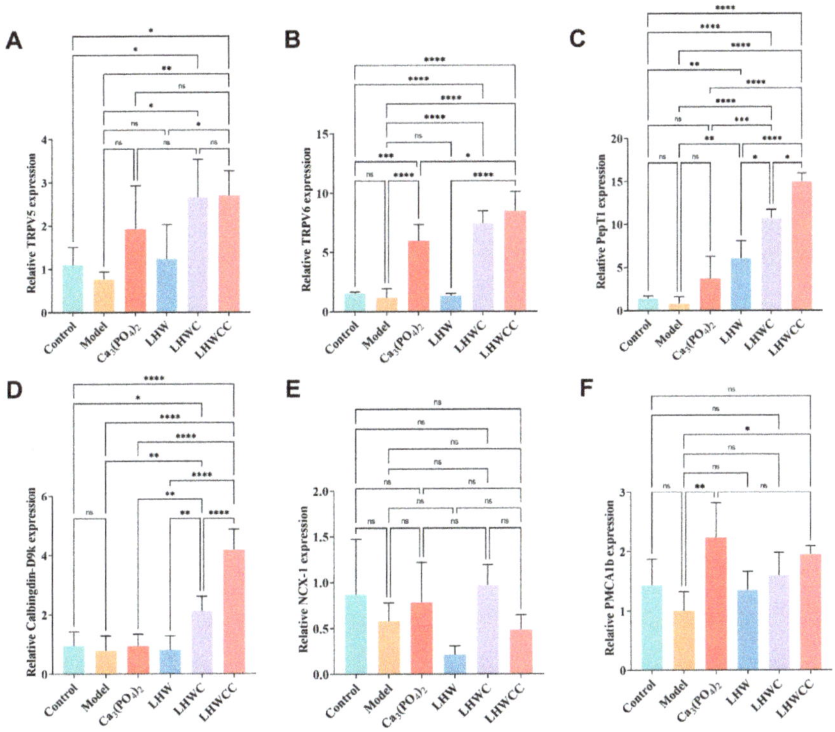

Figure 9. Calcium absorption-related gene expression in intestines of rats (**A**), TRPV5 (**B**), TRPV6 (**C**), PepT1 (**D**), Calbinding-D9k. (**E**), NCX-1 (**F**), PMCA1b. Data are expressed as the mean ± SD (n = 8). ns $p > 0.05$; * $p < 0.05$; ** $p < 0.01$; *** $p < 0.005$; **** $p < 0.001$.

4. Discussion

The FT-IR spectra were used to provide more information on the binding of metal ions with organic ligand groups of LHW, showing that the main binding sites of LHWCC included carboxyl oxygen atoms, amino nitrogen atoms, and phosphate ions, which was similar to CPPH-Ca [10].

Calcium in food can be dissolved into ionic form through gastric acid digestion but it is prone to precipitate in the relatively alkaline environments of the small intestine, leading to a decrease in bioavailability [29]. In vitro models must be created to investigate the calcium release patterns of different calcium supplements [30]. Compared to $Ca_3(PO_4)_2$, LHWCC was less affected by pH, which was similar to the in vitro digestion results of CPP-Ca [31]. Jiang et al. [27] found that most peptide calcium chelates were soluble after digestion, but the dialysis rate was significantly lower than the solubility. Therefore, it is speculated that calcium ions remained in a binding state to macromolecules during in vitro digestion. The pattern of sustained release of calcium and high solubility of LHWCC during simulated intestinal digestion might be partially attributed to the presence of peptides in LHW [15,32] as supported by the upregulation of PepT1 in vivo. Anyway, previous research found that during the simulated in vitro digestion process of the intestine, the solubility of $CaCO_3$ was between 60 and 80% [9], whereas that of $Ca_3(PO_4)_2$ was below 20%, with significant differences in solubility. The low solubility constant of $Ca_3(PO_4)_2$ led to its low calcium solubility during simulated intestinal digestion. However, in vivo experiments showed that the apparent absorption rate in rats of $CaCO_3$ was about 40% [33], which is close to $Ca_3(PO_4)_2$ (45%) in the present study. Our results also indicated that among the calcium absorption-related genes analyzed in the present study, $Ca_3(PO_4)_2$ only upregulated the expression of the TRPV6 channel, similar to the previous study on $CaCO_3$ [34,35]. Therefore, although the two inorganic calcium salts $Ca_3(PO_4)_2$ and $CaCO_3$ had significant differences in solubility in vitro, they shared similarities in both the effect and mechanism of the regulation of calcium absorption in vivo.

Low-calcium diets may cause microarchitectural deterioration of bone tissue, leading to increased bone fragility and risk of fracture [36]. The present study found that $Ca_3(PO_4)_2$, LHWC, and LHWCC significantly restored serum biochemical parameters, bone morphology, and the bone biomechanical property of low-calcium-fed rats, whereas LHW only upregulated the PepT1 expression level to improve serum and bone calcium content in rats. Chelates such as LHWCC showed a stronger influence on trabecular microstructure and calcium absorption than $Ca_3(PO_4)_2$ and the co-administration of LHW and $Ca_3(PO_4)_2$. Bone microstructure, especially trabecular microstructure, plays an important role in monitoring calcium deposition in bone and characterizing bone growth and development levels [37,38]. Bone trabeculae have a certain shape and distance in the bone marrow cavity, cross-linking with each other to form a network structure, and are mainly responsible for maintaining bone strength, bearing loads, and hematopoietic functions [39]. Compared with $Ca_3(PO_4)_2$ and LHWC, LHWCC increased bone mass by promoting the number and thickness of bone trabeculae and making the cross-linking of bone trabeculae denser, highlighting the improvement of efficiency of promotion of bone health through the conversion of inorganic calcium supplements to organic agents, as previously reported [33,40,41].

The small intestine is the main organ responsible for calcium absorption, responsible for over 90% of calcium absorption in the human body [29]. The process of calcium absorption in intestinal cells can be roughly divided into three steps: calcium ions enter the cells through TRPV5/6; calcium binds to Calbindin-D9k for intracellular transport; it is pumped into the bloodstream by NCX-1 and PMCA1b. The main rate-limiting step of the above process is to absorb calcium into cells, which means that the efficiency of active calcium transport is mainly related to channel proteins such as TRPV5/6 [7]. As shown in Figure 10, both LHWCC and CPPH-Ca exerted promotive effects on calcium absorption via regulation of the gene expression of TRPV5, TRPV6, Calbinding-D9k, and PMCA1b. In addition, it is reported that peptide calcium chelates can resist gastric digestion as short peptides enter the intestine. The main pathways currently known to transport peptides through the intestinal cells are the PepT1 pathway and the cell-penetrating peptide pathway, both of which are transcellular pathways. The PepT1 pathway is a widely specific peptide transporter protein that can transport almost all dipeptides and tripeptides [4]. The results have shown that LHWCC also regulated the higher expression level of PepT1 than $Ca_3(PO_4)_2$ and LHWC, which would facilitate the transition of peptides into the intestine and contribute to the enhancement of calcium absorption indirectly due to the increased proportion of oligopeptides in protein hydrolysates after chelating with calcium [42]. Therefore, among the various calcium chelates, protein hydrolysate-calcium chelates are unique as they could upregulate not only the pathway of calcium absorption such as TRPV5, TRPV6, and Calbinding-D9k, but also an indirect pathway potentially beneficial for bone health via PepT1.

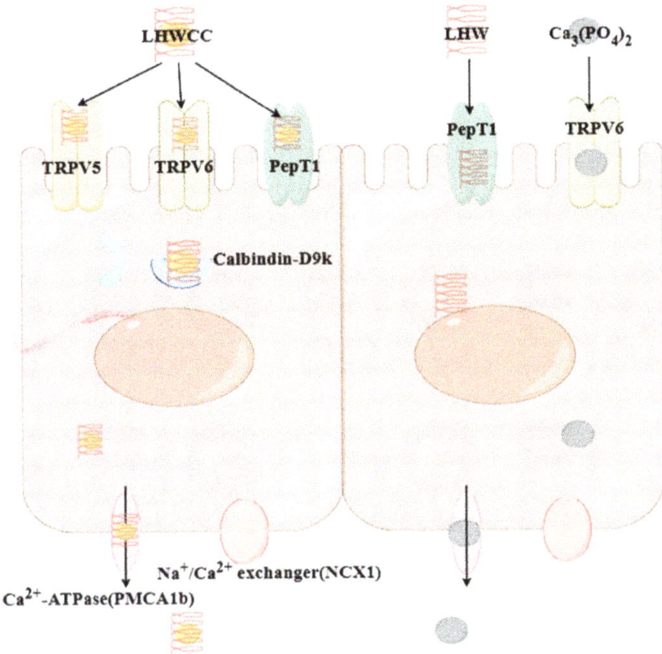

Figure 10. The mechanistic interpretation of intestinal calcium absorption of different calcium agents investigated in the present study.

On the other hand, LHWCC significantly increased calcium absorption in vivo compared to $Ca_3(PO_4)_2$, which may be due to LHWCC significantly upregulating the gene expression of TRPV5 and TRPV6, whereas calcium phosphate can only significantly upregulate the TRPV6 pathway. The expression level of Calbindin-D9k was also higher in LHWCC. TRPV5 and TRPV6 have 75% homology and their main differences are in the N and C terminal tails. Both channels permeate calcium ions, and TRPV5 exhibits stronger ion selectivity. TPPV6 can be regulated by vitamin D_3, as well as Calbindin-D9k and PMCA1b, which may be regulated through interactions with these calcium transporters and enzymes involved in intestinal calcium absorption and increased parathyroid hormone (PTH) [43,44]. Meanwhile, PTH also indirectly affects the content of $1,25(OH)_2D_3$, the hormonal form of vitamin D [45]. Calbindin-D9k is regulated at the transcriptional and post-transcriptional levels by the serum level of $1,25(OH)_2D_3$ [46]. Therefore, the increased expression levels of TRPV6 and Calbindin-D9k in LHWCC may be related to PTH and $1,25(OH)_2D_3$ in the serum of rats. Further experiments in this aspect would be desirable for understanding the mechanism of the effect of LHWCC on calcium absorption and bone health.

5. Conclusions

In conclusion, LHWCC exerted a notable impact on bone health. Compared with inorganic calcium, LHWCC had a higher solubility during in vitro digestion and had promotive effects on serum biochemical parameters, bone microstructure, and calcium absorption in vivo. LHWCC treatment exerted promotive effects on calcium absorption by upregulating TRPV6, TRPV5, PepT1, Calbindin-D9k, and PMCA1b-signaling pathways in intestines, thereby improving serum and bone calcium concentration and restoring bone biomechanical parameters and histomorphometry.

Supplementary Materials: The following supporting information can be downloaded at: https://www.mdpi.com/article/10.3390/nu16081127/s1, Figure S1: changes in body weight, body length, and tail length of rats (A), weight (B), body length (C), tail length.

Author Contributions: W.H. conducted the experiment and wrote the manuscript; W.H., Z.P., A.X. and Y.J. analyzed the data; X.L. designed the study and secured the funding; B.Y., J.Z., H.Z. and W.C. reviewed and edited the manuscript. All authors have read and agreed to the published version of the manuscript.

Funding: This research was funded by the National Natural Science Foundation of China (No. 31871829, 31820103010, and 32021005).

Institutional Review Board Statement: The study was conducted according to the guidelines of the Declaration of Helsinki, and approved by the Animal Ethics and Welfare Committee of Jiangnan University (JN.No 20230530S1200730[247], 8 June 2023).

Informed Consent Statement: Not applicable.

Data Availability Statement: Data are contained within the article and Supplementary Materials.

Conflicts of Interest: The authors declare no conflicts of interest.

References

1. Flynn, A. The Role of Dietary Calcium in Bone Health. *Proc. Nutr. Soc.* **2003**, *62*, 851–858. [CrossRef]
2. Sun, N.; Wu, H.; Du, M.; Tang, Y.; Liu, H.; Fu, Y.; Zhu, B. Food Protein-Derived Calcium Chelating Peptides: A Review. *Trends Food Sci. Technol.* **2016**, *58*, 140–148. [CrossRef]
3. Welch, A.A.; Fransen, H.; Jenab, M.; Boutron-Ruault, M.C.; Tumino, R.; Agnoli, C.; Ericson, U.; Johansson, I.; Ferrari, P.; Engeset, D.; et al. Variation in Intakes of Calcium, Phosphorus, Magnesium, Iron and Potassium in 10 Countries in the European Prospective Investigation into Cancer and Nutrition Study. *Eur. J. Clin. Nutr.* **2009**, *63*, S101–S121. [CrossRef] [PubMed]
4. An, J.; Zhang, Y.; Ying, Z.; Li, H.; Liu, W.; Wang, J.; Liu, X. The Formation, Structural Characteristics, Absorption Pathways and Bioavailability of Calcium–Peptide Chelates. *Foods* **2022**, *11*, 2762. [CrossRef] [PubMed]
5. Lv, Y.; Liu, H.; Ren, J.; Li, X.; Guo, S. The Positive Effect of Soybean Protein Hydrolysates—Calcium Complexes on Bone Mass of Rapidly Growing Rats. *Food Funct.* **2013**, *4*, 1245. [CrossRef] [PubMed]
6. Wang, X.; Gao, A.; Chen, Y.; Zhang, X.; Li, S.; Chen, Y. Preparation of Cucumber Seed Peptide-Calcium Chelate by Liquid State Fermentation and Its Characterization. *Food Chem.* **2017**, *229*, 487–494. [CrossRef]
7. Li, H.; Duan, S.; Yuan, P.; Liu, J.; Wang, X.; Liu, Y.; Peng, Y.; Pan, C.; Xia, K. Preparation of Casein Phosphopeptides Calcium Complex and the Promotion in Calcium Cellular Uptake through Transcellular Transport Pathway. *J. Food Biochem.* **2021**, *45*, e14001. [CrossRef]
8. Tian, L.; Xiong, D.; Jia, J.; Liu, X.; Zhang, Y.; Duan, X. Mechanism Study on Enhanced Emulsifying Properties of Phosvitin and Calcium-Binding Capacity of Its Phosphopeptides by Lactic Acid Bacteria Fermentation. *LWT* **2022**, *155*, 113002. [CrossRef]
9. Lorieau, L.; Le Roux, L.; Gaucheron, F.; Ligneul, A.; Hazart, E.; Dupont, D.; Floury, J. Bioaccessibility of Four Calcium Sources in Different Whey-Based Dairy Matrices Assessed by in Vitro Digestion. *Food Chem.* **2018**, *245*, 454–462. [CrossRef]
10. Hua, P.; Xiong, Y.; Yu, Z.; Liu, B.; Zhao, L. Effect of Chlorella Pyrenoidosa Protein Hydrolysate-Calcium Chelate on Calcium Absorption Metabolism and Gut Microbiota Composition in Low-Calcium Diet-Fed Rats. *Mar. Drugs* **2019**, *17*, 348. [CrossRef]
11. Giraffa, G.; Gatti, M.; Rossetti, L.; Senini, L.; Neviani, E. Molecular Diversity within *Lactobacillus Helveticus* as Revealed by Genotypic Characterization. *Appl. Environ. Microbiol.* **2000**, *66*, 1259–1265. [CrossRef] [PubMed]
12. Sipola, M.; Finckenberg, P.; Santisteban, J.; Korpela, R.; Vapaatalo, H.; Nurminen, M.L. Long-Term Intake of Milk Peptides Attenuates Development of Hypertension in Spontaneously Hypertensive Rats. *J. Physiol. Pharmacol.* **2001**, *52*, 745–754.
13. Jauhiainen, T.; Vapaatalo, H.; Poussa, T.; Kyrönpalo, S.; Rasmussen, M.; Korpela, R. *Lactobacillus Helveticus* Fermented Milk Lowers Blood Pressure in Hypertensive Subjects in 24-h Ambulatory Blood Pressure Measurement. *Am. J. Hypertens* **2005**, *18*, 1600–1605. [CrossRef]
14. Ohsawa, K.; Uchida, N.; Ohki, K.; Nakamura, Y.; Yokogoshi, H. *Lactobacillus Helveticus*-Fermented Milk Improves Learning and Memory in Mice. *Nutr. Neurosci.* **2015**, *18*, 232–240. [PubMed]
15. Gao, S.; Jiang, Y.; Zhang, X.; Cui, S.; Liu, X.; Zhao, J.; Zhang, H.; Chen, W. Comparative Peptidomics Analysis of Milk Fermented by *Lactobacillus Helveticus*. *Foods* **2022**, *11*, 3885. [CrossRef] [PubMed]
16. Wang, J.; Jiang, Y.; Yu, P.; Lee, Y.K.; Liu, X.; Zhao, J.; Zhang, H.; Chen, W. Effect of Carbon Catabolite Repression on Lactose and Galactose Catabolism in *Lacticaseibacillus Paracasei*. *Food Biosci.* **2021**, *40*, 100912. [CrossRef]
17. Lao, L.; He, J.; Liao, W.; Zeng, C.; Liu, G.; Cao, Y.; Miao, J. Casein Calcium-Binding Peptides: Preparation, Characterization, and Promotion of Calcium Uptake in Caco-2 Cell Monolayers. *Process Biochem.* **2023**, *130*, 78–86. [CrossRef]

18. Minekus, M.; Alminger, M.; Alvito, P.; Ballance, S.; Bohn, T.; Bourlieu, C.; Carrière, F.; Boutrou, R.; Corredig, M.; Dupont, D.; et al. A Standardised Static In Vitro Digestion Method Suitable for Food—An International Consensus. *Food Funct.* **2014**, *5*, 1113–1124. [CrossRef]
19. Reeves, P.G.; Nielsen, F.H.; Fahey, G.C. AIN-93 Purified Diets for Laboratory Rodents: Final Report of the American Institute of Nutrition Ad Hoc Writing Committee on the Reformulation of the AIN-76A Rodent Diet. *J. Nutr.* **1993**, *123*, 1939–1951. [CrossRef]
20. Chen, J.; Qiu, X.; Hao, G.; Zhang, M.; Weng, W. Preparation and Bioavailability of Calcium-chelating Peptide Complex from Tilapia Skin Hydrolysates. *J. Sci. Food Agric.* **2017**, *97*, 4898–4903. [CrossRef] [PubMed]
21. Chen, Z.; Liu, D.; Tang, X.; Cui, Y.; Hu, W.; Regenstein, J.M.; Zhou, P. Sea Cucumber Enzymatic Hydrolysates Relieve Osteoporosis through OPG/RANK/RANKL System in Ovariectomized Rats. *Food Biosci.* **2022**, *46*, 101572. [CrossRef]
22. Ye, M.; Zhang, C.; Jia, W.; Shen, Q.; Qin, X.; Zhang, H.; Zhu, L. Metabolomics Strategy Reveals the Osteogenic Mechanism of Yak (Bos Grunniens) Bone Collagen Peptides on Ovariectomy-Induced Osteoporosis in Rats. *Food Funct.* **2020**, *11*, 1498–1512. [CrossRef] [PubMed]
23. Wang, Z.; Wang, K.; Feng, Y.; Jiang, S.; Zhao, Y.; Zeng, M. Preparation, Characterization of L-Aspartic Acid Chelated Calcium from Oyster Shell Source and Its Calcium Supplementation Effect in Rats. *J. Funct. Foods* **2020**, *75*, 104249. [CrossRef]
24. Sun, L.; Liu, J.; Pei, H.; Shi, M.; Chen, W.; Zong, Y.; Zhao, Y.; Li, J.; Du, R.; He, Z. Structural Characterisation of Deer Sinew Peptides as Calcium Carriers, Their Promotion of MC3T3-E1 Cell Proliferation and Their Effect on Bone Deposition in Mice. *Food Funct.* **2024**, *15*, 2587–2603. [CrossRef] [PubMed]
25. Zhai, W.; Lin, D.; Mo, R.; Zou, X.; Zhang, Y.; Zhang, L.; Ge, Y. Process Optimization, Structural Characterization, and Calcium Release Rate Evaluation of Mung Bean Peptides-Calcium Chelate. *Foods* **2023**, *12*, 1058. [CrossRef]
26. Zhang, X.; Jia, Q.; Li, M.; Liu, H.; Wang, Q.; Wu, Y.; Niu, L.; Liu, Z. Isolation of a Novel Calcium-Binding Peptide from Phosvitin Hydrolysates and the Study of Its Calcium Chelation Mechanism. *Food Res. Int.* **2021**, *141*, 110169. [CrossRef]
27. Jiang, Y.; Li, J.; Zhao, H.; Zhao, R.; Xu, Y.; Lyu, X. Preparation of Grape Seed Polypeptide and Its Calcium Chelate with Determination of Calcium Bioaccessibility and Structural Characterisation. *Int. J. Food Sci. Tech.* **2021**, *56*, 166–177. [CrossRef]
28. Dyck, K.V.; Tas, S.; Robberecht, H.; Deelstra, H. The Influence of Different Food Components on the in Vitro Availability of Iron, Zinc and Calcium from a Composed Meal. *Int. J. Food Sci. Nutr.* **1996**, *47*, 499–506. [CrossRef] [PubMed]
29. Bronner, F.; Pansu, D. Nutritional Aspects of Calcium Absorption1. *J. Nutr.* **1999**, *129*, 9–12. [CrossRef] [PubMed]
30. Ménard, O.; Bourlieu, C.; De Oliveira, S.C.; Dellarosa, N.; Laghi, L.; Carrière, F.; Capozzi, F.; Dupont, D.; Deglaire, A. A First Step towards a Consensus Static in Vitro Model for Simulating Full-Term Infant Digestion. *Food Chem.* **2018**, *240*, 338–345. [CrossRef]
31. Wang, Y.; Wang, R.; Bai, H.; Wang, S.; Liu, T.; Zhang, X.; Wang, Z. Casein Phosphopeptide Calcium Chelation: Preparation Optimization, in Vitro Gastrointestinal Simulated Digestion, and Peptide Fragment Exploration. *J. Sci. Food Agric.* **2024**, *104*, 788–796. [CrossRef] [PubMed]
32. Xia, A.; Jiang, Y.; Lee, Y.-K.; Liang, D.; Yang, B.; Liu, X.; Zhao, J.; Zhang, H.; Chen, W. Identification and Validation of Fermented Milk-Derived Osteogenic Peptides via Molecular Docking and Osteoblastic Cell Model. *Food Biosci.* **2024**, *58*, 103698. [CrossRef]
33. Peng, Z.; Hou, H.; Zhang, K.; Li, B. Effect of Calcium-Binding Peptide from Pacific Cod (Gadus Macrocephalus) Bone on Calcium Bioavailability in Rats. *Food Chem.* **2017**, *221*, 373–378. [CrossRef] [PubMed]
34. Shapiro, R.; Heaney, R.P. Co-Dependence of Calcium and Phosphorus for Growth and Bone Development under Conditions of Varying Deficiency. *Bone* **2003**, *32*, 532–540. [CrossRef] [PubMed]
35. Yuan, Y.; Szeto, I.M.-Y.; Li, N.; Yang, H.; Zhou, Y.; Liu, B.; He, F.; Zhang, L.; Duan, S.; Chen, J. Effects of Menaquinone-7 on the Bone Health of Growing Rats under Calcium Restriction: New Insights from Microbiome-Metabolomics. *Nutrients* **2023**, *15*, 3398. [CrossRef]
36. Benzvi, L.; Gershon, A.; Lavi, I.; Wollstein, R. Secondary Prevention of Osteoporosis Following Fragility Fractures of the Distal Radius in a Large Health Maintenance Organization. *Arch. Osteoporos* **2016**, *11*, 20. [CrossRef] [PubMed]
37. Zhang, B.; Yang, L.-L.; Ding, S.-Q.; Liu, J.-J.; Dong, Y.-H.; Li, Y.-T.; Li, N.; Zhao, X.-J.; Hu, C.-L.; Jiang, Y.; et al. Anti-Osteoporotic Activity of an Edible Traditional Chinese Medicine Cistanche Deserticola on Bone Metabolism of Ovariectomized Rats Through RANKL/RANK/TRAF6-Mediated Signaling Pathways. *Front. Pharmacol.* **2019**, *10*, 1412. [CrossRef]
38. Zhao, M.; Ahn, D.U.; Li, S.; Liu, W.; Yi, S.; Huang, X. Effects of Phosvitin Phosphopeptide-Ca Complex Prepared by Efficient Enzymatic Hydrolysis on Calcium Absorption and Bone Deposition of Mice. *Food Sci. Hum. Wellness* **2022**, *11*, 1631–1640. [CrossRef]
39. Keaveny, T.M.; Morgan, E.F.; Niebur, G.L.; Yeh, O.C. Biomechanics of Trabecular Bone. *Annu. Rev. Biomed. Eng.* **2001**, *3*, 307–333. [CrossRef]
40. Chen, D.; Mu, X.; Huang, H.; Nie, R.; Liu, Z.; Zeng, M. Isolation of a Calcium-Binding Peptide from Tilapia Scale Protein Hydrolysate and Its Calcium Bioavailability in Rats. *J. Funct. Foods* **2014**, *6*, 575–584. [CrossRef]
41. Zhao, N.; Hu, J.; Hou, T.; Ma, Z.; Wang, C.; He, H. Effects of Desalted Duck Egg White Peptides and Their Products on Calcium Absorption in Rats. *J. Funct. Foods* **2014**, *8*, 234–242. [CrossRef]
42. Liu, W.-Y.; Lu, J.; Gao, F.; Gu, R.-Z.; Lin, F.; Ren, D.-F.; Cai, M.-Y. Preparation, Characterization and Identification of Calcium-Chelating Atlantic Salmon (*Salmo Salar* L.) Ossein Oligopeptides. *Eur. Food Res. Technol.* **2015**, *241*, 851–860. [CrossRef]
43. Nijenhuis, T.; Hoenderop, J.G.J.; van der Kemp, A.W.C.M.; Bindels, R.J.M. Localization and Regulation of the Epithelial Ca^{2+} Channel TRPV6 in the Kidney. *J. Am. Soc. Nephrol.* **2003**, *14*, 2731–2740. [CrossRef]

44. Zhang, Y.; Dong, X.-L.; Leung, P.-C.; Che, C.-T.; Wong, M.-S. Fructus Ligustri Lucidi Extract Improves Calcium Balance and Modulates the Calciotropic Hormone Level and Vitamin D-Dependent Gene Expression in Aged Ovariectomized Rats. *Menopause* **2008**, *15*, 558–565. [CrossRef] [PubMed]
45. Sassi, F.; Tamone, C.; D'Amelio, P. Vitamin D: Nutrient, Hormone, and Immunomodulator. *Nutrients* **2018**, *10*, 1656. [CrossRef]
46. Goda, T.; Kishi, K.; Ezawa, I.; Takase, S. The Maltitol-Induced Increase in Intestinal Calcium Transport Increases the Calcium Content and Breaking Force of Femoral Bone in Weanling Rats. *J. Nutr.* **1998**, *128*, 2028–2031. [CrossRef]

nutrients

MDPI

Article

Yogurt Alleviates Cyclophosphamide-Induced Immunosuppression in Mice through D-Lactate

Xinru Du [1,2,*], Yongheng Yan [3,*], Yufeng Dai [1,2] and Ruijie Xu [4]

1 State Key Laboratory of Food Science and Resources, Jiangnan University, Wuxi 214122, China; 7200112055@stu.jiangnan.edu.cn
2 School of Food Science and Technology, Jiangnan University, Wuxi 214122, China
3 School of Public Health, Shandong First Medical University, Jinan 271016, China
4 Global Health Institute, School of Public Health, Xi'an Jiaotong University, Xi'an 710061, China; xurj0087@xjtu.edu.cn
* Correspondence: 6210113016@stu.jiangnan.edu.cn (X.D.); yhyan@sdfmu.edu.cn (Y.Y.)

Abstract: Numerous studies have investigated the immunomodulatory effects of yogurt, but the underlying mechanism remained elusive. This study aimed to elucidate the alleviating properties of yogurt on immunosuppression and proposed the underlying mechanism was related to the metabolite D-lactate. In the healthy mice, we validated the safety of daily yogurt consumption (600 μL) or D-lactate (300 mg/kg). In immunosuppressed mice induced by cyclophosphamide (CTX), we evaluated the immune regulation of yogurt and D-lactate. The result showed that yogurt restored body weight, boosted immune organ index, repaired splenic tissue, recovered the severity of delayed-type hypersensitivity reactions and increased serum cytokines (IgA, IgG, IL-6, IFN-γ). Additionally, yogurt enhanced intestinal immune function by restoring the intestinal barrier and upregulating the abundance of Bifidobacterium and Lactobacillus. Further studies showed that D-lactate alleviated immunosuppression in mice mainly by promoting cellular immunity. D-lactate recovered body weight and organ development, elevated serum cytokines (IgA, IgG, IL-6, IFN-γ), enhanced splenic lymphocyte proliferation and increased the mRNA level of T-bet in splenic lymphocyte to bolster Th1 differentiation. Finally, CTX is a chemotherapeutic drug, thus, the application of yogurt and D-lactate in the tumor-bearing mouse model was initially explored. The results showed that both yogurt (600 μL) and D-lactate (300 mg/kg) reduced cyclophosphamide-induced immunosuppression without promoting tumor growth. Overall, this study evaluated the safety, immune efficacy and applicability of yogurt and D-lactate in regulating immunosuppression. It emphasized the potential of yogurt as a functional food for immune regulation, with D-lactate playing a crucial role in its immunomodulatory effects.

Keywords: yogurt; D-lactate; cyclophosphamide (CTX); immunosuppression; gut microbiota

1. Introduction

Cyclophosphamide (CTX) is a broad-spectrum anticancer drug. It exerts the effects by interfering with the DNA synthesis of tumor cells, thereby inhibiting their proliferation and survival. However, while killing tumor cells, CTX also exhibits toxic side effects of immunosuppression [1,2]. CTX suppresses the immune system through diverse mechanisms, including encompassing the inhibition of immune cell functionality, attenuation of immune responses in T cells and B cells, as well as modulation of immune globulins, chemokines, and cytokines [3]. Immunosuppression is correlated with various chronic diseases, such as infections and cancers [4]. Furthermore, an imbalance of immune regulation results in gastrointestinal inflammation and intestinal flora disorders [5,6]. Therefore, it is imperative to identify effective strategies for preventing and alleviating immunosuppression.

Yogurt is a typical functional food. Epidemiological studies have revealed that yogurt can decrease the incidence of type 2 diabetes, metabolic syndrome and heart disease [7–10].

Previous researches on the immunoregulation of yogurt have focused on bioactive nutrients, such as fat acids, phytosterols, proteins, vitamins and probiotics [7,11,12]. However, D-lactate has been almost ignored as a byproduct of bacteria fermentation in yogurt. D-lactate is a configuration of chiral lactate. D-lactate typically has two origins in the human body. A portion is the dietary intake digested by bacteria in conventional foods, such as yogurt or pickles [13,14]. Lactobacillus bulgaricus can convert 90% of pyruvate into D-lactate [14] during yogurt manufacturing. Endogenous D-lactate is processed by closely related gut bacteria [15]. According to prevailing research, it is widely accepted that the human body exclusively harbors L-lactate dehydrogenase, which possesses rapid metabolic capacity towards L-lactate, while lacking D-lactate dehydrogenase. Consequently, the elevated concentration of D-lactate in plasma results in the acidosis. However, our recent research has demonstrated the daily intake of 2000 mg/kg of D-lactate does not affect the normal growth of mice. Furthermore, in comparison to L-lactate, D-lactate exhibits stronger anti-inflammatory properties due to its pharmacokinetic advantages [16]. Additionally, the recent study also reports that D-lactate plays a crucial role in preventing colitis-associated colon cancer in yogurt [17]. Hence, D-lactate is plausibly a potential dietary nutrient factor.

This research studies the actions of yogurt on immunosuppression by constructing three animal models (healthy mice, immunosuppressive mice and tumor-bearing mice), through D-lactate-dependent mechanisms. This study provides novel insights into alleviating immunosuppression and supports the benefits of traditional fermented foods and the development of D-lactate.

2. Materials and Methods

2.1. Chemicals and Reagents

Cyclophosphamide and Levamisole hydrochloride (LM) were sourced from Aladdin. D-sodium lactate, ConA and LPS were purchased from Sigma-Aldrich Co., St. Louis, MO, USA. Kits for measuring creatinine (CRE), urea nitrogen (BUN), aspartate aminotransferase (AST), and alanine aminotransferase (ALT) were acquired from the Nanjing Jiancheng Institute of Biological Engineering (Nanjing, China). Sheep red blood cells (SRBC) were obtained from Nanjing Senbeijia Biological Co., Ltd. (Nanjing, China). Spleen lymphocyte extraction kit was purchased from Beijing Solarbio Science & Technology Co., Ltd. (Beijing, China). CCK-8 Cell Counting Kit was purchased from Nanjing Vazyme Biotech Co., Ltd. (Nanjing, China). IgA, IgG, IL-4, IL-6, and IFN-γ Elisa kits were purchased from R&D systems. The CT26 cell line was derived from the American Type Culture Collection (ATCC) (maintained in a humidified incubator at 37 °C and 5% CO_2).

2.2. Yogurt Preparation

A simulated commercial yogurt was prepared according to a previous study [18,19]. Lactobacillus bulgaricus and Streptococcus thermophilus bacterial strains were mixed in a 1:1 ratio and incubated at 39 °C for 18 h in 10% skim milk, followed by a 24h incubation at 4 °C. At the end of this process, the total viable count was 9.16 lg (CFU/mL) consistent with the former research [20].

2.3. Determination of D-Lactate in Yogurt by High-Performance Liquid Chromatography (HPLC)

The sample pretreatment was drawing upon established approache with moderate modification [21]. Samples were centrifuged at 12,000 r/min for 15 min. Subsequently, 10% trichloroacetic acid was added to the samples and allowed to react for two hours before being centrifuged at 12,000 r/min for 20 min. Following this, the samples were filtered using a 0.22 μm filtration membrane and degassed through ultrasonic means before analysis with HPLC. The separation of L-lactate and D-lactate was achieved by Chirex 3126 (D) penicillamine LC Column [21,22].

2.4. Animal Experiment

Female SPF BALB/c mice weighing approximately 20.0 ± 2.0 g and aged 7 weeks were procured from Beijing Vital River Laboratory Animal Technology Co., Ltd. (Beijing, China). The mice were housed in cage and a controlled environment with a temperature of 22 ± 2 °C, a humidity of 50 ± 10%, and a 12-light-dark cycle, following the Guidelines for Keeping Experimental Animals issued by the Chinese government. The Experimental Animal Welfare and Ethics Committee of Jiangnan University approved the study (license numbers JN.No20220315c0900425(012), JN.No20220615c0801001(198) and JN.No20221130b07002209467).

2.4.1. Animal Experiment I

After seven days of adaptive feeding, total of 42 mice aged 5-week-old were randomly assigned to 6 groups, with 7 mice per group. Daily records were maintained for the baseline condition and body weight of the mice for 22 days. Based on animal welfare principles, at the end of the experiment, the liver, spleen, and thymus were extracted and weighed for calculation. The toxicological evaluation of yogurt and D-lactate was conducted by assessing hepatic function (represented by ALT and AST) and renal function (represented by BUN and CRE). CRE, BUN, AST, and ALT levels were measured using appropriate kits and following the manufacturer's instructions.

2.4.2. Animal Experiment II

After seven days of adaptive feeding, total of 108 mice aged 7-week-old mice were randomly assigned to 9 groups, with 12 mice per group. In each treatment group, immunosuppression was induced by intraperitoneal injection of CTX (80 mg/kg) for 3 days. The successful establishment of an immunosuppression model was recognized when the body weight of the mice decreased by 15% of the original. Different doses of yogurt and D-lactate were supplied during the following days. Based on animal welfare principles, on day 17 of the experiment, 6 mice were randomly selected to inject intraperitoneally with 0.2 mL of 5% (v/v) sheep red blood cells (SRBC). After four days, serum was collected from the eye orbit for the HC_{50} value assessment. Simultaneously, 20 μL of 20% (v/v) SRBC was injected into the right hindfoot pad for the measurement of the delayed-type hypersensitivity (DTH) reaction. Serum, spleen, thymus, and fecal samples were collected for biochemical analysis at the end of the experiment.

2.4.3. Animal Experiment III

After seven days of adaptive feeding, total of 70 mice aged 7-week-old mice were randomly assigned to 7 groups, with 10 mice per group. For the tumor-bearing model, after adjusting the CT26 cell at the logarithmic growth phase suspension to a concentration of 1×10^6 cells/mL with PBS, the cell suspension was inoculated subcutaneously into the right axilla of mice, with a dose of 0.2 mL per mouse. The mice were then bred for seven days, and those who developed a tumor volume of about 50 ± 16 mm^3 were deemed to have successfully established models [23]. Subsequently, the mice were injected with CTX every three days and orally administered yogurt and D-lactate daily. Daily observations were made of the behavior, body weight, and tumor size of all mice. At the end of the test, the tumor volume did not exceed the ethical limits. Based on animal welfare principles, serum, spleen, thymus, and tumor tissues were collected for biochemical analysis at the end of the experiment.

2.5. Methods for Physiological and Pathological Analysis

2.5.1. ELISA Assay

The IL-4, IL-6, IFN-γ, IgA, and IgG cytokines were measured using a commercial ELISA kit and following the manufacturer's protocols.

2.5.2. Histopathological Staining

The sample tissues were fixed overnight at room temperature with 10% formaldehyde, washed with distilled water, subjected to dehydration using a gradient of alcohol, and embedded in paraffin wax. Paraffin-embedded slices were stained. Images were taken using a light microscope.

2.5.3. RT-qPCR Analysis

Total RNA was extracted using a Trizol reagent and assessed for purity and integrity through NanoDrop and gel electrophoresis. RNA was converted to cDNA using a reverse transcription kit. Gene expression levels were evaluated using a real-time quantitative PCR system. Gene-specific primers were listed in Table 1. The relative quantification of the target gene was determined by comparing it to β-actin and calculating the results using the $2^{-\Delta\Delta Ct}$ method [24].

Table 1. Primer sequences.

Genes	Primer Forward	Primer Reverse
MUC-2	GATTCGAAGTGAAGAGCAAG	CACTTGGAGGAATAAACTGG
Claudin5	GAGAGGAACTACCCTTATGCC	ATTGAGTAATTAAACGGGACAGG
T-bet	CGTTTCTACCCCGACCTTCC	ATGCTCACAGCTCGGAACTC
GATA-3	AAGCTCAGTATCCGCTGACG	GATACCTCTGCACCGTAGCC
Bax	ACAGATCATGAAGACAGGGG	CAAAGTAGAAGAGGGCAACC
Bcl-2	ATGTGTGTGGAGAGCGTCAAC	AGACAGCCAGGAGAAATCAAAC
β-actin	TGCTCTCCCTCACGCCATC	GAGGAAGAGGATGCGGCAGT

2.5.4. Proliferation Assay of Splenic Lymphocytes

Mouse spleens were aseptically removed, and lymphocytes were collected using the Animal Splenic Lymphocyte Isolation Kit from Beijing Solarbio Science & Technology Co., Ltd. (Beijing, China). [25]. Cells were incubated in 96-well plates with ConA (10 μg/mL) and LPS (5 μg/mL) for 24 h, followed by treatment with CCK-8 solution and another 2 h incubation [26]. The absorbance measurement at 450 nm was quantified using a Thermo Scientific Varioskan Flash spectrophotometer (Waltham, Massachusetts, America).

2.5.5. Delayed-Type Hypersensitivity (DTH)

On day 17 of the experiment, 0.2 mL of 5% (*v*/*v*) SRBC was injected intraperitoneally into the mice, and the thickness of the right hindfoot pad was measured utilizing vernier calipers. Four days after the initial injection, 20 μL of 20% (*v*/*v*) SRBC was administered to the right hindfoot pad. The resulting increase in footpad thickness was determined 24 h after the second injection and utilized as an indicator of DTH.

2.5.6. Serum Hemolysin

Mice were received an injection of 0.2 mL of 5% (*v*/*v*) SRBC, and after four days, serum was obtained from blood collected from their eye orbit. The serum was diluted with SA buffer (1:5) and added to a 96-well culture plate with a control buffer. Then, SRBC and guinea pig serum were added to each well, and the supernatant was mixed with Drabkin's solution. After resting for 10 min, the optical density of each well was measured at 540 nm using an automatic microplate reader to evaluate serum hemolysin levels.

2.5.7. Gut Microbiota Analysis

DNA was extracted from the cecal contents using the FastDNA™ Spin Kit for Feces. Agarose electrophoresis was used to detect gDNA integrity and nucleic acid concentration. PCR was performed using universal primer pairs on the V3–V4 high variant region of the bacterial 16S rRNA gene [27]. The 16SrDNA sequence data were processed using QIME V19.1 to remove any raw sequences that did not meet specific criteria. High-quality reads were selected for bioinformatics analysis, and operational taxonomic units (OTUs) were formed by clustering all valid reads with similarities greater than 97%. OTUs were classified according to the Greengenes database, and the R package was utilized for α-diversity, β-diversity, and species screening based on the abundance of OTUs.

2.6. Statistical Analyses

Statistical analyses were performed using GraphPad Prism 8.0. A one-way analysis of variance (ANOVA), followed by the Bonferroni procedure, was applied to compare means for multiple group comparisons. At the same time, a Student's *t*-test was used to compare two independent groups. The data were expressed as mean ± SEM, with a significance level set at $p \leq 0.05$.

3. Results

3.1. Detection of D-Lactate in Yogurt

The findings indicated a total lactate content of 15.43 mg/mL in yogurt, with the specific D-lactate content measured at 5.90 mg/mL. After conversion, the proportion of total lactate in yogurt was 1.50%, with the proportion of D-lactate being 0.57%. Additional details concerning the dosage of yogurt and D-lactate were found in the supporting information (Figure S1, Table S1).

3.2. Animal Experiment I: Toxicity Evaluation of Yogurt and D-Lactate in Healthy Mice

In Table 2, mice treated with yogurt and D-lactate maintained stable body weights within the normal range. Yogurt (600 μL) and D-lactate (300 mg/kg) increased immune organ indexes of the spleen and thymus without causing any toxic effects on the hepatic (represented by ALT and AST) and renal function (represented by BUN and CRE). Comparable results were observed in the Positive Control group treated with LM, a recognized immunoregulatory compound [28]. The findings showed the oral safety of yogurt (600 μL) and D-lacate (300 mg/kg) in healthy mice.

Table 2. Evaluation of immune efficacy and toxicity of yogurt and D-lactate in healthy mice.

	Normal Control	Positive Control	Yogurt (200 μL)	Yogurt (600 μL)	D-Lactate (75 mg/kg)	D-Lactate (300 mg/kg)
Body weight (g)	28.01 ± 0.8	29.11 ± 1.2	28.31 ± 0.7	29.21 ± 0.5	27.26 ± 1.9	28.09 ± 1.1
Thymus index (%)	0.27 ± 0.06	0.36 ± 0.09 *	0.28 ± 0.12	0.32 ± 0.03 *	0.28 ± 0.04	0.38 ± 0.02 *
Spleen index (%)	0.32 ± 0.05	0.42 ± 0.12 *	0.38 ± 0.17 *	0.40 ± 0.19 *	0.32 ± 0.09	0.40 ± 0.10 *
Liver index (%)	4.31 ± 0.21	4.51 ± 0.09	4.33 ± 0.19	4.68 ± 0.16	4.53 ± 0.14	4.61 ± 0.08
BUN (mmol/L)	10.09 ± 0.19	10.13 ± 0.31	10.01 ± 0.46	10.32 ± 0.36	10.16 ± 0.21	10.11 ± 0.31
CRE (μmol/L)	44.03 ± 1.91	45.21 ± 2.31	42.91 ± 3.33	44.19 ± 2.98	42.98 ± 1.08	43.26 ± 0.09
ALT (IU/L)	38.21 ± 3.41	42.87 ± 2.12	40.23 ± 3.61	41.87 ± 1.97	42.09 ± 2.71	40.98 ± 3.01
AST (IU/L)	129.23 ± 23.12	136.21 ± 11.21	132.98 ± 31.21	138.12 ± 29.12	119.21 ± 38.24	129.12 ± 31.36

* $p < 0.05$ vs. Normal Control.

3.3. Animal Experiment II: Evaluation of Immune Efficacy of Yogurt and D-Lactate in Immunosuppressive Mice Induced by CTX

3.3.1. Yogurt Supplementation Ameliorated CTX-Induced Immunosuppression in Mice

The experimental design was displayed (Figure 1A). Yogurt dose-dependently recovered the body weight (Figure 1B) and facilitated the growth of spleen and thymus compared to the MC group (Figure 1C). The spleen of the MC group exhibited the reduced number of splenic corpuscles and lymphocytes, dispersed germinal centers, and the unclear distinction between the red and white pulp. However, this trend was reversed upon yogurt administration (Figure 1D). Besides these analyses, the yogurt administration resulted in a dose-dependent increase in serum IgA, IgG, IFN-γ, and IL-6 levels (Figure 1E–H). The DTH reaction exhibited similar alterations. Treatment with medium or high dosages of yogurt resulted in a significant increase in footpad thickness compared to the MC group (Figure 1I).

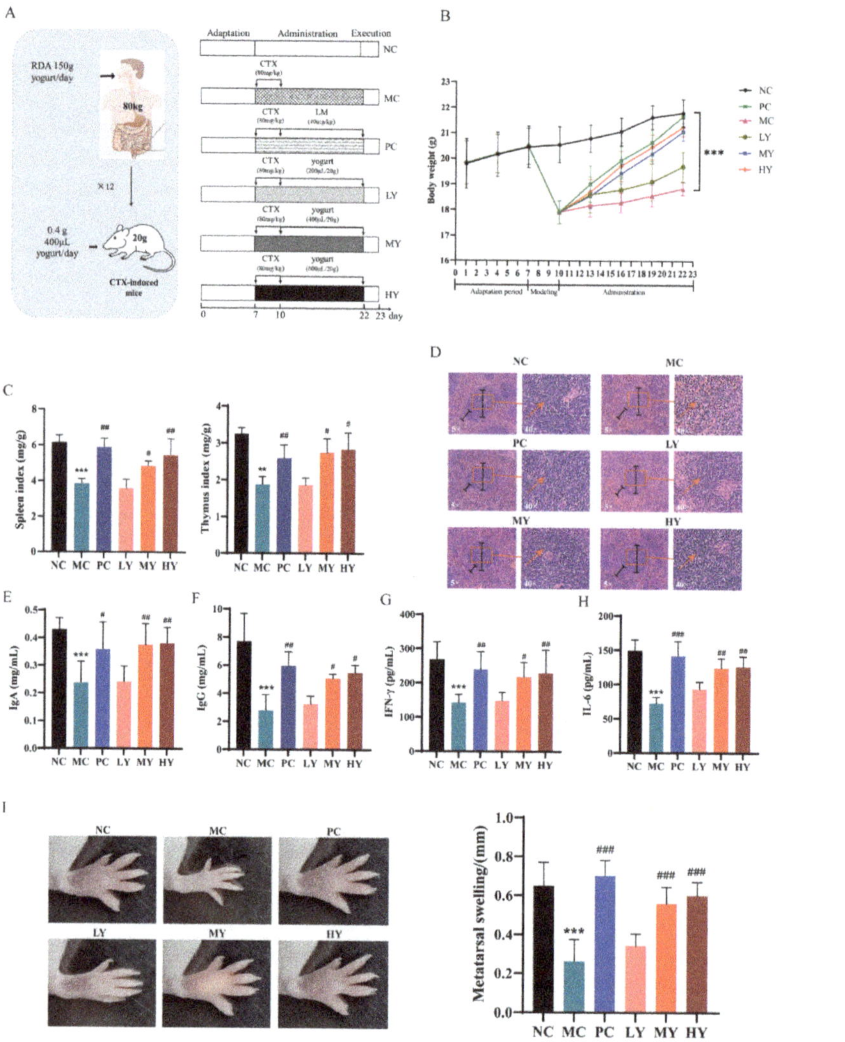

Figure 1. Yogurt supplementation ameliorated CTX-induced immunosuppression in mice. (**A**) Experimental design. NC: the normal control group; MC: the model control group (cyclophosphamide, 80 mg/kg bw); PC: the positive control group (levamisole hydrochloride, 40 mg/kg bw); LY: Low-dose of yogurt group (200 μL); MY: Medium-dose of yogurt group (400 μL); HY: High-dose of yogurt group (600 μL). (**B**) Body weight. (**C**) Spleen and thymus indexes. (**D**) Histopathology observation of the spleen (original magnification: ×5 and ×40). (**E–H**) Serum cytokines of IgA, IgG, IL-6 and IFN-γ. (**I**) DTH reaction and Metatarsal swelling, ** $p < 0.01$ and *** $p < 0.005$ vs. NC group. # $p < 0.05$, ## $p < 0.01$ and ### $p < 0.005$ vs. MC group.

3.3.2. Yogurt Supplementation Regulated Intestinal Immunity and Gut Microbiota in CTX-Induced Mice

As was showed in Figure 2, the standard group showed typical glandular structures and slender villi arranged tightly and completely in the intestines. In contrast, the MC group suffered from significant injury to the intestinal wall, featuring shortened and detached villi. However, the medium and high dosage of yogurt groups exhibited restored villi length (Figure 2A). Yogurt upregulated the expression of MUC-2 (Figure 2B) and claudin5

(Figure 2C), enhancing the integrity of the intestinal barrier. The detected biomarkers of the ratio of IL-4 and IFN-γ related to immune responses in the intestine were significantly improved by yogurt (Figure 2D). Data from the α-diversity (Figure 2E) of Chao1, Shannon, Simpson and ACE index indicated that yogurt modulated the overall diversity of gut microbiota. The β-diversity analysis showed that the gut microbiota composition in yogurt group was distinct from the NC and MC groups (Figure 2F), characterized by 4187 unique OTUs (Figure 2G). At the phylum level, the ratio of Firmicutes to Bacteroidetes (F/B) was a biomarker to assess pathological status. F/B tended to increase moderately by yogurt supplementation (Figure 2H). At the genus level, according to the heat map analysis (Figure 2I), yogurt consumption resulted in a dominate abundance of beneficial bacteria of Lactobacillus, Streptococcus, Bifidobacterium, Akkermansia and Ruminococcus. Yogurt especially increased the abundance of Bifidobacterium and Lactobacillaceae (Figure 2I,J). In addition, it mitigated the harmful bacteria such as Desulfovibrio, Staphylococcus, and Escherichia. We examined the D-lactate level by HPLC in the gut contents to assess the potential involvement of D-lactate in intestinal immunity. The results showed high D-lactate levels in the feces of yogurt groups but minimal changes in D-lactate groups (Figure 2K).

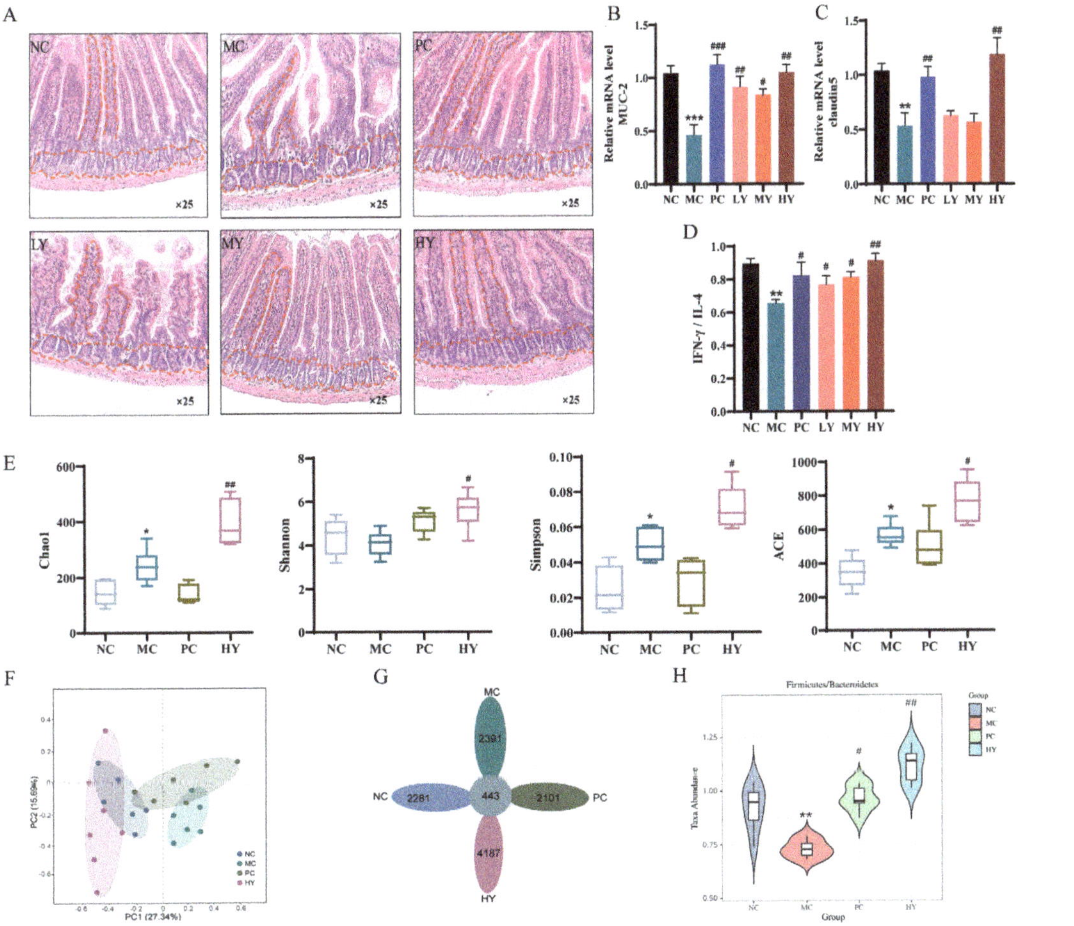

Figure 2. *Cont.*

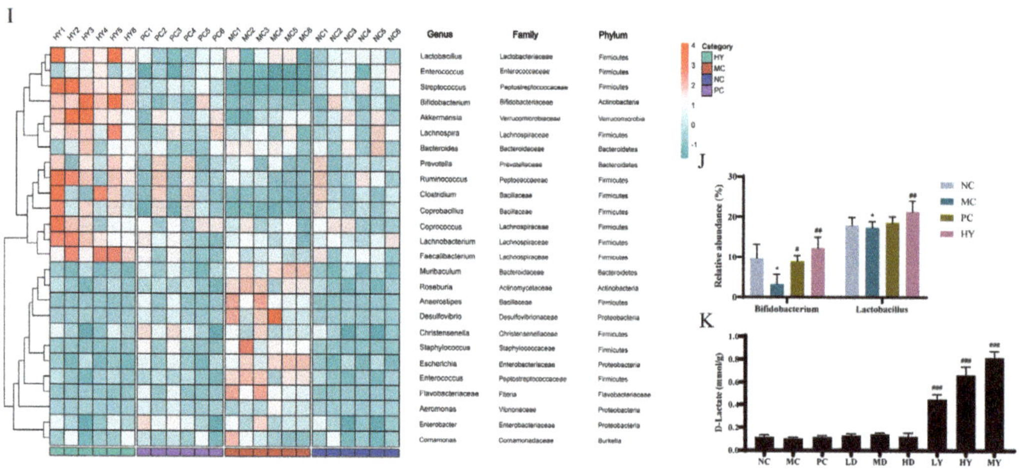

Figure 2. Yogurt supplementation regulated intestinal immunity and gut microbiota in CTX-induced mice. NC: the normal control group; MC: the model control group (cyclophosphamide, 80 mg/kg bw); PC: the positive control group (levamisole hydrochloride, 40 mg/kg bw); LY: Low-dose of yogurt group (200 µL); MY: Medium-dose of yogurt group (400 µL); HY: High-dose of yogurt group (600 µL); LD: Low-dose of D-lactate group (75 mg/kg bw); MD: Medium-dose of D-lactate group (150 mg/kg bw); HD: High-dose of D-lactate group (300 mg/kg bw). (**A**) Histopathology observation of the ileum tissue (original magnification: ×25). (**B**) Relative mRNA level of MUC-2. (**C**) Relative mRNA level of claudin5. (**D**) Cytokines of IFN-γ/IL-4 in ileum tissue. (**E**) Alpha diversity of Chao 1, Shannon, Simpson and ACE indexes. (**F**,**G**) PCA and Venn diagram of gut microbiota. (**H**) The ratio of Firmicutes to Bacteroidetes abundance. (**I**) Heatmap. (**J**) The relative abundance of Bifidobacterium and Lactobacillus. (**K**) The D-lactate concentration in feces. * $p < 0.05$, ** $p < 0.01$ and *** $p < 0.005$ vs. NC group. # $p < 0.05$, ## $p < 0.01$ and ### $p < 0.005$ vs. MC group.

3.3.3. D-Lactate Supplementation Ameliorated Immunosuppression in CTX-Induced Mice

The experimental design was displayed (Figure 3A). The mice administered with D-lactate showed a significant increase in body weight (Figure 3B) and organ development (Figure 3C) dose-dependently. D-lactate ameliorated splenic tissue damage induced by CTX (Figure 3D). Furthermore, splenic lymphocytes were isolated and stimulated by ConA and LPS in vitro to assess transformation capacity of T cells and B cells respectively. The splenic lymphocyte proliferation was measured by SI values. The result indicated that treatment with D-lactate significantly boosted the ConA-stimulated proliferation responses of T cells in immunosuppressive mice (Figure 3E). No similar results were observed in LPS-stimulated proliferation responses of B cells. The results demonstrated that CTX caused a decrease in the relative mRNA expression levels of T-bet, GATA3, Foxp3, and RORγt in splenic lymphocytes mice. The medium and high dosage of D-lactate increased T-bet mRNA level (Figure 3F), while only the high dosage of D-lactate increased GATA3 mRNA level in splenic lymphocytes (Figure 3G). However, no alteration was observed in the expression level of Foxp3 (Figure 3H) and RORγt (Figure 3I). CTX inhibited immune cell cytokine production and resulting in immunosuppression. However, the suppression of cytokine levels (Figure 3J–M) was significantly eased by D-lactate. The HC_{50} values were used to assess murine humoral immune function, as reflected by the serum hemolysin index [29]. The levels of HC_{50} were not differentially affected by the three D-lactate treatments (Figure 3N).

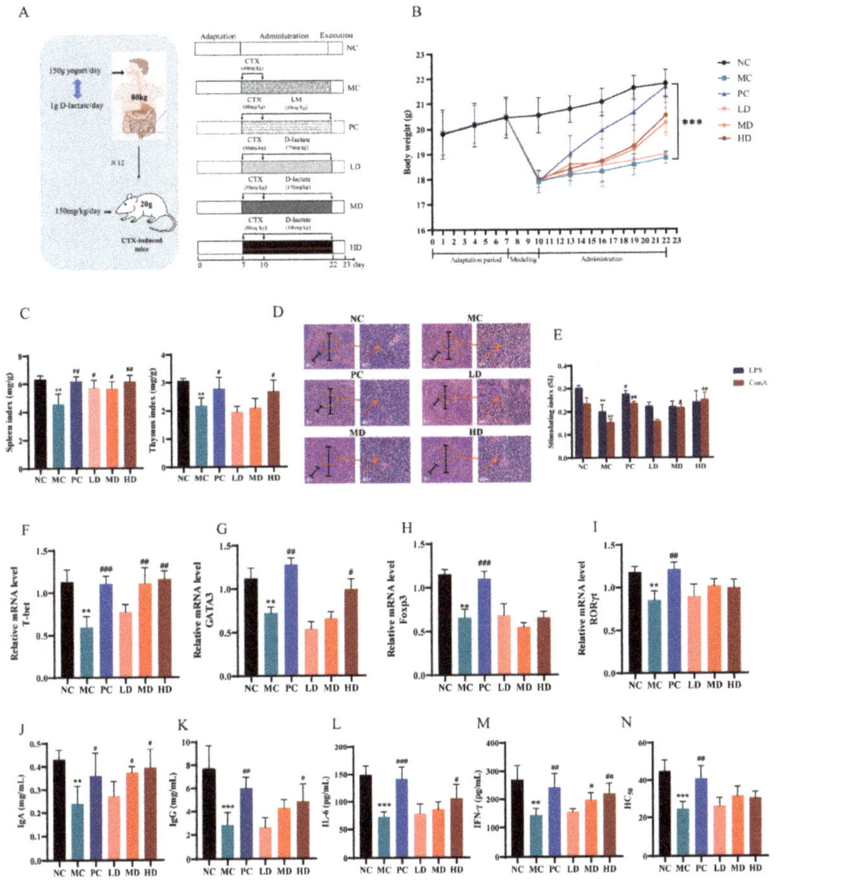

Figure 3. D-lactate supplementation ameliorated immunosuppression in CTX-induced mice. (**A**) Experimental design. NC: the normal control group; MC: the model control group (cyclophosphamide, 80 mg/kg bw); PC: the positive control group (levamisole hydrochloride, 40 mg/kg bw); LD: Low-dose of D-lactate group (75 mg/kg bw); MD: Medium-dose of D-lactate group (150 mg/kg bw); HD: High-dose of D-lactate group (300 mg/kg bw). (**B**) Body weight. (**C**) Spleen and thymus indexes. (**D**) Histopathology observation of the spleen (original magnification: ×5 and ×40). (**E**) Stimulating index (SI). (**F–I**) Relative mRNA level of T-bet, GATA3, Foxp3 and RORγt. (**J–M**) Serum cytokines of IgA, IgG, IL-6 and IFN-γ. (**N**) Serum half hemolysis value (HC_{50}), ** $p < 0.01$ and *** $p < 0.005$ vs. NC group. # $p < 0.05$, ## $p < 0.01$ and ### $p < 0.005$ vs. MC group.

3.4. Animal Experiment III: Evaluation of Immune Efficacy of Yogurt and D-Lactate in CT26 Tumor-Bearing Mice

The experimental design was displayed (Figure 4A). Yogurt effectively ameliorated CTX-induced body weight loss in CT26 tumor-bearing mice (Figure 4B). Yogurt restored the organ development (Figure 4C) and promoted the cytokine secretion of IL-6 and IFN-γ (Figure 4D) in tumor-bearing mice treated with CTX. The tumor tissue (Figure 4E) and the analysis of tumor weight on the day 20 (Figure 4F) revealed that the tumor inhibition rates of the CTX and C + Y groups were 68.02 ± 5.6% and 71.34 ± 4.8%, respectively. The Bax/Bcl-2 ratio expression of colorectal cancer was enhanced with the statistical difference in the CTX and C + Y groups compared to the control group (Figure 4G). This observation suggests that yogurt consumption did not compromise the antitumor efficacy of CTX. Similarly, the experimental design of D-lactate was displayed (Figure 4H). Significant variations in body weight were observed among the groups (Figure 4I). The C + D group enhanced organ index (Figure 4J) and cytokine secretion levels (Figure 4K) compared to the CTX group. D-lactate did not impact the antitumor effectiveness of CTX, as evidenced by tumor growth inhibition rates of 70.28% ± 2.6% for the C + D group (Figure 4L,M) and the promotion of tumor apoptosis (Figure 4N). In summary, yogurt and D-lactate alleviated the immunosuppressive effect of CTX in tumor-bearing mice and did not affect the antitumor efficacy of CTX.

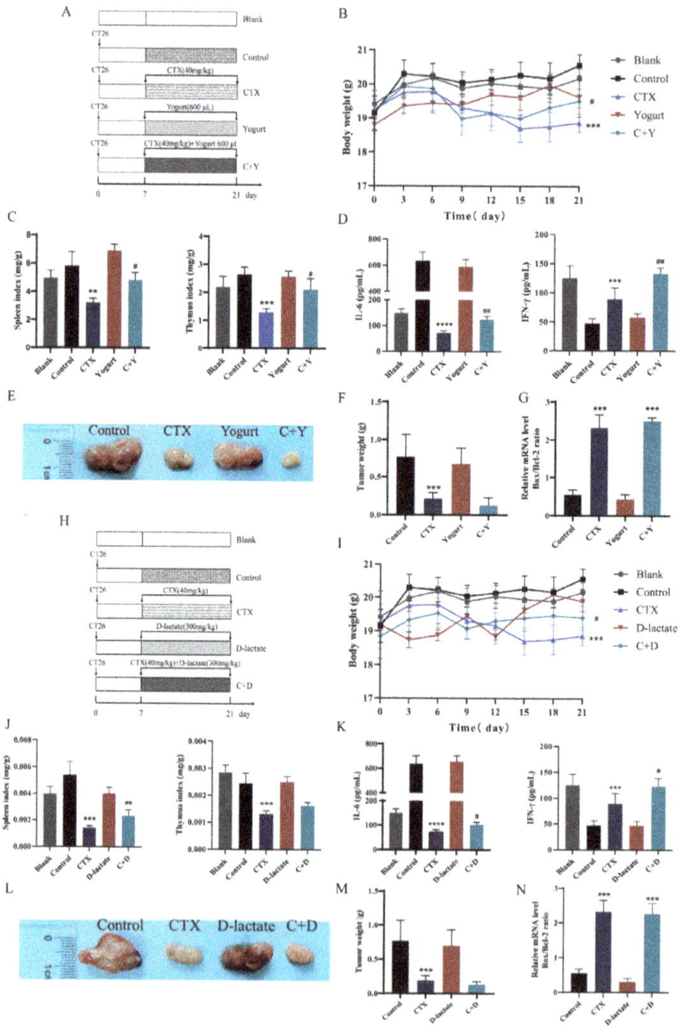

Figure 4. Evaluation of immune efficacy of yogurt and D-lactate in CT26 tumor-bearing mice. (**A**,**H**) Experimental design, Blank: healthy mice; Control: tumor model group; CTX: cyclophosphamide (40 mg/kg bw); C + Y: cyclophosphamide + yogurt (cyclophosphamide, 40 mg/kg bw; yogurt, 600 μL); C + D: cyclophosphamide + D-lactate (cyclophosphamide, 40 mg/kg bw; D-lactate, 300 mg/kg bw). (**B**,**I**) Body weight. (**C**,**J**) Immune Organ index. (**D**,**K**) Serum cytokines of IL6 and IFN-γ. (**E**,**L**) Images of tumor tissues at treatment termination. (**F**,**M**) tumor weight at 20 d. (**G**,**N**) Relative mRNA level of Bax/Bcl-2 ratio, ** $p < 0.01$, *** $p < 0.001$ vs. control group. # $p < 0.05$, ## $p < 0.01$ vs. CTX group. **** $p < 0.0001$.

4. Discussion

The present study provided direct evidence of yogurt to alleviate the CTX-induced immunosuppression. Furthermore, D-lactate was identified as a potential substance responsible for the immunomodulatory effects of yogurt. Although the results appeared promising, some statements and discussion still required to be supplied.

The first question was regard to the dosage information of yogurt and D-lactate. Figures S1 and S2 displayed the lactate concentration in simulated commercial yogurt. The data illustrated that the total lactate content in yogurt was 1.50% and D-lactate content was 0.57%. According to FDA, the recommended daily intake of yogurt for a human weighed 80 kg was 150–200 g, which was converted to 300–400 μL per day in mice. Accordingly, a human weighing 80 kg consuming 200 g yogurt a day was equivalent to a mouse weighing 20 g ingested with about 4 mg D-lactate per day. This served as the basis for the dosage of yogurt and D-lactate in the experimental design.

The second question revolved the modulation of gut microbiota in immunosuppressive mice by yogurt. From the data of α-diversity, the increase of Chaos, Simpson and ACE indexes in the model group mice were possibly attributed to the upregulated abundance of pathogenic microbiota [30] (Figure S2). It was speculated that the increased indexes of Chaos, Shannon, Simpson and ACE in yogurt group might contribute to the enhanced diversity of beneficial gut bacteria [7,31]. Further β-diversity analysis of the gut microbiota has validated that hypothesis (Figure S3). The findings of β-diversity coincided precisely with the α-diversity results. Particularly, Lactobacillus and Bifidobacterium showed a notable increase, which are potentially considered to hydrolyze carbohydrates in the intestine to produce D-lactate [32]. Correlational probiotic strains, including Lactobacillus reuteri ATCC 55730 [33], Lactobacillus johnsonii La [34], and *L. reuteri* DSM 17938 [35,36] have been reported to produce D-lactate. The results of D-lactate detection in intestinal contents provided further inference. Therefore, it was reasonable to speculate that the increasing D-lactate concentration in feces was potentially associated with the remodeling of the intestinal flora. Furthermore, studies have demonstrated that microbial D-lactate can affect macrophage function locally and maintain mucosal integrity within the gut [37]. Thus, yogurt consumption enhanced the intestinal immune function by hypothetically reshaping the gut microbiota to boost beneficial probiotics producing D-lactate in the intestine. Nevertheless, it cannot be ruled out that the gut immunity might be modulated by the oral administration of D-lactate through other pathways.

The third question was to discuss the mechanism by which D-lactate alleviated immunosuppression. Immunocytes can be categorized into T cells and B cells. Our findings demonstrated that D-lactate enhanced the immune response of splenic T cells stimulated by ConA, thereby augmenting their capacity for lymphocyte transformation. However, no significant differences were observed regarding the immune response of splenic B cells. Consequently, we further examined the expression levels of nuclear transcription factors of the T cell family in the mouse spleen. T-bet was a nuclear transcription factor specifically expressed in Th1 cells, regulating cellular immune function. GATA3 was a key transcription factor involved in the development of Th2 cells, regulating humoral immunity. A delicate balance between Th1 and Th2 cells was crucial for the healthy host [38,39]. Foxp3 was a transcriptional regulatory factor that was critical for the development and suppressive function of regulatory T cells. RORγt was a lineage-specific transcription factor for T helper 17 cells. The results demonstrated that the ingestion of medium and high doses of D-lactate resulted in an increase in the expression level of T-bet, while only a high dose of D-lactate elevated the expression level of GATA3. This indicated that D-lactate regulated the differentiation of Th cells towards Th1 cells and alleviated immunosuppressive by enhancing cellular immunity. These findings were consistent with the negative results of HC_{50} (an indicator for measuring humoral immunity) and positive results of DTH (the vivo detection of cellular immunity) [40]. Therefore, D-lactate exerted its mitigating effect on immunosuppression by promoting Th cell differentiation to Th1 and enhancing the cellular immunity of splenic lymphocytes.

The fourth question addressed why the tumor model was constructed. In healthy mice and immunosuppression mice, we verified the safety and immune efficacy of daily intake of 600 μL yogurt or 300 mg/kg D-lacate in mice. However, whether yogurt or D-lactate could be applied to clinical cancer chemotherapy patients remains debatable. In the tumor model, we conducted preliminary exploration of the therapeutic effects of yogurt and D-lactate on CTX chemotherapy. Our research findings demonstrated that yogurt and D-lactate can alleviate CTX-induced immunosuppression to a certain extent in the mouse tumor model, and they had no detrimental effects on the antitumor efficacy of CTX. The findings from this study have provided preliminary data support for the clinical application of yogurt and D-lactate in alleviating immunosuppressive.

Although our research has successfully assessed the mitigating effects of yogurt and D-lactate on immunosuppression, several limitations remain. The immune efficacy of other bioactive ingredients in yogurt cannot be denied, but this study focuses on evaluating the benefits of D-lactate in yogurt, aiming to develop D-lactate as a new type of food functional factor. The potential benefits of other components in yogurt should be explored in the future. Additionally, further exploration of the specific production of D-lactate by gut microbiota was valuable for developing D-lactate into a new type of food nutrient factor. Furthermore, mechanistic investigations at the molecular level have elucidated that lactate exerted its effects through specific binding to its receptor GPR81 [41]. Using flow cytometry to subtype lymphocytes might be advantageous for investigating the involvement of GPR81 in immune responses at a more advanced scientific level. On the other hand, despite our research findings has demonstrated the positive adjunctive effect of D-lactate on chemotherapy, clinical trials were warranted to validate these findings and establish the utility of yogurt as an immunomodulatory food product. D-lactate remained to determine whether it was comparable to the clinical drug Mesna.

5. Conclusions

In summary, this study effectively demonstrated the mitigating effects of yogurt on immunosuppression. The alleviation of yogurt on immunosuppression is partially attributed to the enhanced cellular immunity of D-lactate on splenic lymphocytes. This article provides a new interpretation of yogurt as a functional food exerting physiological effects, making a positive contribution to the functional food segment.

Supplementary Materials: The following supporting information can be downloaded at: https://www.mdpi.com/article/10.3390/nu16091395/s1, Figure S1. The chromatogram of lactate concentration in simulated commercial yogurt detected by high-performance liquid chromatography (HPLC). Table S1. The lactate concentration in simulated commercial yogurt. Figure S2. The relative abundance of Escherichia coli, Desulfovibrio and Staphylococcus in the fecal of CTX-induced mice. Statistical significance was evaluated by performing a one-way ANOVA followed by the Tukey test on the values presented as mean ± SEM. * $p < 0.05$, ** $p < 0.01$, *** $p < 0.001$ vs. normal control group (NC). # $p < 0.05$, ## $p < 0.01$, ### $p < 0.001$ vs. model control group (MC). Figure S3.The relative abundance of Streptococcus, Akkermansia and Ruminococcus in the fecal of CTX-induced mice. Statistical significance was evaluated by performing a one-way ANOVA followed by the Tukey test on the values presented as mean ± SEM (n = 10). * $p < 0.05$, ** $p < 0.01$, *** $p < 0.001$ vs. normal control group (NC). # $p < 0.05$, ## $p < 0.01$, ### $p < 0.001$ vs. model control group (MC).

Author Contributions: Conceptualization, X.D.; methodology, Y.D. and R.X.; software, X.D.; validation, X.D.; formal analysis, X.D.; investigation, Y.Y.; data curation, X.D. and Y.Y.; writing—original draft preparation, X.D.; writing—review and editing, Y.D.; visualization, Y.Y.; supervision, Y.Y. All authors have read and agreed to the published version of the manuscript.

Funding: This research was funded by the National Natural Science Foundation of China (grant no. 32272290 and 31972973).

Institutional Review Board Statement: The Institutional Animal Ethics Committee of Jiangnan University approved all animal experimental procedures (protocol numbers JN.No20220315c0900425(012), JN.No20220615c0801001(198)and JN.No20221130b0700220(467).

Informed Consent Statement: Not applicable.

Data Availability Statement: Data will be made available on request.

Acknowledgments: We would like to express our sincere appreciation to Haitao Li for his invaluable guidance and support. We also appreciate the assistance provided by colleagues and teachers throughout this research.

Conflicts of Interest: The authors declare no conflicts of interest.

References

1. Li, K.; Cao, Y.X.; Jiao, S.M.; Du, G.H.; Du, Y.G.; Qin, X.M. Structural Characterization and Immune Activity Screening of Polysaccharides with Different Molecular Weights from Astragali Radix. *Front. Pharmacol.* **2020**, *11*, 582091. [CrossRef]
2. Xie, H.; Fang, J.; Farag, M.A.; Li, Z.; Sun, P.; Shao, P. Dendrobium officinale leaf polysaccharides regulation of immune response and gut microbiota composition in cyclophosphamide-treated mice. *Food Chem. X* **2022**, *13*, 100235. [CrossRef]
3. Douglas, A.; Stevens, B.; Lynch, L. Interleukin-17 as a key player in neuroimmunometabolism. *Nat. Metab.* **2023**, *5*, 1088–1100. [CrossRef] [PubMed]
4. Martin, T.D.; Patel, R.S.; Cook, D.R.; Choi, M.Y.; Patil, A.B.; Liang, A.C.; Li, M.Z.; Haigis, K.M.; Elledge, S.J. The adaptive immune system is a major driver of selection for tumor suppressor gene inactivation. *Science* **2021**, *373*, 1327–1335. [CrossRef] [PubMed]
5. Schluter, J.; Peled, J.U.; Taylor, B.P.; Markey, K.A.; Smith, M.; Taur, Y.; Niehus, R.; Staffas, A.; Dai, A.; Fontana, E.; et al. The gut microbiota is associated with immune cell dynamics in humans. *Nature* **2020**, *588*, 303–307. [CrossRef] [PubMed]
6. Kempen, J.H.; Newcomb, C.W.; Washington, T.L.; Foster, C.S.; Sobrin, L.; Thorne, J.E.; Jabs, D.A.; Suhler, E.B.; Rosenbaum, J.T.; Sen, H.N.; et al. Use of Immunosuppression and the Risk of Subsequent Overall or Cancer Mortality. *Ophthalmology* **2023**, *130*, 1258–1268. [CrossRef] [PubMed]
7. Daniel, N.; Nachbar, R.; Tran, T.T.T.; Ouellette, A.; Varin, T.V.; Cotillard, A.; Quinquis, L.; Gagné, A.; St-Pierre, P.; Trottier, J.; et al. Gut microbiota and fermentation-derived branched chain hydroxy acids mediate health benefits of yogurt consumption in obese mice. *Nat. Commun.* **2022**, *13*, 1343. [CrossRef] [PubMed]
8. Kok, C.R.; Hutkins, R. Yogurt and other fermented foods as sources of health-promoting bacteria. *Nutr. Rev.* **2018**, *76*, 4–15. [CrossRef] [PubMed]
9. Barengolts, E.; Smith, E.D.; Reutrakul, S.; Tonucci, L.; Anothaisintawee, T. The Effect of Probiotic Yogurt on Glycemic Control in Type 2 Diabetes or Obesity: A Meta-Analysis of Nine Randomized Controlled Trials. *Nutrients* **2019**, *11*, 671. [CrossRef]
10. Wu, L.; Sun, D. Consumption of Yogurt and the Incident Risk of Cardiovascular Disease: A Meta-Analysis of Nine Cohort Studies. *Nutrients* **2017**, *9*, 315. [CrossRef]
11. Aslam, H.; Marx, W.; Rocks, T.; Loughman, A.; Chandrasekaran, V.; Ruusunen, A.; Dawson, S.L.; West, M.; Mullarkey, E.; Pasco, J.A.; et al. The effects of dairy and dairy derivatives on the gut microbiota: A systematic literature review. *Gut Microbes* **2020**, *12*, 1799533. [CrossRef]
12. Başpinar, B.; Güldaş, M. Traditional plain yogurt: A therapeutic food for metabolic syndrome? *Crit. Rev. Food Sci. Nutr.* **2020**, *61*, 3129–3143. [CrossRef] [PubMed]
13. Adeva-Andany, M.M.; López-Ojén, M.; Funcasta-Calderón, R.; Ameneiros-Rodríguez, E.; Donapetry-García, C.; Vila-Altesor, M.; Rodríguez-Seijas, J. Comprehensive review on lactate metabolism in human health. *Mitochondrion* **2014**, *17*, 76–100. [CrossRef] [PubMed]
14. Jia, B.; Pu, Z.J.; Tang, K.; Jia, X.; Kim, K.H.; Liu, X.; Jeon, C.O. Catalytic, Computational, and Evolutionary Analysis of the d-Lactate Dehydrogenases Responsible for d-Lactic Acid Production in Lactic Acid Bacteria. *J. Agric. Food Chem.* **2018**, *66*, 8371–8381. [CrossRef] [PubMed]
15. Blake, A.B.; Guard, B.C.; Honneffer, J.B.; Lidbury, J.A.; Steiner, J.M.; Suchodolski, J.S. Altered microbiota, fecal lactate, and fecal bile acids in dogs with gastrointestinal disease. *PLoS ONE* **2019**, *14*, e0224454. [CrossRef] [PubMed]
16. Yan, Y.; Li, X.-x.; Yang, Q.; Zhang, H.; Hettinga, K.A.; Li, H.; Chen, W. Dietary D-Lactate Intake Facilitates Inflammatory Resolution by Modulating M1 Macrophage Polarization. *Mol. Nutr. Food Res.* **2022**, *66*, e2200196. [CrossRef] [PubMed]
17. Li, X.; Yan, Y.; Du, X.; Zhang, H.; Li, H.; Chen, W. Yogurt Prevents Colitis-Associated Colorectal Cancer in Mice. *Mol. Nutr. Food Res.* **2023**, *67*, e2300444. [CrossRef]
18. Cho, W.-Y.; Hong, G.-E.; Lee, H.-J.; Yeon, S.-J.; Paik, H.-D.; Hosaka, Y.Z.; Lee, C.-H. Effect of Yogurt Fermented by Lactobacillus Fermentum TSI and L. Fermentum S2 Derived from a Mongolian Traditional Dairy Product on Rats with High-Fat-Diet-Induced Obesity. *Foods* **2020**, *9*, 594. [CrossRef]
19. Tang, C.; Zhao, H.; Kong, L.; Meng, F.; Zhou, L.; Lu, Z.; Lu, Y. Probiotic Yogurt Alleviates High-Fat Diet-Induced Lipid Accumulation and Insulin Resistance in Mice via the Adiponectin Pathway. *J. Agric. Food. Chem.* **2023**, *71*, 1464–1476. [CrossRef]
20. Fan, X.; Shi, Z.-Q.; Xu, J.; Li, C.; Li, X.; Jiang, X.; Du, L.; Tu, M.; Zeng, X.; Wu, Z.; et al. Characterization of the effects of binary probiotics and wolfberry dietary fiber on the quality of yogurt. *Food Chem.* **2022**, *406*, 135020. [CrossRef]
21. Yan, Y.; Xu, R.; Li, X.-x.; Yao, Z.; Zhang, H.; Li, H.; Chen, W. Unexpected immunoregulation effects of D-lactate, different from L-lactate. *Food Agric. Immunol.* **2022**, *33*, 286–301. [CrossRef]

22. Zhu, Z.; Neirinck, L.G. Chiral separation and determination of R-(-)- and S-(+)-baclofen in human plasma by high-performance liquid chromatography. *J. Chromatogr. B Anal. Technol. Biomed. Life Sci.* **2003**, *785*, 277–283. [CrossRef] [PubMed]
23. Park, J.; Kim, J.S.; Yang, G.; Lee, H.-H.; Shim, G.; Lee, J.; Oh, Y.K. Lysyl oxidase-responsive anchoring nanoparticles for modulation of the tumor immune microenvironment. *J. Control. Release* **2023**, *360*, 376–391. [CrossRef] [PubMed]
24. Schmittgen, T.D.; Livak, K.J. Analyzing real-time PCR data by the comparative CT method. *Nat. Protoc.* **2008**, *3*, 1101–1108. [CrossRef]
25. Bai, Z.; Yang, P.; Yu, F.; Li, Z.; Yao, Z.; Martinez, J.; Li, M.; Xu, H. Combining adoptive NK cell infusion with a dopamine-releasing peptide reduces senescent cells in aged mice. *Cell Death Dis.* **2022**, *13*, 305. [CrossRef] [PubMed]
26. Xu, D.; Hu, J.-l.; Zhong, Y.; Zhang, Y.; Liu, W.; Nie, S.; Xie, M. Effects of Rosa roxburghii & edible fungus fermentation broth on immune response and gut microbiota in immunosuppressed mice. *Food Sci. Hum. Wellness* **2023**, *13*, 154–165.
27. Zhang, Y.; Tang, Y.; Cai, L.; He, J.; Chen, L.; Ouyang, K.; Wang, W. Chimonanthus nitens Oliv Polysaccharides Modulate Immunity and Gut Microbiota in Immunocompromised Mice. *Oxidative Med. Cell. Longev.* **2023**, *2023*, 6208680. [CrossRef] [PubMed]
28. Wang, J.; Liu, J.; Wang, M.; Zhao, F.; Ge, M.; Liu, L.; Jiang, E.; Feng, S.; Han, M.; Pei, X.; et al. Levamisole Suppresses CD4(+) T-Cell Proliferation and Antigen-Presenting Cell Activation in Aplastic Anemia by Regulating the JAK/STAT and TLR Signaling Pathways. *Front. Immunol.* **2022**, *13*, 907808. [CrossRef]
29. Yu, Q.; Nie, S.; Wang, J.; Liu, X.; Yin, P.-F.; Huang, D.; Li, W.; Gong, D.; Xie, M. Chemoprotective effects of Ganoderma atrum polysaccharide in cyclophosphamide-induced mice. *Int. J. Biol. Macromol.* **2014**, *64*, 395–401. [CrossRef]
30. Yin, H.; Li, R.; Liu, J.; Sun, Y.; Zhao, L.; Mou, J.; Yang, J. Fucosylated chondroitin sulfate from sea cucumber Stichopus chloronotus alleviate the intestinal barrier injury and oxidative stress damage in vitro and in vivo. *Carbohydr. Polym.* **2024**, *328*, 121722. [CrossRef]
31. Hasegawa, Y.; Pei, R.; Raghuvanshi, R.; Liu, Z.; Bolling, B.W. Yogurt Supplementation Attenuates Insulin Resistance in Obese Mice by Reducing Metabolic Endotoxemia and Inflammation. *J. Nutr.* **2023**, *153*, 703–712. [CrossRef] [PubMed]
32. Łukasik, J.; Salminen, S.; Szajewska, H. Rapid review shows that probiotics and fermented infant formulas do not cause d-lactic acidosis in healthy children. *Acta Paediatr.* **2018**, *107*, 1322–1326. [CrossRef] [PubMed]
33. Connolly, E.; Abrahamsson, T.R.; Björkstén, B. Safety of D(-)-Lactic Acid Producing Bacteria in the Human Infant. *J. Pediatr. Gastroenterol. Nutr.* **2005**, *41*, 489–492. [CrossRef] [PubMed]
34. Haschke-Becher, E.; Brunser, O.; Cruchet, S.; Gotteland, M.; Haschke, F.; Bachmann, C. Urinary D-Lactate Excretion in Infants Receiving Lactobacillus johnsonii with Formula. *Ann. Nutr. Metab.* **2008**, *53*, 240–244. [CrossRef] [PubMed]
35. Papagaroufalis, K.; Fotiou, A.; Egli, D.; Tran, L.-A.; Steenhout, P.G. A Randomized Double Blind Controlled Safety Trial Evaluating d-Lactic Acid Production in Healthy Infants Fed a Lactobacillus reuteri-containing Formula. *Nutr. Metab. Insights* **2014**, *7*, 19–27. [CrossRef] [PubMed]
36. Li, M.; Laura, B.L.; Chen, X.; Wang, M.; Kuhlenschmidt, T.B.; Kuhlenschmidt, M.S.; Fahey, G.C.; Donovan, S.M. Microbial composition and in vitro fermentation patterns of human milk oligosaccharides and prebiotics differ between formula-fed and sow-reared piglets. *FASEB J.* **2012**, *142*, 681–689. [CrossRef] [PubMed]
37. Morita, N.; Umemoto, E.; Fujita, S.; Hayashi, A.; Kikuta, J.; Kimura, I.; Haneda, T.; Imai, T.; Inoue, A.; Mimuro, H.; et al. GPR31-dependent dendrite protrusion of intestinal CX3CR1+ cells by bacterial metabolites. *Nature* **2019**, *566*, 110–114. [CrossRef] [PubMed]
38. Min, F.; Hu, J.-l.; Huang, T.; Huang, Y.; Nie, S.; Xiong, T.; Xie, M. Effects of Lactobacillus casei NCU011054 on immune response and gut microbiota of cyclophosphamide induced immunosuppression mice. *Food Chem. Toxicol.* **2023**, *174*, 113662. [CrossRef]
39. Kim, J.; Lee, H.; You, S. Dried Ginger Extract Restores the T Helper Type 1/T Helper Type 2 Balance and Antibody Production in Cyclophosphamide-Induced Immunocompromised Mice after Flu Vaccination. *Nutrients* **2022**, *14*, 1984. [CrossRef]
40. Bai, R.-b.; Zhang, Y.; Fan, J.-m.; Jia, X.; Li, D.; Wang, Y.; Zhou, J.; Yan, Q.; Hu, F. Immune-enhancement effects of oligosaccharides from Codonopsis pilosula on cyclophosphamide induced immunosuppression in mice. *Food Funct.* **2020**, *11*, 3306–3315. [CrossRef]
41. Colucci, A.; Tassinari, I.D.Á.; Loss, E.d.S.; Fraga, L.S.d. History and Function of the Lactate Receptor GPR81/HCAR1 in the Brain: A Putative Therapeutic Target for the Treatment of Cerebral Ischemia. *Neuroscience* **2023**, *526*, 144–163. [CrossRef] [PubMed]

nutrients

MDPI

Systematic Review

Antioxidant Lipid Supplement on Cardiovascular Risk Factors: A Systematic Review and Meta-Analysis

Sitong Wan [1,2,†], Wenbin Wu [2,†], Yan Zhang [1,†], Jian He [3], Xiaoping Wang [4], Peng An [2], Junjie Luo [5,*], Yinhua Zhu [6,*] and Yongting Luo [1,2,*]

1 College of Food Science and Engineering, Gansu Agricultural University, Lanzhou 730070, China; adeline7wan@163.com (S.W.); zhangyan@gsau.edu.cn (Y.Z.)
2 Key Laboratory of Precision Nutrition and Food Quality, Department of Nutrition and Health, China Agricultural University, Beijing 100193, China; wwb091828@163.com (W.W.); an-peng@cau.edu.cn (P.A.)
3 National Center of Technology Innovation for Dairy, Hohhot 010110, China; hejian@yili.com
4 Zhejiang Medicine Co., Ltd., Shaoxing 312366, China; wangxiaoping@zmc.top
5 Food Laboratory of Zhongyuan, Luohe 462300, China
6 State Key Laboratory for Quality Ensurance and Sustainable Use of Dao-di Herbs, Artemisinin Research Center, and Institute of Chinese Materia Medica, China Academy of Chinese Medical Sciences, Beijing 100700, China
* Correspondence: luojj@cau.edu.cn (J.L.); zhuyinhua@cau.edu.cn (Y.Z.); luo.yongting@cau.edu.cn (Y.L.)
† These authors contributed equally to this work.

Abstract: The efficacy of functional lipids with antioxidant properties in reducing cardiovascular risk has not been consistent. Randomized controlled trials (RCTs) reporting estimates for the effects of antioxidant functional lipid supplementations on cardiometabolic risk factors were searched up to 1 May 2024. Overall, antioxidant lipid supplementations, compared with placebo, had favorable effects on systolic blood pressure (lycopene: −1.95 [−3.54, −0.36] mmHg), low-density lipoprotein cholesterol (n6 fatty acid: −0.39 [−0.71, −0.06] mmol/L; astaxanthin: −0.11 [−0.21, −0.01] mmol/L), high-density lipoprotein cholesterol (n3 fatty acid: 0.20 [0.13, 0.27] mmol/L; n6 fatty acid: 0.08 [0.01, 0.14] mmol/L; astaxanthin: 0.13 [0.05, 0.21] mmol/L), total cholesterol (n6 fatty acid: −0.24 [−0.37, −0.11] mmol/L; astaxanthin: −0.22 [−0.32, −0.12] mmol/L; beta-carotene: −0.13 [−0.23, −0.04] mmol/L), triglyceride (n3 fatty acid: −0.37 [−0.47, −0.28] mmol/L; astaxanthin: −0.46 [−0.83, −0.10] mmol/L), and fasting blood insulin (astaxanthin: −2.66 [−3.98, −1.34] pmol/L). The benefits of antioxidant lipid supplementations appeared to be most evident in blood pressure and blood lipids in participants with different cardiometabolic health statuses. Notably, n9 fatty acid increased triglyceride and hemoglobin A1C in the total population, which increases CVD risk. Antioxidant lipid supplementations ameliorate cardiometabolic risk factors, while their effect may depend on type and cardiometabolic health status. Long-term RCTs are needed to corroborate risk–benefit ratios across different antioxidant functional lipid supplementation settings.

Keywords: antioxidant functional lipids; cardiovascular disease; meta-analysis

1. Introduction

Cardiovascular diseases (CVDs) continue to be a major cause of morbidity and mortality worldwide despite advances in preventive and therapeutic medicine [1]. High levels of blood glucose, blood pressure, and lipids, including low-density lipoprotein cholesterol, total cholesterol, and triglyceride, have been identified over the past 50 years as modifiable risk factors that act as predictors of CVD events and are thus key targets for the primary prevention of CVDs [2–5].

Of the deaths or disabilities associated with CVDs and type 2 diabetes (T2D), a significant proportion is attributable to suboptimal dietary habits, with different types of functional lipids garnering substantial attention [6–8]. Functional lipids refer to a class of lipids with specific physiological functions, defined as fat-soluble substances required for the maintenance of human nutrition and health, as well as the prevention and treatment of certain consequential nutrient deficiencies and endogenous diseases, especially hypertension, T2D, and other CVDs [9]. Functional lipids mainly include polyunsaturated fatty acids such as linoleic acid, linolenic acid, eicosapentaenoic acid, and eicosahexaenoic acid, as well as phytosterols [9]. Polyunsaturated fatty acids are the mainstay of functional lipids research and are generally defined as fatty acids containing either two or more double carbons with a carbon length of 18 or more. Phytosterols are active components that are widely found in roots, stems, leaves, fruits, and seeds of plants and possess favorable antioxidant properties and anti-inflammatory effects [9].

Oxidative stress is a contributing factor to CVDs, which has long been recognized as being involved in the pathogenesis of CVDs [10]. The adverse effects of oxidative stress on the cardiovascular system are attributed to decreased nitric oxide availability, inflammatory responses, and lipid peroxidation through which reactive oxygen species disrupt the homeostasis of the vascular wall, leading to defective endothelium-dependent vasodilatation [11]. Once formed, ROS activates nuclear factor-kappa B, leading to transcriptional activation of more than 100 genes involved in the immune system and inflammatory response, such as tumor necrosis factor-α, interleukin-1β, and interleukin-6. Macrophages absorb oxidized low-density lipoprotein and then convert it to foam cells in vascular endothelial cells, leading to the development of atherosclerotic lesions [10,11]. Preclinical and epidemiological studies have suggested that dietary antioxidants such as vitamin E, carotenoids, and polyphenols inhibit oxidative stress, thereby providing cardiovascular protection. Physiologically, unsaturated fatty acids, phytosterols, and other functional lipids with antioxidant properties may contribute to cardiometabolic health by removing free radicals and decreasing inflammation and platelet activity while preserving endothelial cell homeostasis and cardiac function. Further, free radicals impair beta cell function and insulin sensitivity, resulting in hyperglycemia and insulin resistance, thereby predisposing to CVDs [12,13].

However, randomized clinical trials (RCTs) investigating the efficacy of antioxidant functional lipid supplementations in reducing cardiometabolic risk factors displayed inconsistent findings. Unsaturated fatty acid supplementations have been shown to have certain beneficial effects on blood glucose [14] and lipids [15–17] among patients with T2D in some but not all studies [18,19]. Moreover, lycopene [20,21], astaxanthin [22,23], and beta-carotene [24,25] showed inconsistent results in CVD risk factors. To reconcile the inconsistencies in the literature regarding the role of antioxidant functional lipid supplementations in the development of health outcomes, we conducted a systematic review and meta-analysis of all available RCTs to investigate the effect of interventions with functional lipids with antioxidant properties on CVD risk factors.

2. Methods

Per the Preferred Reporting Items for Systematic Reviews and Meta-Analyses guidelines [26], we registered the study protocol in the International Prospective Register of Systematic Reviews (PROSPERO CRD42024536111). The included RCTs in this meta-analysis received ethics approval from relevant institutional review boards.

2.1. Search Strategy

The PubMed, Web of Science, and Embase databases were searched for RCTs published up to the 1st of May 2024. To conduct the systematic search, the following terms were used: ("N3 fatty acid." OR "n-6 fatty acid" OR "n-9 fatty acid" OR "EPA" OR "Eicosapentaenoic Acid" OR "DHA" OR "Docosahexaenoic Acid" OR "linoleic acid" OR "gamma-linolenic acid" OR "oleic acid" OR "lycopene" OR "astaxanthin" OR "beta-carotene") AND ("Blood glucose" OR "Blood sugar" OR "glycemic" OR "Blood lipids" OR "triglyceride" OR "cholesterol" OR "Blood pressure").

2.2. Inclusion and Exclusion Criteria

RCTs assessing the effect of antioxidant functional lipid supplementations on blood pressure (systolic blood pressure [SBP]; diastolic blood pressure [DBP]), blood lipids (total cholesterol [TC]; high-density lipoprotein cholesterol [HDL-C]; low-density lipoprotein cholesterol [LDL-C]; and triglyceride [TG]), and glycemic parameters (fasting blood glucose [FBG]; hemoglobin [A1C]; and fasting blood insulin [FBI]) were included for further review.

Trials without randomization, relevant cardiometabolic outcomes, a corresponding placebo or control substance, or viable mean change and standard deviation (SD) were excluded. Additionally, studies with intervention durations of less than 1 week or included participants with severe cardiovascular diseases, mental disorders, or other severe diseases at baseline were excluded.

2.3. Study Selection

The literature search was conducted independently by two reviewers and relevant published articles were identified. All selected studies were re-examined by a third reviewer and discrepancies were resolved through group discussions.

2.4. Data Extraction

Information extracted from eligible studies included the last name of the first author, publication year, geographic location of the study population, study design, participant characteristics (number of participants, mean age, sex, and health status), intervention substance, control substance, intervention dose, and intervention duration. For studies that did not report the SD of the mean difference between the baseline and endpoint cardiometabolic risk factors, the SD of the mean difference was estimated by the formula SDchange = square root [(SDbaseline2 + SDendpoint2)/2] [27]. If the outcome data were presented as graphs, we used WebPlotDigitizer (https://automeris.io/WebPlotDigitizer/, accessed on 1 January 2024.) to estimate the values.

2.5. Quality Assessment

The evaluation of the risk of bias in the included trials was conducted per the recommendations of the Cochrane Collaboration Handbook [28], which included six domains: selection bias (random sequence generation and allocation concealment); performance bias (blinding of participants and personnel); detection bias (blinding of outcome assessment); attrition bias (incomplete outcome data); reporting bias (selective reporting), and other bias.

The GRADE (Grading of Recommendations, Assessment, Development, and Evaluation) approach was used to assess the quality of evidence, graded as high, moderate, low, or very low [29]. The initial GRADE quality score defaults to high and would then be downgraded according to pre-specified fields, including the risk of bias (over 20%), inconsistency ($I^2 > 50\%$ and Pheterogeneity < 0.1), indirectness (presence of limitations to the universalization of the results), imprecision (95% confidence intervals (CIs) overlapped with the minimally important difference, i.e., 2 mmHg for blood pressure [30], 0.1 mol/L for blood lipids [31], 0.5% for A1C [32], 0.56 mmol/L or 10 mg/dL for FBG [33], and 5 pmol/L for FBI [34]), and publication bias (significant evidence of small study effects).

2.6. Statistical Analysis

The mean differences in specific cardiometabolic risk factors between intervention and control groups and the SDs were used as the basis for each trial comparison. The effect size was evaluated according to the Cochrane guidelines [27]. The random effects model was used to generate an effect size for cardiometabolic risk factors, expressed as the weighted mean difference and 95% CI. Heterogeneity was estimated among the included studies using I2 statistics. The significance for heterogeneity was set at $p < 0.05$, with an I2 > 50%, which was considered to be evidence of substantial heterogeneity [35,36]. Subgroup analyses were performed based on different cardiometabolic health statuses of the participants included in the trials. Possible publication bias was evaluated by visual inspection of funnel plots and Egger's linear regression test ($p < 0.05$ indicates the presence of publication bias [37]). Sensitivity analyses were performed to assess the effect of individual studies on pooled effect sizes by omitting one study at a time [38]. RevMan (version 5.4) and Stata/SE (version 17.0) software were applied to all statistical analyses.

3. Results

3.1. Study Selection and Characteristics of Included Trials

The selection process of this study is summarized as a flow chart in Figure 1. A total of 5853 articles were identified through the combined search. Of the remaining 2545 articles, 2107 were identified as unrelated after reviewing for titles and abstracts, while 438 were reviewed and evaluated for suitability. Studies lacking randomization (*n* = 97), relevant outcomes (*n* = 136), or consisting of participants with severe disorders (*n* = 51) were excluded, leaving 130 articles (161 studies) from which to extract and analyze data. Characteristics of covered trials are outlined in Supplementary Materials.

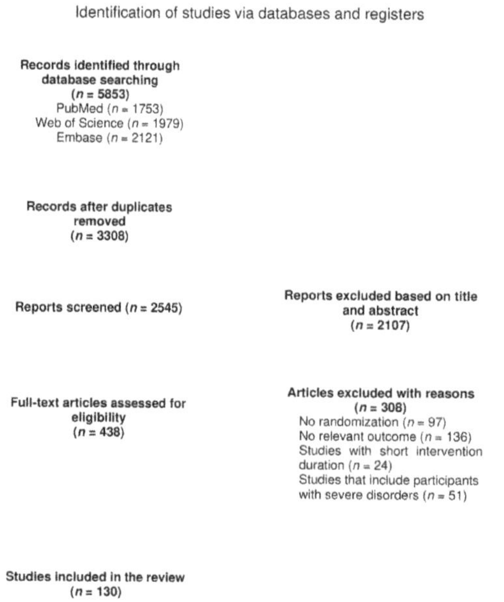

Figure 1. Flow chart of study selection.

The current analysis involved 161 studies with a total of 12,307 participants aged 18–75 years (median age: 49.0 years). The included studies were conducted in participants intervened with n-3 fatty acid (*n* = 89), n-6 fatty acid (*n* = 23), n-9 fatty acid (*n* = 16), lycopene (*n* = 15), astaxanthin (*n* = 9), and beta-carotene (*n* = 6). The intervention lasted from 2 weeks to 5 years.

3.2. Effect of Antioxidant Lipid Supplementations on Blood Pressure

Ninety-seven eligible RCTs involving 8576 participants were included to investigate the effects of antioxidant lipid supplementations on blood pressure (Figure 2). Lycopene supplementation decreased systolic blood pressure (−1.95 [−3.54, −0.36] mmHg) in the total population. No other lipid supplementations displayed an effect on blood pressure in the total population.

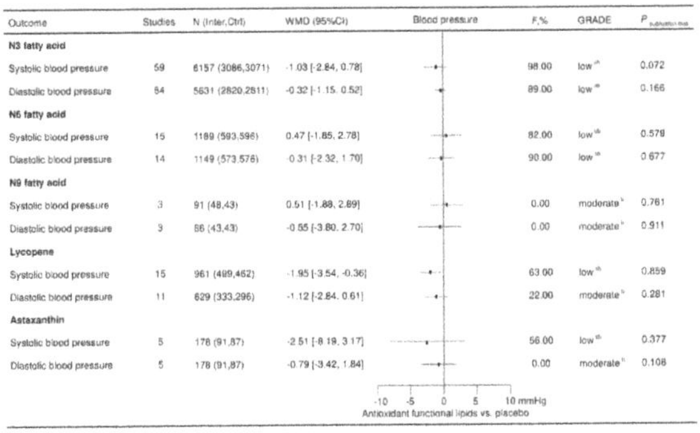

Figure 2. Effects of antioxidant lipid supplementations on blood pressure. Ctrl—control group; Inter—intervention group; SBP—systolic blood pressure; DBP—diastolic blood pressure; WMD—weighted mean difference; I^2—values for between-study heterogeneity; [a]—rated down for inconsistency; and [b]—rated down for imprecision.

3.3. Effect of Antioxidant Lipid Supplementations on Blood Lipids

A total of 119 eligible RCTs involving 8001 participants were included to assess the effects of antioxidant lipid supplementations on blood lipids (Figure 3). In the total population, n3 fatty acid significantly decreased TG (−0.37 [−0.47, −0.28] mmol/L); n6 fatty acid significantly improved LDL-C (−0.39 [−0.71, −0.06] mmol/L), HDL-C (0.08 [0.01, 0.14] mmol/L), and TC (−0.24 [−0.37, −0.11] mmol/L); astaxanthin significantly improved LDL-C (−0.11 [−0.21, −0.01] mmol/L), HDL-C (0.13 [0.05, 0.21] mmol/L), TC (−0.22 [−0.32, −0.12] mmol/L), and TG (−0.46 [−0.83, −0.10] mmol/L); beta-carotene significantly decreased TC (−0.13 [−0.23, −0.04] mmol/L); and notably, n9 fatty acid improved TG (0.06 [0.01, 0.11] mmol/L) in the total population.

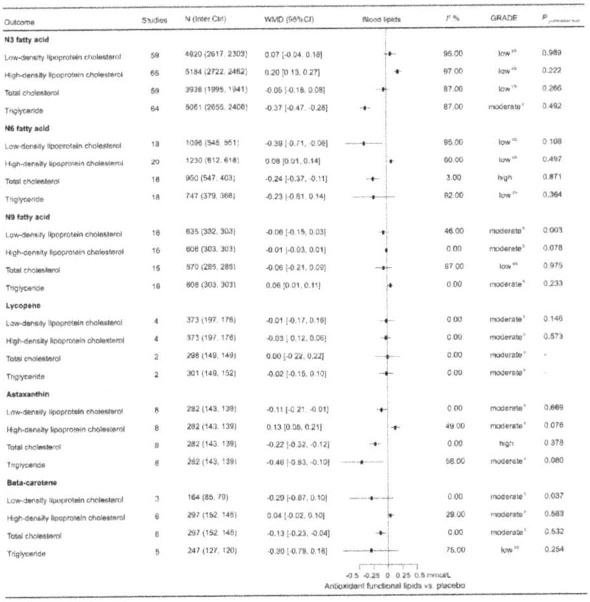

Figure 3. Effects of antioxidant lipid supplementations on blood pressure. Ctrl—control group; Inter—intervention group; SBP—systolic blood pressure; DBP—diastolic blood pressure; WMD—weighted mean difference; I^2—values for between-study heterogeneity; [a]—rated down for inconsistency; and [b]—rated down for imprecision.

3.4. *Effect of Antioxidant Lipid Supplementations on Glycemic Status*

Seventy-six eligible RCTs involving 4518 participants were included to assess the effect of antioxidant functional lipid supplementations on glycemic status (Figure 4). Astaxanthin improved FBI (−2.66 [−3.98, −1.34] pmol/L) in the total population. Notably, n9 fatty acid increased A1C (0.04 [0.02, 0.06] %) in the total population. No other lipid supplementations displayed an effect on glycemic status in the total population.

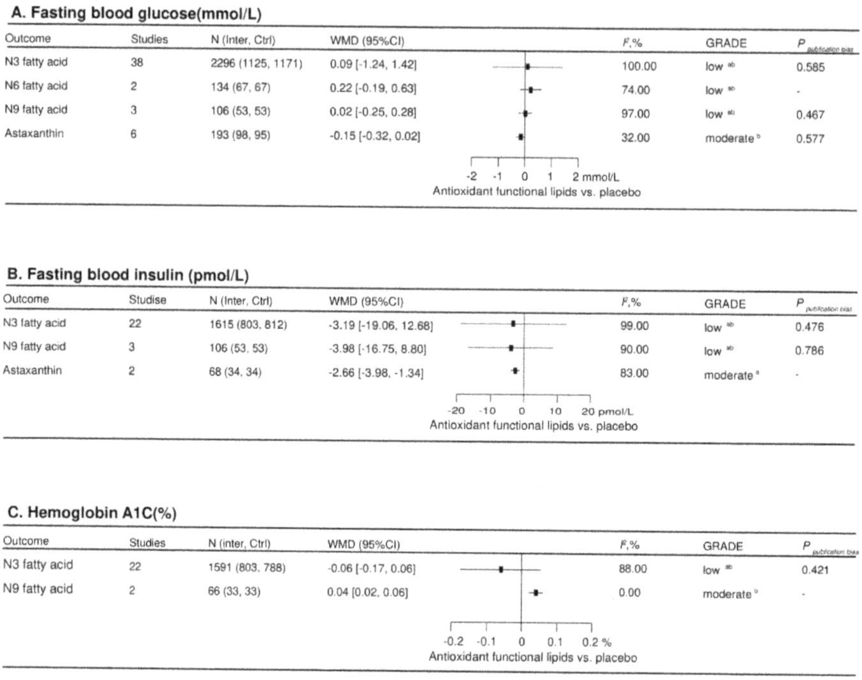

Figure 4. Effects of antioxidant lipid supplementations on glycemic control. Ctrl—control group; Inter—intervention group; FBG—fasting blood glucose; A1C—hemoglobin A1c; FBI—fasting blood insulin; WMD—weighted mean difference; I^2—values for between-study heterogeneity; [a]—rated down for inconsistency; and [b]—rated down for imprecision.

3.5. *Effect of Antioxidant Lipid Supplementations among Participants with Different Cardiometabolic Health Statuses*

Subgroup analysis of antioxidant lipid supplementations was performed in participants with different cardiometabolic health statuses (Figure 5). For healthy populations, antioxidant functional lipid supplementations improved HDL-C (0.03 [0.00, 0.06] mmol/L) and TG (−0.15 [−0.25, −0.06] mmol/L). For participants with pre-diabetes or T2D, antioxidant lipid supplementations improved HDL-C (0.28 [0.07,0.50] mmol/L) and TG (−0.26 [−0.27, −0.15] mmol/L). For hypertensive participants, antioxidant lipid supplementations improved TC (−0.40 [−0.68, −0.12] mmol/L). For dyslipidemia participants, antioxidant lipid supplementations improved DBP (−0.81 [−1.51, −0.10] mmHg), HDL-C (0.16 [0.08, 0.24] mmol/L), and TG (−0.56 [−0.81, −0.30] mmol/L). For participants with overweight or obesity, antioxidant lipid supplementations improved HDL-C (0.06 [0.02, 0.10] mmol/L) and TG (−0.13 [−0.24, −0.02] mmol/L). Lastly, antioxidant lipid supplementations improved DBP (−3.00 [−4.15, −1.85] mmHg) in participants with metabolic syndrome.

Cardiometabolic health	Blood pressure		Blood lipid				Blood glucose		
	SBP	DBP	LDL-C	HDL-C	TC	TG	FBG	FBI	A1C
Healthy	-0.80 [-2.99, 1.38]	0.64 [-0.80, 2.08]	-0.06 [-0.25, 0.12]	0.03 [0.00, 0.06]	-0.02 [-0.07, 0.04]	-0.15 [-0.25, -0.06]	0.16 [-0.05, 0.37]	-3.60 [-11.91, 4.71]	
Pre-T2D/T2D	0.54 [-2.45, 3.53]	-0.36 [-1.10, 0.37]	-0.02 [-0.04, 0.00]	0.29 [0.07, 0.50]	-0.21 [-0.54, 0.13]	-0.26 [-0.37, -0.15]	0.03 [-0.32, 0.38]	-7.37 [-24.11, 9.38]	-0.09 [-0.23, 0.06]
Hypertension	-1.81 [-4.14, 0.53]	-1.22 [-2.79, 0.35]	-0.28 [-0.60, 0.03]	-0.04 [-0.16, 0.08]	-0.40 [-0.68, -0.12]	-0.04 [-0.24, 0.15]			
Dyslipidemia	0.01 [-2.64, 2.66]	-0.81 [-1.51, -0.10]	-0.01 [-0.25, 0.22]	0.16 [0.08, 0.24]	0.01 [-0.14, 0.16]	-0.56 [-0.81, -0.30]	-0.58 [-2.46, 1.30]	-5.49 [-11.71, 0.73]	
Overweight/Obesity	-2.65 [-6.19, 0.89]	-1.57 [-5.58, 2.45]	-0.08 [-0.21, 0.06]	0.06 [0.02, 0.10]	-0.21 [-0.64, 0.22]	-0.13 [-0.24, -0.02]	-1.10 [-3.79, 1.60]	-4.45 [-16.84, 7.94]	
Metabolic syndrome	-2.76 [-7.60, 2.09]	-3.00 [-4.15, -1.85]	0.04 [-0.05, 0.13]	-0.00 [-0.04, 0.03]	-0.03 [-0.47, 0.40]	-0.55 [-1.24, 0.14]			

Benefit | Neutral

GRADE | High | Moderate | Low

Figure 5. Effects of antioxidant lipid supplementations on participants with different cardiometabolic health statuses. Subgroup analysis of antioxidant lipid supplementations was performed in healthy participants and participants with pre-type 2 diabetes (Pre-T2D)/T2D, hypertension, dyslipidemia, overweight/obesity, or metabolic syndrome.

4. Discussion

This study intended to provide a comprehensive analysis and identify appropriate antioxidant lipid supplementations to improve cardiometabolic health. Overall, our results suggest that n3 fatty acid, n6 fatty acid, lycopene, astaxanthin, and beta-carotene significantly improve cardiovascular risk factors, including SBP, all lipid profiles, and FBI in the total population (Figure 6). The benefits of antioxidant lipid supplementations appeared to be more pronounced in blood pressure and blood lipids in participants with different cardiometabolic health statuses. Particularly, n9 fatty acid was identified to increase TG and A1C in the total population in our results, which increases CVD risk and is not suggested to be over-consumed. This is probably attributed to excessive n9 fatty acid enhancing oxidative damage and inducing oxidative stress [39,40], though its specific molecular mechanism has not yet been elucidated.

Fatty acids	Blood pressure		Blood lipid				Blood glucose		
	SBP	DBP	LDL-C	HDL-C	TC	TG	FBG	FBI	A1C
N-3	•	•	•	•	•	▼	•	•	•
N-6	•	•	▼	▲	▼	•	•		
N-9	•	•	•	•	•	▲	•	•	▲
Lycopene	▼	•	•	•	•	•			
Astaxanthin	•	•	▼	▲	▼	▼	•	▼	
Beta-carotene			•	•	▼	•			

Benefit | Neutral | Harm

GRADE | High | Moderate | Low

▼ Decrease | ▲ Increase | • Unchange

Figure 6. An evidence-based map of antioxidant lipid supplementations on cardiometabolic health.

It has been reported that dietary intervention focused on n6 and n3 fatty acids may improve cardiovascular risk factors [41], which is consistent with our results. The current meta-analysis still supports that n3 fatty acid supplementation improves HDL-C and TG levels, probably through regulating the coding of different genes involved in lipid metabolic hemostasis at transcriptional and post-transcriptional levels [42]. For example, consumption of n3 fatty acid suppresses the transcription of the sterol regulatory element-binding protein gene, thereby inhibiting the de novo synthesis of TGs [43]. Similarly, n6 fatty acid supplementation improves HDL-C and TC levels, probably by contributing to cholesterol catabolism through upregulating the expression of the cholesterol 7α-hydroxylase gene, which encodes an enzyme that regulates the pathway for cholesterol to bile acids, via peroxisome proliferator-activated receptors [44]. In this study, n9 supplementation was found to increase TGs and A1C, which is inconsistent with previous findings [45].

Lycopene supplementation decreased SBP, which is consistent with previous findings [46,47]. The antihypertensive properties of lycopene are thought to derive from the stimulation of nitric oxide production by the vascular endothelium [48]. Nitric oxide exerts a complex effect on the modulation of local and systemic vascular resistance, blood flow distribution, as well as arterial pressure [49]. Previous studies reported a beneficial effect of astaxanthin on preventing diabetes and atherosclerosis [22,50]. This analysis underscores the protective role of astaxanthin supplementation in improving lipid profiles and insulin metabolism. As for blood lipids, astaxanthin increases hepatic LDL receptor levels and sterol regulatory element-binding protein 2, which modulates cholesterol metabolism [51]. Moreover, astaxanthin could improve insulin secretion by modulating impaired glucose metabolism and beta cell dysfunction through glucose transporter 4 regulation [52,53].

In this study, beta-carotene supplementation showed a beneficial effect on TC in the total population. However, some studies demonstrated that beta-carotene had potentially harmful effects on CVD mortality and cancer incidence in smokers. The potential explanation is that beta-carotene offers several therapeutic effects as a provitamin A, including an antioxidant effect to neutralize reactive oxygen species and regulate connexin expression, thereby improving communication through gap junctions [54]. However, in some conditions, such as high oxygen concentrations in smokers, beta-carotene turns into a pro-oxidant, generating beta-carotene radical cations that require vitamin C for repair [55]. Due to low serum levels of vitamin C in smokers, beta-carotene radicals may contribute to an increased risk of CVDs and cancer [56].

The association between antioxidant supplementation and cardiovascular disease prevention has been controversial. To date, analyses of certain well-designed studies and some preclinical studies have led to the hypothesis that supplementation with pure free radical scavengers may not be sufficient to produce beneficial effects in pre-protective models [57]. Therefore, only compounds that are capable of influencing oxidative stress through more than one pathway or have pleiotropic properties can produce significant clinical effects. This is supported by a number of basic studies that suggest that the heavy use of certain free radical scavengers may exacerbate, rather than alleviate, oxidative stress [45,57]. The results of previous studies suggest that the preventive effect of supplements on cardiovascular disease will be proportional to the pleiotropic level of the substance administered [45]. Specifically, n-3 fatty acids, followed by folic acid and coenzyme Q10, showed beneficial effects, whereas scavengers with lower pleiotropic effects, such as vitamins C and E, did not alter the results, whereas some pure free radical scavengers with minimal cardiovascular pleiotropic effects, such as beta-carotene, worsened the results, which is also consistent with our findings.

5. Study Limitations and Conclusions

Several limitations need to be considered when interpreting results from current analyses. First, in this study, there was a lack of evidence regarding the improvement in cardiovascular outcome events and incidence of T2D, which leaves uncertainty as to whether antioxidant functional lipid supplementations also ameliorated the occurrence of CVD events. Second, the heterogeneity of included studies was high due to limitations of the number and sample size, variation in intervention duration between studies, wide study time range, as well as the low-quality evidence of some RCTs, although trials with intervention durations of less than 1 week were excluded from our analysis. Thirdly, owing to the lack of RCTs, some antioxidant functional lipid supplementations were not included in the current analysis, including dietary β-ketones with biologically relevant antioxidant activity and palmitoleic acid (16:1 n-7), known to reduce atherosclerotic lesions. Moreover, since the intervention period of the existing RCTs is short (median 12 weeks), it is unknown whether long-term administration will cause health hazards. At present, there are still many uncertainties and controversies regarding the recommendation of antioxidant functional lipid supplementations for the adjunct treatment of patients with T2D due to inconsistent and insufficient clinical results. Well-designed, high-quality, large, and long-term studies are needed to strengthen the existing evidence on the efficacy of antioxidant functional lipid supplementations in modulating cardiometabolic risk factors.

Ultimately, antioxidant functional lipid supplementations, except n9 fatty acid, exert beneficial effects on blood pressure, blood lipids, and glycemic parameters in the total population. The benefits of antioxidant functional lipid supplementations appeared to be most evidenced in blood pressure and blood lipids in participants with different cardiometabolic health statuses. Our findings highlight the importance of antioxidant functional lipid diversity and the balance of benefits and risks. Considerations should also be given to administering higher doses and longer durations when designing personalized intervention strategies aimed at enhancing cardiometabolic health. From the perspective of research, it should be noted that although current information opens up the prospect of consolidating the role of antioxidant lipids in preventive cardiology in the future, there is still a long way to go in providing evidence. In terms of routine clinical practice, these results are beginning to open up space for incorporating new tools into the therapeutic armory aimed at preventing cardiovascular disease in specific populations.

Supplementary Materials: The following supporting information can be downloaded at: https://www.mdpi.com/article/10.3390/nu16142213/s1.

Author Contributions: All authors contributed to the study's conception and design. Y.L., Y.Z. (Yinhua Zhu) and J.L. conceived and designed the study. S.W., W.W., Y.Z. (Yan Zhang), J.H., X.W. and P.A. were involved in the data collection. S.W., W.W. and Y.Z. (Yan Zhang) compiled the data before analysis. S.W., W.W. and J.H. conducted data analysis. S.W., W.W., J.H. and X.W. drafted the manuscript. Y.L., Y.Z. (Yinhua Zhu), J.L. and P.A. revised the manuscript. All authors have read and agreed to the published version of the manuscript.

Funding: This work was supported by the National Key R&D Program of China (2023YFF1103501).

Data Availability Statement: The original contributions presented in the study are included in the article/Supplementary Materials, further inquiries can be directed to the corresponding authors.

Acknowledgments: We thank those who conducted the data collection and our collaborators who contributed to this study.

Conflicts of Interest: Author X.W. was employed by the company Zhejiang Medicine Co., Ltd. The remaining authors declare that the research was conducted in the absence of any commercial or financial relationships that could be construed as potential conflicts of interest.

References

1. Powell-Wiley, T.M.; Poirier, P.; Burke, L.E.; Després, J.-P.; Gordon-Larsen, P.; Lavie, C.J.; Lear, S.A.; Ndumele, C.E.; Neeland, I.J.; Sanders, P.; et al. Obesity and Cardiovascular Disease: A Scientific Statement from the American Heart Association. *Circulation* **2021**, *143*, e984–e1010. [CrossRef] [PubMed]
2. Stefan, N.; Schulze, M.B. Metabolic health and cardiometabolic risk clusters: Implications for prediction, prevention, and treatment. *Lancet Diabetes Endocrinol.* **2023**, *11*, 426–440. [CrossRef] [PubMed]
3. Vo, V.; Lopez, G.; Malay, S.; Roman, Y.M. Cardiovascular Risk Factors Among Asian Americans: Perspectives on the Role of Acculturation in Cardiovascular Diseases Health Disparities. *J. Immigr. Minor. Health* **2024**, *26*, 409–420. [CrossRef]
4. Rosei, C.A.; Del Pinto, R.; Grassi, G.; Muiesan, M.L.; Ferri, C. Prevalence of Cardiovascular Risk Factors and Related Medical and Lifestyle Interventions Among Italian Cardiovascular Specialists: A Proof-of-Concept Study. *High Blood Press. Cardiovasc. Prev.* **2023**, *30*, 255–264. [CrossRef] [PubMed]
5. Chen, J.X.; Zhou, Y.F.; Geng, T.; Chen, S.; Chen, S.; Wang, G.; Zhang, Y.-B.; Wang, Y.; Tu, Z.-Z.; Liu, G.; et al. Low Concordance Between Blood Pressures Measured in Periodic Health Examinations and in a Workplace-Based Hypertension Management Program. *Phenomics* **2022**, *2*, 419–429. [CrossRef] [PubMed]
6. GBD 2017 Diet Collaborators. Health effects of dietary risks in 195 countries, 1990–2017: A systematic analysis for the Global Burden of Disease Study 2017. *Lancet* **2019**, *393*, 1958–1972. [CrossRef]
7. García-Lluch, G.; Pardo, J.; Moreno, L.; Peña-Bautista, C.; Baquero, M.; Cháfer-Pericás, C. Cardiovascular Risk Scales Association with Cerebrospinal Fluid Alzheimer's Disease Biomarkers in Cardiovascular Low Cardiovascular Risk Regions. *J. Prev. Alzheimer's Dis.* **2024**, *11*, 453–462. [CrossRef] [PubMed]

8. Deng, X.; Wang, J.; Yu, S.; Tan, S.; Yu, T.; Xu, Q.; Chen, N.; Zhang, S.; Zhang, M.; Hu, K.; et al. Advances in the treatment of atherosclerosis with ligand-modified nanocarriers. *Exploration* **2023**, *4*, 20230090. [CrossRef] [PubMed]
9. Alabdulkarim, B.; Bakeet, Z.A.N.; Arzoo, S. Role of some functional lipids in preventing diseases and promoting health. *J. King Saud Univ. Sci.* **2012**, *24*, 319–329. [CrossRef]
10. Hu, Q.; Fang, Z.; Ge, J.; Li, H. Nanotechnology for cardiovascular diseases. *Innovation* **2022**, *3*, 100214. [CrossRef] [PubMed]
11. Zhang, B.; Luo, W.; Cai, Y.; Liu, L.; Ma, X.; Yang, W.; Meng, S.; Zhao, G.; Sun, A.; Ge, J.; et al. Global burden of adolescent and young adult cardiovascular diseases and risk factors: Results from Global Burden of Disease Study 2019. *Innov. Med.* **2024**, *2*, 100063. [CrossRef]
12. Tribble, D.L. AHA Science Advisory. Antioxidant consumption and risk of coronary heart disease: Emphasison vitamin C.; vitamin E.; and beta-carotene: A statement for healthcare professionals from the American Heart Association. *Circulation* **1999**, *99*, 591–595. [CrossRef] [PubMed]
13. Aune, D.; Keum, N.; Giovannucci, E.; Fadnes, L.T.; Boffetta, P.; Greenwood, D.C.; Tonstad, S.; Vatten, L.J.; Riboli, E.; Norat, T. Dietary intake and blood concentrations of antioxidants and the risk of cardiovascular disease, total cancer, and all-cause mortality: A systematic review and dose-response meta-analysis of prospective studies. *Am. J. Clin. Nutr.* **2018**, *108*, 1069–1091. [CrossRef] [PubMed]
14. Samimi, M.; Jamilian, M.; Asemi, Z.; Esmaillzadeh, A. Effects of omega-3 fatty acid supplementation on insulin metabolism and lipid profiles in gestational diabetes: Randomized, double-blind, placebo-controlled trial. *Clin. Nutr.* **2015**, *34*, 388–393. [CrossRef] [PubMed]
15. Ide, K.; Koshizaka, M.; Tokuyama, H.; Tokuyama, T.; Ishikawa, T.; Maezawa, Y.; Takemoto, M.; Yokote, K. N-3 polyunsaturated fatty acids improve lipoprotein particle size and concentration in Japanese patients with type 2 diabetes and hypertriglyceridemia: A pilot study. *Lipids Health Dis.* **2018**, *17*, 51. [CrossRef] [PubMed]
16. Miller, E.R., 3rd; Juraschek, S.P.; Anderson, C.A.; Guallar, E.; Henoch-Ryugo, K.; Charleston, J.; Turban, S.; Bennett, M.R.; Appel, L.J. The effects of n-3 long-chain polyunsaturated fatty acid supplementation on biomarkers of kidney injury in adults with diabetes: Results of the GO-FISH trial. *Diabetes Care* **2013**, *36*, 1462–1469. [CrossRef] [PubMed]
17. Huang, Q.; Hu, Z.; Zheng, Q.; Mao, X.; Lv, W.; Wu, F.; Fu, D.; Lu, C.; Zeng, C.; Wang, F.; et al. A Proactive Intervention Study in Metabolic Syndrome High-Risk Populations Using Phenome-Based Actionable P4 Medicine Strategy. *Phenomics* **2024**, *4*, 91–108. [CrossRef] [PubMed]
18. SCEND Study Collaborative Group. Effects of n-3 Fatty Acid Supplements in Diabetes Mellitus. *N. Engl. J. Med.* **2018**, *379*, 1540–1550. [CrossRef] [PubMed]
19. Limonte, C.P.; Zelnick, L.R.; Ruzinski, J.; Hoofnagle, A.N.; Thadhani, R.; Melamed, M.L.; Lee, I.-M.; Buring, J.E.; Sesso, H.D.; Manson, J.E.; et al. Effects of long-term vitamin D and n-3 fatty acid supplementation on inflammatory and cardiac biomarkers in patients with type 2 diabetes: Secondary analyses from a randomised controlled trial. *Diabetologia* **2021**, *64*, 437–447. [CrossRef] [PubMed]
20. McEneny, J.; Wade, L.; Young, I.S.; Masson, L.; Duthie, G.; McGinty, A.; McMaster, C.; Thies, F. Lycopene intervention reduces inflammation and improves HDL functionality in moderately overweight middle-aged individuals. *J. Nutr. Biochem.* **2013**, *24*, 163–168. [CrossRef]
21. Thies, F.; Masson, L.F.; Rudd, A.; Vaughan, N.; Tsang, C.; Brittenden, J.; Simpson, W.G.; Duthie, S.; Horgan, G.W.; Duthie, G. Effect of a tomato-rich diet on markers of cardiovascular disease risk in moderately overweight, disease-free, middle-aged adults: A randomized controlled trial. *Am. J. Clin. Nutr.* **2012**, *95*, 1013–1022. [CrossRef] [PubMed]
22. Saeidi, A.; Nouri-Habashi, A.; Razi, O.; Ataeinosrat, A.; Rahmani, H.; Mollabashi, S.S.; Bagherzadeh-Rahmani, B.; Aghdam, S.M.; Khalajzadeh, L.; Al Kiyumi, M.H.; et al. Astaxanthin Supplemented with High-Intensity Functional Training Decreases Adipokines Levels and Cardiovascular Risk Factors in Men with Obesity. *Nutrients* **2023**, *15*, 286. [CrossRef] [PubMed]
23. Coombes, J.S.; Sharman, J.E.; Fassett, R.G. Astaxanthin has no effect on arterial stiffness, oxidative stress, or inflammation in renal transplant recipients: A randomized controlled trial (the XANTHIN trial). *Am. J. Clin. Nutr.* **2016**, *103*, 283–289. [CrossRef] [PubMed]
24. Asemi, Z.; Alizadeh, S.-A.; Ahmad, K.; Goli, M.; Esmaillzadeh, A. Effects of beta-carotene fortified synbiotic food on metabolic control of patients with type 2 diabetes mellitus: A double-blind randomized cross-over controlled clinical trial. *Clin. Nutr.* **2016**, *35*, 819–825. [CrossRef] [PubMed]
25. Ribaya-Mercado, J.D.; Ordovas, J.M.; Russell, R.M. Effect of beta-carotene supplementation on the concentrations and distribution of carotenoids, vitamin E, vitamin A, and cholesterol in plasma lipoprotein and non-lipoprotein fractions in healthy older women. *J. Am. Coll. Nutr.* **1995**, *14*, 614–620. [CrossRef] [PubMed]
26. Shamseer, L.; Moher, D.; Clarke, M.; Ghersi, D.; Liberati, A.; Petticrew, M.; Shekelle, P.; Stewart, L.A.; The PRISMA-P Group. Preferred reporting items for systematic review and meta-analysis protocols (PRISMA-P) 2015: Elaboration and explanation. *BMJ* **2015**, *350*, g7647. [CrossRef] [PubMed]
27. Riley, R.D.; Lambert, P.C.; Abo-Zaid, G. Meta-analysis of individual participant data: Rationale, conduct, and reporting. *BMJ* **2010**, *340*, c221. [CrossRef] [PubMed]
28. Cumpston, M.; Li, T.; Page, M.J.; Chandler, J.; Welch, V.A.; Higgins, J.P.; Thomas, J. Updated guidance for trusted systematic reviews: A new edition of the Cochrane Handbook for Systematic Reviews of Interventions. *Cochrane Database Syst. Rev.* **2019**, *10*, Ed000142. [CrossRef] [PubMed]
29. Guyatt, G.H.; Oxman, A.D.; Vist, G.E.; Kunz, R.; Falck-Ytter, Y.; Alonso-Coello, P.; Schünemann, H.J. GRADE: An emerging consensus on rating quality of evidence and strength of recommendations. *BMJ* **2008**, *336*, 924–926. [CrossRef]
30. Appel, L.J.; Brands, M.W.; Daniels, S.R.; Karanja, N.; Elmer, P.J.; Sacks, F.M. Dietary approaches to prevent and treat hypertension: A scientific statement from the American Heart Association. *Hypertension* **2006**, *47*, 296–308. [CrossRef]

31. Langsted, A.; Freiberg, J.J.; Nordestgaard, B.G. Fasting and nonfasting lipid levels: Influence of normal food intake on lipids.; lipoproteins, apolipoproteins.; and cardiovascular risk prediction. *Circulation* **2008**, *118*, 2047–2056. [CrossRef] [PubMed]
32. Lenters-Westra, E.; Schindhelm, R.K.; Bilo, H.J.G.; Groenier, K.H.; Slingerland, R.J. Differences in interpretation of haemoglobin A1c values among diabetes care professionals. *Neth. J. Med.* **2014**, *72*, 462–466. [PubMed]
33. Wei, M.; Gibbons, L.W.; Mitchell, T.L.; Kampert, J.B.; Stern, M.P.; Blair, S.N. Low fasting plasma glucose level as a predictor of cardiovascular disease and all-cause mortality. *Circulation* **2000**, *101*, 2047–2052. [CrossRef] [PubMed]
34. Chiavaroli, L.; Lee, D.; Ahmed, A.; Cheung, A.; Khan, T.A.; Mejia, S.B.; Mirrahimi, A.; Jenkins, D.J.A.; Livesey, G.; Wolever, T.M.S.; et al. Effect of low glycaemic index or load dietary patterns on glycaemic control and cardiometabolic risk factors in diabetes: Systematic review and meta-analysis of randomised controlled trials. *BMJ* **2021**, *374*, n1651. [CrossRef] [PubMed]
35. Higgins, J.P.; Thompson, S.G.; Deeks, J.J.; Altman, D.G. Measuring inconsistency in meta-analyses. *BMJ* **2003**, *327*, 557–560. [CrossRef] [PubMed]
36. Jackson, D.; White, I.R.; Riley, R.D. Quantifying the impact of between-study heterogeneity in multivariate meta-analyses. *Stat. Med.* **2012**, *31*, 3805–3820. [CrossRef] [PubMed]
37. Egger, M.; Smith, G.D.; Schneider, M.; Minder, C. Bias in meta-analysis detected by a simple, graphical test. *BMJ* **1997**, *315*, 629–634. [CrossRef] [PubMed]
38. Tobias, A. Assessing the influence of a single study in the meta-analysis estimate. *Stata Tech. Bull.* **1998**, *47*, 15–17.
39. Yu, Q.; Liu, Y.; Wu, Y.; Chen, Y. Dihydrocurcumin ameliorates the lipid accumulation.; oxidative stress and insulin resistance in oleic acid-induced L02 and HepG2 cells. *Biomed. Pharmacother.* **2018**, *103*, 1327–1336. [CrossRef] [PubMed]
40. Zhang, H.; Wang, J.; Yang, L.; Yang, W.; Luo, T.; Yuan, Y.; Gu, J.; Zou, H.; Bian, J.; Liu, Z.; et al. Effect of oleic acid on induction of steatosis and cytotoxicity in BRL 3A cells. *J. Cell. Biochem.* **2019**, *120*, 19541–19554. [CrossRef] [PubMed]
41. Lee, S.P.S.; Dart, A.M.; Walker, K.Z.; O'Dea, K.; Chin-Dusting, J.P.F.; Skilton, M.R. Effect of altering dietary *n*-6:*n*-3 PUFA ratio on cardiovascular risk measures in patients treated with statins: A pilot study. *Br. J. Nutr.* **2012**, *108*, 1280–1285. [CrossRef] [PubMed]
42. Gnoni, A.; Giudetti, A.M. Dietary long-chain unsaturated fatty acids acutely and differently reduce the activities of lipogenic enzymes and of citrate carrier in rat liver. *J. Physiol. Biochem.* **2016**, *72*, 485–494. [CrossRef] [PubMed]
43. Tang, M.; Floyd, S.; Cai, H.; Zhang, M.; Yang, R.; Dang, R. The status of ω-3 PUFAs influence chronic unpredicted mild stress-induced metabolic side effects in rats through INSIG/SREBP pathway. *Food Funct.* **2019**, *10*, 4649–4660. [CrossRef] [PubMed]
44. Froyen, E.; Burns-Whitmore, B. The Effects of Linoleic Acid Consumption on Lipid Risk Markers for Cardiovascular Disease in Healthy Individuals: A Review of Human Intervention Trials. *Nutrients* **2020**, *12*, 2329. [CrossRef] [PubMed]
45. An, P.; Wan, S.; Luo, Y.; Luo, J.; Zhang, X.; Zhou, S.; Xu, T.; He, J.; Mechanick, J.I.; Wu, W.-C.; et al. Micronutrient Supplementation to Reduce Cardiovascular Risk. *J. Am. Coll. Cardiol.* **2022**, *80*, 2269–2285. [CrossRef]
46. Gajendragadkar, P.R.; Hubsch, A.; Mäki-Petäjä, K.M.; Serg, M.; Wilkinson, I.B.; Cheriyan, J. Effects of oral lycopene supplementation on vascular function in patients with cardiovascular disease and healthy volunteers: A randomised controlled trial. *PLoS ONE* **2014**, *9*, e99070. [CrossRef] [PubMed]
47. Wolak, T.; Sharoni, Y.; Levy, J.; Linnewiel-Hermoni, K.; Stepensky, D.; Paran, E. Effect of Tomato Nutrient Complex on Blood Pressure: A Double Blind, Randomized Dose-Response Study. *Nutrients* **2019**, *11*, 950. [CrossRef] [PubMed]
48. Umans, J.G.; Levi, R. Nitric oxide in the regulation of blood flow and arterial pressure. *Annu. Rev. Physiol.* **1995**, *57*, 771–790. [CrossRef]
49. Förstermann, U.; Sessa, W.C. Nitric oxide synthases: Regulation and function. *Eur. Heart J.* **2012**, *33*, 829–837. [CrossRef] [PubMed]
50. Urakaze, M.; Kobashi, C.; Satou, Y.; Shigeta, K.; Toshima, M.; Takagi, M.; Takahashi, J.; Nishida, H. The Beneficial Effects of Astaxanthin on Glucose Metabolism and Modified Low-Density Lipoprotein in Healthy Volunteers and Subjects with Prediabetes. *Nutrients* **2021**, *13*, 4381. [CrossRef] [PubMed]
51. Yang, Y.; Seo, J.M.; Nguyen, A.; Pham, T.X.; Park, H.J.; Park, Y.; Kim, B.; Bruno, R.S.; Lee, J. Astaxanthin-rich extract from the green alga *Haematococcus pluvialis* lowers plasma lipid concentrations and enhances antioxidant defense in apolipoprotein E knockout mice. *J. Nutr.* **2011**, *141*, 1611–1617. [CrossRef] [PubMed]
52. Bhuvaneswari, S.; Anuradha, C.V. Astaxanthin prevents loss of insulin signaling and improves glucose metabolism in liver of insulin resistant mice. *Can. J. Physiol. Pharmacol.* **2012**, *90*, 1544–1552. [CrossRef] [PubMed]
53. Ishiki, M.; Nishida, Y.; Ishibashi, H.; Wada, T.; Fujisaka, S.; Takikawa, A.; Urakaze, M.; Sasaoka, T.; Usui, I.; Tobe, K. Impact of divergent effects of astaxanthin on insulin signaling in L6 cells. *Endocrinology* **2013**, *154*, 2600–2612. [CrossRef] [PubMed]
54. Chen, Q.H.; Wu, B.K.; Pan, D.; Sang, L.X.; Chang, B. Beta-carotene and its protective effect on gastric cancer. *World J. Clin. Cases* **2021**, *9*, 6591–6607. [CrossRef] [PubMed]
55. Palozza, P. Prooxidant actions of carotenoids in biologic systems. *Nutr. Rev.* **1998**, *56*, 257–265. [CrossRef] [PubMed]
56. Truscott, T.G. Beta-carotene and disease: A suggested pro-oxidant and anti-oxidant mechanism and speculations concerning its role in cigarette smoking. *J. Photochem. Photobiol. B* **1996**, *35*, 233–235. [CrossRef] [PubMed]
57. Gormaz, J.G.; Carrasco, R. Antioxidant Supplementation in Cardiovascular Prevention: New Challenges in the Face of New Evidence. *J. Am. Coll. Cardiol.* **2022**, *80*, 2286–2288. [CrossRef] [PubMed]

nutrients

MDPI

Article

Sex and Age Differences in the Effects of Food Frequency on Metabolic Parameters in Japanese Adults

Katsumi Iizuka [1,2,*], Kotone Yanagi [3], Kanako Deguchi [1], Chihiro Ushiroda [1], Risako Yamamoto-Wada [1], Kazuko Kobae [3], Yoshiko Yamada [3] and Hiroyuki Naruse [3,4]

1 Department of Clinical Nutrition, Fujita Health University, Toyoake 470-1192, Japan; kanasakuran@gmail.com (K.D.); chihiro.ushiroda@fujita-hu.ac.jp (C.U.); risako.wada@fujita-hu.ac.jp (R.Y.-W.)
2 Food and Nutrition Service Department, Fujita Health University Hospital, Toyoake 470-1192, Japan
3 Health Management Center, Fujita Health University, Toyoake 470-1192, Japan; yanagi-k@fujita-hu.ac.jp (K.Y.); kobae@fujita-hu.ac.jp (K.K.); yoshiko.yamada@fujita-hu.ac.jp (Y.Y.); hnaruse@fujita-hu.ac.jp (H.N.)
4 Department of Medical Laboratory Science, Fujita Health University Graduate School of Health Sciences, Toyoake 4470-1192, Japan
* Correspondence: katsumi.iizuka@fujita-hu.ac.jp; Tel.: +81-562-93-2329

Abstract: Owing to differences in dietary preferences between men and women, the associations between dietary intake frequency and metabolic parameters may differ between the sexes. A retrospective observational study of the checkup findings of 3147 Japanese individuals (968 men, 2179 women) aged 20–59 years was conducted to examine differences in dietary habits and associations between food frequency and blood parameters (eGFR, HbA1c, uric acid, and lipids) by sex and age. Males were more likely to consume meat, fish, soft drinks, and alcohol, whereas women were more likely to consume soybeans, dairy products, vegetables, fruits, and snacks. Multivariate linear regression models adjusted for age and BMI revealed that meat intake frequency was positively associated with HbA1c ($\beta = 0.007$, $p = 0.03$) and negatively associated with eGFR ($\beta = -0.3$, $p = 0.01$) only in males, whereas fish intake frequency was positively associated with eGFR ($\beta = 0.4$, $p = 0.005$) only in females. Egg and soy intake frequencies were positively and negatively associated with non-HDL-C (egg: $\beta = 0.6$, $p = 0.02$; soy: $\beta = -0.3$, $p = 0.03$) only in females. Alcohol consumption frequency was associated with uric acid (M: $\beta = 0.06$, $p < 0.001$; F: $\beta = 0.06$, $p < 0.001$) and HDL-C (M: $\beta = 1.0$, $p < 0.001$; F: $\beta = 1.3$, $p < 0.001$) in both sexes. Future research is needed to determine whether varying the emphasis of dietary guidance by sex and age group is effective, since the effects of dietary preferences on metabolic parameters vary by age and sex.

Keywords: dietary preference; food frequency; BMI; uric acid; HbA1c; eGFR; triglyceride; HDL-C; non-HDL-C

1. Introduction

Eating habits and food preferences affect cognitive function, learning, body size, and the development of lifestyle-related diseases [1–12]. Eating habits included the frequency of meals, meal content, time taken to eat a meal, and the number of times the food was chewed. Dietary variety has been reported to be associated with cognitive function, chronic kidney disease, dental health, and all-cause mortality [13,14]. Dietary variety also reflects diet quality. Therefore, the greater the dietary variety is, the more types of nutrients are consumed.

Food preferences are influenced by many factors, including culture, age, and sex. The relationship between food preference and sex has also been documented [3–11]. Men prefer red and processed meats, whereas women tend to prefer vegetables, whole grains, tofu, and dark chocolate with a high cacao content, which is consistent with healthier food choices [1]. Women prefer whole grains, vegetables, and salty foods, whereas men consume more meat [2]. In terms of sugar intake, women tend to consume more sugar in their diets than men do [15]. In contrast, men consumed more alcoholic beverages than women did. Age is also an important factor that affects food preferences. Older adults tend to consume fewer energy-dense sweets and fast foods and consume more energy-dilute grains, vegetables, and fruits. The daily volume of food and beverages also decreases with age [16]. Therefore, dietary counseling for patients should consider differences in dietary preferences based on sex and age.

Dietary education in the workplace has not yet been adequately implemented in Japan. In France, work engagement has a positive relationship with the daily consumption of healthy food items [17]. However, in recent years, the concept of human capital has spread throughout Japan, creating a climate where companies are actively involved in disease prevention. The concept of health management emphasizes the importance of sleep debt [18,19]. Sleep debt worsens glucose tolerance, decreases thyrotropin levels, elevates cortisol levels in the evening, and decreases sympathetic tone [20].

The Food Frequency Questionnaire on Food Groups (FFQg), which was specifically created for the Japanese population, has often been used in Japan [21]. However, it has been used without considering sex differences in food preferences. Sex- and age-specific advice on the consumption of these 10 foods would compensate for the shortcomings of the guidelines, which arise from sex and age differences in food preferences.

The aim of this study was to determine the effects of food frequency on metabolic parameters, in terms of sex and age. For three thousand individuals aged 20–59 years, we first compared the differences in dietary preferences by age and sex. To clarify whether sex differences in food preference affect glucose and lipid metabolism, we examined the associations between food preference and blood parameters. This study not only reveals differences in food preferences by sex and age among health checkup recipients but also provides dietary guidance on the basis of sex differences in eating habits.

2. Materials and Methods

2.1. Study Design and Participants

This retrospective cross-sectional observational study aimed to clarify the associations between food frequency and metabolic parameters with reference to sex and age. The target population consisted of 968 men and 2179 women who had undergone a medical checkup by 2023 and had responded to the dietary questionnaire. The physical data and food frequency questionnaire were provided by the healthcare center at our university in a fully anonymized form, such that they were depersonalized (accessed on 26 March 2024).

2.2. Food Frequency Questionnaire on Food Groups

During the medical examination, the FFQg was used for dietary questions [21]. The FFQg is one of the most widely used food intake frequency questionnaires in Japan [22–25]. The FFQg included information on the frequency of eating 10 different food types (meat, fish, eggs, dairy products, soya, green vegetables, soya, green vegetables, seaweed, fruits, potatoes, oils, and fats), the frequency of drinking sugar-sweetened coffee and tea, and the frequency of consuming soft sweets, colas, and other soft drinks and alcohol [21]. For the ten food types, the subjects simply listed how many times per week they had consumed each type of food. The number of times snacks, sugar-sweetened coffee/tea, soft drinks, and alcoholic beverages were consumed every 7 days. The snacks included rice crackers, potato chips, cookies, cakes, and candies. Soft drinks included sweetened sugar beverages such as cola, cider, and fruit juice.

2.3. Physical Examination

Age (years), sex, body mass index (BMI, kg/m^2), waist circumference (cm), handgrip strength (kg), sleep duration (h), and blood-sampling data (glycated hemoglobin A1c (HbA1c,%), estimated glomerular filtration rate (eGFR, mL/min/cm^2), uric acid (UA, mg/dL), triglycerides (TG, mg/dL), high-density lipoprotein cholesterol (HDL-C, mg/dL), total cholesterol (TC, mg/dL), and non-HDL-C, mg/dL)) at the health checkup were obtained from the Health Management Department in the form of anonymized data linked to the FFQg. Height, weight, waist circumference (cm), and handgrip strength (kg) were measured in the presence of a nurse. BMI was automatically calculated from height and weight. Sleep duration was self-monitored, and the subjects simply listed the average sleep duration per week (e.g., six hours). The plasma creatinine, UA, and lipid concentrations (TC, TG, and HDL-C) were measured via a Hitachi LABOSPECT008 (Hitachi High-Tech Corporation, Tokyo, Japan), and HbA1c was measured via an A1c HA-8190 (Arkray, Kyoto, Japan). The eGFR was automatically calculated via the plasma creatinine level, age, and sex. Non-HDL-C concentrations were calculated from the TC and HDL-C concentrations. Blood samples were collected from nonfasting participants at approximately 16:00–17:00. As this was a hospital staff medical checkup, it was set at 3:30 p.m. when the medical staff had finished seeing the outpatients. The data are presented as the means (SDs).

2.4. Statistical Analysis

For comparisons by sex, t tests or Mann–Whitney U tests were used to compare men and women. Similarly, each individual was grouped as 20–29 years old (yo), 30–39 yo, 40–49 yo, or 50–59 yo, and we compared the food frequency of 20–29 yo with those of other age groups. Comparisons of the frequency of intake of the ten foods among the age groups were performed via the Kruskal–Wallis test followed by the Bonferroni method. To determine the effects of the frequency of eating the 10 food types, the frequency of sugar and alcohol intake, and sleep duration on body size and blood-sampling data (HbA1c, eGFR, UA, TG, HDL-C, and non-HDL-C levels), multivariate linear regression models adjusted for age and BMI were constructed. The data are presented as the means ± standard deviations (SDs). Statistical significance was set at $p < 0.05$. Statistical analyses were performed via SPSS version 28.0.0.0 for Mac software (IBM Corp., Armonk, NY, USA).

3. Results

3.1. Background of the Study Sample

Among the 3345 individuals (1057 men and 2268 women) who underwent all of the health examinations, those who were 20–59 years old and fully answered the dietary questionnaire were included in the study. The total number of individuals evaluated in this study was 3147 (M: 968, F: 2179), and the average age of the individuals (mean ± SD) was 35.1 ± 11.3 years (M: 37.9 ± 10.9, F: 33.9 ± 11.2) (Table 1). In men, age (yo) (mean ± SD), BMI (mean ± SD), waist circumference (cm) (mean ± SD), and handgrip strength (kg) (mean ± SD) were significantly greater than those in females (23.3 ± 3.4 vs. 21.3 ± 3.3, $p < 0.001$; 81.2 ± 9.1 vs. 70.8 ± 9.1, $p < 0.001$; 41.1 ± 9.1 vs. 24.5 ± 7.1, $p < 0.001$, respectively). Blood HbA1c (%) (mean ± SD), TG (mg/dL) (mean ± SD), non-HDL-C (mg/dL) (mean ± SD), and UA (mg/dL) (mean ± SD) levels were greater in men than in women (5.46 ± 0.42 vs. 5.40 ± 0.35, $p < 0.001$; 131.5 ± 95.6 vs. 87.8 ±55.8, $p < 0.001$; 139.19 ± 33.83 vs. 124.33 ±29.91, $p < 0.001$; 6.0 ± 1.2 vs. 4.2 ± 0.9, $p < 0.001$, respectively). In contrast, HDL-C (mean ± SD) and the eGFR (mean ± SD) were significantly lower in men than in women (53.7 ± 12.4 vs. 65.8 ± 13.6, $p < 0.001$; 84.7 ± 15.8 vs. 92.8 ± 17.7, $p < 0.001$, respectively). In males, sleep duration (h) (mean ± SD) was significantly shorter (6.3 ± 1.0 vs. 6.4 ± 1.0, $p = 0.001$). The frequencies of eating meat and fish (time per week; mean ± SD) were significantly greater in males (8.8 ± 4.5 vs. 7.8 ± 4.1, $p < 0.001$; 3.8 ± 3.0 vs. 3.3 ± 2.6, $p = 0.001$, respectively). In contrast, the frequencies of eating soybeans, dairy products, vegetables, and fruits (times per week; mean ± SD) in males were significantly lower than those in females (5.5 ± 4.3 vs. 5.9 ± 4.3, $p = 0.002$; 2.9 ± 2.8 vs. 3.3 ± 2.8, $p < 0.001$; 8.9 ± 4.8 vs. 9.3 ± 4.7, $p = 0.029$; 2.7 ± 2.7 vs. 3.1 ± 2.5 $p < 0.001$, respectively). Despite significant differences, both men and women consumed meat and vegetables almost daily; fish, dairy products, and eggs once every two days (four times per week) and soybeans, seaweed, and potatoes once every three or four days (three times per week) (Table 1).

Table 1. Background of the subjects.

	Total (n = 3147)	Male (n = 968)	Female (n = 2179)	p
Age	35.1 (11.3)	37.9 (10.9)	33.9 (11.2)	**<0.001** *
BMI	21.9 (3.4)	23.3 (3.4)	21.3 (3.3)	**<0.001**
Waist circumference	74.0 (10.3)	81.2 (9.1)	70.8 (9.1)	**<0.001**
Handgrip strength	29.6 (10.9)	41.1 (9.1)	24.5 (7.1)	**<0.001**
HbA1c	5.42 (0.38)	5.46 (0.42)	5.40 (0.35)	**<0.001**
Triglyceride	101.3 (73.3)	131.5 (95.6)	87.8 (55.8)	**<0.001** *
HDL-C	62.1 (14.4)	53.7 (12.4)	65.8 (13.6)	**<0.001**
Non-HDL-C	128.9 (31.9)	139.2 (33.8)	124.4 (29.9)	**<0.001**
eGFR	90.3 (17.6)	84.7 (15.8)	92.8 (17.7)	**<0.001**
Uric acid	4.8 (1.3)	6.0 (1.2)	4.2 (0.9)	**<0.001**
Hours of sleep	6.4 (1.0)	6.3 (1.0)	6.4 (1.0)	**0.001**
Meat (/week)	8.2 (4.2)	8.8 (4.5)	7.8 (4.1)	**<0.001** *
Fish (/week)	3.5 (2.7)	3.8 (3.0)	3.3 (2.6)	**0.001** *
Egg (/week)	4.2 (2.7)	4.2 (3.0)	4.2 (2.5)	0.58 *
Soybeans(/week)	5.8 (4.3)	5.5 (4.3)	5.9 (4.3)	**0.002** *
Dairy products (/week)	3.2 (2.8)	2.9 (2.8)	3.3 (2.8)	**<0.001** *
Seaweed (/week)	2.0 (2.1)	1.9 (2.2)	2.0 (2.0)	0.72 *
Vegetables (/week)	9.2 (4.7)	8.9 (4.8)	9.3 (4.7)	**0.029** *
Fruits (/week)	2.9 (2.6)	2.7 (2.7)	3.1 (2.5)	**<0.001** *
Potatoes (/week)	2.1 (1.7)	2.0 (1.8)	2.1 (1.7)	0.24 *
Oils and fats (/week)	10.0 (5.5)	10.1 (5.5)	9.9 (5.6)	0.11 *
Snacks (/week)	11.0 (12.0)	9.4 (11.9)	11.7 (12.0)	**<0.001** *
Coffee/tea with sugar (/week)	0.9 (2.7)	0.9 (2.8)	0.9 (2.7)	0.057 *
Soft drinks (/week)	1.3 (2.6)	1.9 (3.0)	1.0 (2.3)	**<0.001** *
Alcohol (/week)	1.3 (2.1)	1.7 (2.4)	1.1 (1.9)	**<0.001** *

The data are presented as the mean (SD). * Mann–Whitney U test. Bold letters indicate significance ($p < 0.05$ vs. male). Abbreviations: BMI, body mass index; HbA1c, glycated hemoglobin A1c; HDL-C, high-density lipoprotein cholesterol; eGFR, estimated glomerular filtration rate.

Finally, men consumed soft drinks and alcohol more frequently per week (1.9 ± 3.0 vs. 1.0 ± 2.3, $p < 0.001$; 1.7 ± 2.4 vs. 1.1 ± 1.9, $p < 0.001$, respectively). In contrast, the frequency of eating snacks was greater among women (9.4 ± 11.9 vs. 11.7 ± 12.0, $p < 0.001$) (Table 1). The frequency of drinking coffee/tea with sugar was not significantly different (0.9 ± 2.8 vs. 0.9 ± 2.7, $p = 0.057$). Sex differences in the consumption of beverages and snacks are related to preferences.

3.2. Effects of Sex and Age on Food Frequency

We then compared food frequency across age groups (20–29, 30–39, 40–49, and 50–59 years) divided by sex (Table 2). No differences in the frequency of meat or egg intake were found between the 30-, 39-, 40–49-, and 50–59-year-old age groups and the 20–29-year-old group in either men or women. According to the results of the Bonferroni correction after the Kruskal–Wallis test, the consumption of fish, soybeans, dairy products, seaweed, fruits, potatoes, and oils and fats significantly increased in the 40 to 49-year-old and 50 to 59-year-old groups for men and women compared with the 20 to 29-year-old group (men:fish: 3.3 (3.0) vs. 3.7 (2.9) vs. 4.7 (3.3), $p < 0.01$; soybeans: 4.8 (4.2) vs. 6.0 (4.4) vs. 5.9 (4.1), $p < 0.01$; dairy products: 2.5 (2.4) vs. 3.2 (2.9) vs. 3.4 (2.8), $p < 0.01$; seaweed: 1.4 (1.5) vs. 2.2 (2.5) vs. 2.6 (2.0), $p < 0.001$; fruits: 1.9 (2.2) vs. 2.7 (2.4) vs. 3.9 (2.9), $p < 0.001$ The consumption of vegetables significantly increased in the 50 to 59-year-old groups for men and in the 40 to 49-year-old and 50 to 59-year-old groups for women compared with the 20 to 29-year-old group (men: 8.0 (4.4) vs. 10.1 (5.2), $p < 0.001$; women: 8.8 (0.1) vs. 9.4 (0.2) vs. 10.7 (0.3), $p < 0.001$). In contrast, the consumption of meat and eggs did not differ between the 40 to 49-year-old and 50 to 59-year-old groups for women compared with the 20 to 29-year-old group (men: meat: 8.7 (4.0) vs. 9.1 (4.8) vs. 8.9 (4.8), $p = 0.76$; egg: 4.3 (2.8) vs. 4.3 (3.7) vs. 4.2 (2.9), $p = 0.4$; women: meat: 7.7 (0.1) vs. 8.3 (0.2) vs. 7.5 (0.2),

$p = 0.02$; egg: 4.1 (0.1) vs. 4.3 (0.1) vs. 4.2 (0.1), $p = 0.9$). Thus, most food frequencies differ according to age and sex, with the exceptions of eggs and meat.

Table 2. Frequency of the intake of ten food items by sex and age group.

	Male			Female		
Foods	**Age**	**Mean (SD)**	***p***	**Age**	**Mean (SD)**	***p***
Meat	20 yo (n = 303) 30 yo (n = 253) 40 yo (n = 222) 50 yo (n = 190)	8.7(4.0) 8.6(4.4) 9.1(4.8) 8.9(4.8)	0.76	20 yo (n = 1091) 30 yo (n = 399) 40 yo (n = 383) 50 yo (n = 306)	7.7(0.1) 8.2(0.2) 8.3(0.2) 7.5(0.2)	**0.02**
Fish	20 yo (n = 303) 30 yo (n = 253) 40 yo (n = 221) 50 yo (n = 189)	3.3(3.0) 3.7(2.9) 3.7(2.9) * 4.7(3.3) ***	**<0.001**	20 yo (n = 1091) 30 yo (n = 399) 40 yo (n = 383) 50 yo (n = 306)	3.0(0.1) 3.4(0.1) *** 3.6(0.1) *** 4.0(0.1) ***	**<0.001**
Egg	20 yo (n = 303) 30 yo (n = 253) 40 yo (n = 221) 50 yo (n = 189)	4.3(2.8) 4.1(2.8) 4.3(3.7) 4.2(2.9)	0.4	20 yo (n = 1091) 30 yo (n = 399) 40 yo (n = 383) 50 yo (n = 306)	4.1(0.1) 4.2(0.1) 4.3(0.1) 4.2(0.1)	0.9
Soybean	20 yo (n = 303) 30 yo (n = 253) 40 yo (n = 221) 50 yo (n = 189)	4.8(4.2) 5.4(4.3) 6.0(4.4) ** 5.9(4.1) **	**<0.001**	20 yo (n = 1091) 30 yo (n = 399) 40 yo (n = 383) 50 yo (n = 306)	5.2(0.1) 6.0(0.2) ** 6.8(0.2) *** 7.3(0.3) ***	**<0.001**
Dairy product	20 yo (n = 303) 30 yo (n = 253) 40 yo (n = 221) 50 yo (n = 189)	2.5(2.4) 2.7(3.1) 3.2(2.9) * 3.4(2.8) **	**<0.001**	20 yo (n = 1091) 30 yo (n = 399) 40 yo (n = 383) 50 yo (n = 306)	2.9(0.1) 3.4(0.1) ** 3.5(0.1) *** 4.0(0.2) ***	**<0.001**
Seaweed	20 yo (n = 303) 30 yo (n = 253) 40 yo (n = 221) 50 yo (n = 189)	1.4(1.5) 1.9(2.5) * 2.2(2.5) *** 2.6(2.0) ***	**<0.001**	20 yo (n = 1091) 30 yo (n = 399) 40 yo (n = 383) 50 yo (n = 306)	1.6(0.06) 1.9(0.09) ** 2.5(0.1) *** 2.6(0.1) ***	**<0.001**
Vegetable	20 yo (n = 303) 30 yo (n = 253) 40 yo (n = 221) 50 yo (n = 189)	8.0(4.4) 8.6(4.6) * 9.4(4.8) *** 10.1(5.2) ***	**<0.001**	20 yo (n = 1091) 30 yo (n = 399) 40 yo (n = 383) 50 yo (n = 306)	8.8(0.1) 9.3(0.2) 9.4(0.2) 10.7(0.3) ***	**<0.001**
Fruit	20 yo (n = 303) 30 yo(n = 253) 40 yo(n = 221) 50 yo(n = 189)	1.9(2.2) 2.6(3.0) ** 2.7(2.4) *** 3.9(2.9) ***	**<0.001**	20 yo (n = 1091) 30 yo (n = 399) 40 yo (n = 383) 50 yo (n = 306)	2.6(0.07) 3.4(0.1) *** 3.4(0.1) *** 3.9(0.1) ***	**<0.001**
Potatoes	20 yo (n = 303) 30 yo (n = 253) 40 yo (n = 221) 50 yo (n = 189)	1.8(1.6) 2.1(2.4) 2.2(1.7)* 2.1(1.6) *	**0.022**	20 yo (n = 1091) 30 yo (n = 399) 40 yo (n = 383) 50 yo (n = 306)	1.9(0.1) 2.3(0.1) ** 2.3(0.1) *** 2.2(0.1) ***	**<0.001**
Oils and fats	20 yo (n = 303) 30 yo (n = 253) 40 yo (n = 221) 50 yo (n = 189)	8.8(4.7) 9.7(5.4) 11.1(5.5) *** 11.7(6.1) ***	**<0.001**	20 yo (n = 1091) 30 yo (n = 399) 40 yo (n = 383) 50 yo (n = 306)	8.3(0.1) 10.6(0.3) *** 11.5(0.3) *** 12.8(0.3) ***	**<0.001**

The data are presented as the mean (SD). Bold letters indicate significance (* $p < 0.05$ vs. 20 yo, ** $p < 0.01$ vs. 20 yo, *** $p < 0.001$ vs. 20 yo).

3.3. Effect of Age on the Frequency of Consuming Snacks, Soft Drinks, and Alcoholic Beverages

We examined the effects of age on the frequency of consumption of snacks, sugar-sweetened coffee/tea, soft drinks, and alcohol according to sex (Table 3). The frequency of eating snacks increased significantly among men and women 40–49 years and 50–59 years of age (men: 8.0 (10.0) vs. 10.9 (10.5) vs. 10.2 (9.0), $p < 0.001$; women: 10.5 (10.3) vs. 13.5 (14.7) vs. 14.8 (14.6), $p < 0.001$) (Table 3). In contrast, the habits of drinking sugar-sweetened coffee, tea, or soft drinks were not significantly affected by age. The frequency of alcohol consumption increased significantly in both men and women aged 40--49 and 50--59 years (men: 1.3 (2.4) vs. 2.3 (2.6) vs. 2.2 (2.5), $p < 0.001$; women: 0.8 (1.2) vs. 1.6 (2.3) vs. 1.9 (2.6), $p < 0.001$). Thus, the frequency of eating snacks and drinking alcohol significantly increased at 40–49 and 50–59 years of age (Table 3).

Table 3. Food preferences by age and sex groups.

	Male			Female		
Foods	**Age**	**Mean (SE)**	***p***	**Age**	**Mean (SE)**	***p***
Snacks	20 yo (n = 303) 30 yo (n = 253) 40 yo (n = 221) 50 yo (n = 189)	8.0 (10.0) 9.1 (16.1) 10.9 (10.5) ** 10.2 (9.0) **	**<0.001**	20 yo (n = 1091) 30 yo (n = 399) 40 yo (n = 383) 50 yo (n = 306)	10.5 (10.3) 10.9 (0.8) 13.5 (14.7) ** 14.8 (14.6) **	**<0.001**
Coffee/Tea with sugars	20 yo (n = 303) 30 yo (n = 253) 40 yo (n = 221) 50 yo (n = 189)	0.5 (1.4) 1.0 (3.5) 1.3 (3.2) 0.9 (2.8)	0.42	20 yo (n = 1091) 30 yo (n = 399) 40 yo (n = 383) 50 yo (n = 306)	0.7 (1.9) 1.3 (3.8) 1.0 (2.7) 0.9 (3.0)	0.15
Soft Drink	20 yo (n = 303) 30 yo (n = 253) 40 yo (n = 221) 50 yo (n = 189)	2.0 (3.1) 2.0 (3.5) 1.7 (2.5) 1.7 (2.5)	0.32	20 yo (n = 1091) 30 yo (n = 399) 40 yo (n = 383) 50 yo (n = 306)	1.0 (2.3) 1.1 (2.0) 1.0 (2.9) 0.8 (1.7)	0.09
Alcohol	20 yo (n = 303) 30 yo (n = 253) 40 yo (n = 221) 50 yo (n = 189)	1.3 (2.4) 1.5 (2.0) 2.3 (2.6) *** 2.2 (2.5) ***	**<0.001**	20 yo (n = 1091) 30 yo (n = 399) 40 yo (n = 383) 50 yo (n = 306)	0.8 (1.2) 1.1 (2.0) 1.6 (2.3) ** 1.9 2.6) ***	**<0.001**

The data are presented as the mean (SD). Bold letters indicate significance (** $p < 0.01$ vs. 20 yo, *** $p < 0.001$ vs. 20 yo).

3.4. Effects of Food Intake and Sugar-Sweetened Drink, Snack, and Alcohol Consumption on BMI, Waist Circumference, and Grip Strength

With age and BMI as covariates, the frequency of food intake and the frequency of food intake as independent variables, and waist circumference and grip strength as dependent variables, we conducted a multivariate linear regression analysis to determine the effect of the frequency of preferred food intake on waist circumference and grip strength. In males, waist circumference was positively associated with age (0.09 (0.05, 0.12), $p < 0.001$), BMI (2.1 (2.0, 2.2), $p < 0.001$), and the frequency of oil and fat intake ($p = 0.014$) and negatively correlated with the frequency of soybean intake (−0.05 (−0.09, 0.02), $p = 0.004$). In females, waist circumference was positively associated with age (0.24 (0.21, 0.26), $p < 0.001$), BMI (1.66 (1.58, 1.75), $p < 0.001$), hours of sleep (0.29 (0.03, 0.54), $p = 0.03$), frequency of meat intake (0.09 (0.02, 0.16), $p = 0.01$), and frequency of egg intake (−0.17 (0.07, 0.30), $p = 0.001$) and negatively associated with the frequency of soybean intake (−0.34 (−0.17, 0.03), $p = 0.007$) (Table 4).

In males, handgrip strength was associated with age (−0.1 (−0.15, −0.04), $p < 0.001$) and BMI (0.7 (0.5,0.8), $p < 0.001$). In females, handgrip strength was associated with BMI (0.14 (0.05, 0.23), $p = 0.003$), the frequency of seaweed intake (0.23 (0.07, 0.4), $p = 0.005$), and alcohol intake (0.23 (0.06, 0.39), $p = 0.007$). Thus, the effects of the frequency of food intake on body size and grip strength were more potent in women than in men (Table 4).

Table 4. The effects of food frequency on circumference and handgrip strength.

	Waist Circumference				Handgrip Strength			
	Male		Female		Male		Female	
	B	*p*	B	*p*	B	*p*	B	*p*
Meat	0.05 (−0.04,0.13)	0.27	**0.09 (0.02, 0.16)**	**0.01**	−0.04 (−0.18, 0.10)	0.56	−0.01 (−0.09, 0.07)	0.74
Fish	−0.09 (−0.21, 0.04)	0.16	−0.11(−0.23,0.003)	0.06	-0.05 (−0.26, 0.17)	0.67	-0.07 (−0.2, 0.06)	0.31
Egg	−0.004 (−0.12, 0.11)	0.95	**0.19 (0.07, 0.30)**	**0.001**	0.07 (−0.13, 0.27)	0.5	0.12 (−0.004, 0.25)	0.058
Soybeans	0.02 (-0.07, 0.10)	0.74	**−0.17 (−0.17, −0.03)**	**0.007**	0.08 (−0.07, 0.23)	0.3	−0.001 (−0.08, 0.08)	0.98
Dairy products	**−0.17 (−0.3, −0.04)**	**0.01**	0.05 (−0.06, 0.15)	0.37	0.06 (−0.07, 0.29)	0.61	0.11 (−0.004, 0.22)	0.058
Seaweed	−0.03 (−0.22, 0.15)	0.72	0.14 (−0.003,0.39)	0.055	0.07 (−0.25, 0.38)	0.69	**0.23 (0.07, 0.4)**	**0.005**
Vegetables	−0.02 (−0.1, 0.1)	0.67	−0.02 (−0.09, 0.04)	0.49	0.004 (−0.14, 0.15)	0.96	−0.05 (−0.13, 0.02)	0.17
Fruits	0.1 (−0.1, 0.2)	0.52	−0.03 (−0.15, 0.09)	0.67	0.21 (−0.5, 0.46)	0.11	−0.085 (−0.22, 0.05)	0.21
Potatoes	0.02 (−0.2, 0.3)	0.85	0.13 (−0.05, 0.3)	0.15	−0.39 (−0.79, 0.01)	0.054	−0.1 (−0.3, 0.1)	0.32
Oils and fats	**0.08 (0.01, 0.15)**	**0.02**	0.05 (−0.002,0.11)	0.057	0.05 (−0.07, 0.17)	0.41	0.03 (−0.03, 0.09)	0.37
Snacks	0.002 (−0.03, 0.04)	0.92	−0.01 (−0.03, 0.02)	0.51	−0.03 (−0.09, 0.03)	0.33	0.011 (−0.01, 0.04)	0.39
Coffee/tea with sugar	0.05 (−0.08, 0.18)	0.42	0.04 (−0.07, 0.14)	0.49	−0.13 (−0.35, 0.09)	0.23	0.01 (−0.11, 0.12)	0.89
Soft drinks	0.03 (−0.1, 0.15)	0.68	0.12 (−0.001, 0.23)	0.052	−0.05 (−0.26, 0.15)	0.61	0.05 (−0.09, 0.18)	0.5
Alcohol	-0.05 (−0.19, 0.09)	0.48	−0.05 (−0.19, 0.10)	0.54	0.22 (−0.02, 0.46)	0.07	**0.23 (0.06, 0.39)**	**0.007**
Age	**0.09 (0.05, 0.12)**	**<0.001**	**0.24 (0.21, 0.26)**	**<0.001**	**−0.1 (−0.15, −0.04)**	**<0.001**	0.01 (−0.02, 0.04)	0.48
BMI	**2.1 (2.0, 2.2)**	**<0.001**	**1.66 (1.58, 1.75)**	**<0.001**	**0.7 (0.5, 0.8)**	**<0.001**	**0.14 (0.05, 0.23)**	**0.003**
Hours of sleep	0.3 (−0.1, 0.6)	0.13	**0.29 (0.03, 0.54)**	**0.03**	−0.2 (−0.8, 0.4)	0.5	−0.2 (−0.5, 0.1)	0.27

The gray areas (letters in bold) indicate significance ($p < 0.05$).

3.5. Effects of Food Intake Frequency and Sugar-Sweetened Drink, Sweet Drink, and Alcohol Consumption on HbA1c, eGFR and UA

Next, we conducted multivariate analyses to clarify the effects of the frequency of food intake on HbA1c, eGFR, and UA levels. The HbA1c level in males was positively associated with age (β (95% CI): 0.011 (0.009, 0.014), $p < 0.001$), BMI (0.031 (0.024,0.038), $p < 0.001$), and the frequency of meat intake (0.007 (0.001,0.013), $p = 0.03$) and negatively associated with hours of sleep (−0.04 (−0.064, −0.016), $p = 0.001$). In females, HbA1c was positively associated with age (0.01 (0.009, 0.012), $p < 0.001$) and BMI (0.02 (0.016, 0.024), $p < 0.001$) and negatively associated with hours of sleep (−0.03 (−0.04, −0.01), $p < 0.001$) and the frequency of alcohol intake (−0.018 (−0.025, −0.01), $p < 0.001$). Thus, age, BMI, and sleep duration affected HbA1c levels in both men and women, whereas the frequency of meat intake and alcohol intake affected HbA1c levels only in men and women (Table 5).

eGFR in males was positively associated with seaweed intake (0.8 (0.3, 1.2), $p = 0.004$) and negatively correlated with age (−0.8 (−0.9, −0.7), $p < 0.001$), frequency of meat intake (−0.3 (−0.5, −0.1), $p = 0.008$), and frequency of potato intake (−0.9 (−1.4, −0.3), $p = 0.004$). In females, the eGFR was positively associated with the frequency of fish intake

(0.4 (0.1, 0.7), $p = 0.001$) and negatively correlated with age (−0.82 (−0.89, −0.76); $p < 0.01$), frequency of dairy product intake (−0.3 (−4.80, −0.47), $p = 0.02$), and frequency of snack intake (−0.66 (−1.01, −0.31), $p < 0.001$) (Table 5).

UA in males was positively associated with BMI (0.11 (0.09, 0.13); $p < 0.001$) and the frequency of alcohol intake (0.06 (0.03, 0.09) $p < 0.001$). In females, UA was positively associated with BMI (0.084 (0.073, 0.096), $p < 0.001$), the frequency of soybean intake (0.013 (0.003, 0.023), $p = 0.009$), and the frequency of alcohol intake (0.06 (0.04, 0.08), $p < 0.001$) and negatively associated with the frequency of dairy product intake (−0.01 (−0.03, 0), $p = 0.048$) and the frequency of oil and fat intake (−0.01 (−0.02, −0.002), $p = 0.01$). Thus, BMI and alcohol consumption were positively correlated with UA levels. The frequency of soybean, dairy products, and oil and fat intake was positively associated with UA only in women, whereas the frequency of dairy products and oil and fat intake was negatively associated with UA (Table 5).

Table 5. The effects of food frequency on HbA1c, eGFR, and uric acid.

	HbA1c				eGFR			
	Male		Female		Male		Female	
	B	*p*	B	*p*	B	*p*	B	*p*
Meat	**0.007 (0.001, 0.013)**	**0.03**	0.003 (0, 0.007)	0.09	**−0.3 (−0.5, −0.1)**	**0.01**	−0.09 (−0.25, 0.08)	0.32
Fish	0.004 (−0.005, 0.013)	0.35	−0.001 (−0.006, 0.005)	0.83	−0.01 (−0.3, 0.3)	0.97	**0.4 (0.1, 0.7)**	**0.005**
Egg	−0.007 (−0.016, 0.001)	0.097	0 (−0.005, 0.006)	0.87	0.2 (−0.1, 0.5)	0.15	0.1 (−0.1, 0.4)	0.31
Soybeans	−0.006 (−0.012, 0.001)	0.08	0.001 (−0.003, 0.004)	0.76	0.1 (−0.1, 0.3)	0.29	−0.08 (−0.25, 0.09)	0.37
Dairy products	0.007 (−0.003, 0.016)	0.18	0.003 (−0.002, 0.008)	0.21	0.2 (−0.1, 0.6)	0.15	**−0.3 (−0.5, −0.02)**	**0.03**
Seaweed	−0.005 (−0.019, 0.009)	0.49	−0.005 (−0.012, 0.002)	0.19	**0.8 (0.3, 1.2)**	**0.001**	−0.07 (−0.4, 0.3)	0.69
Vegetables	0.004 (−0.002, 0.01)	0.19	−0.001 (−0.005, 0.002)	0.45	−0.1 (−0.3, 0.2)	0.63	−0.01 (−0.17, 0.15)	0.9
Fruits	−0.004 (−0.015, 0.007)	0.47	0.004 (−0.002, 0.010)	0.22	−0.04 (−0.4, 0.3)	0.82	−0.05 (−0.3, 0.2)	0.73
Potatoes	0.014 (−0.003, 0.031)	0.11	0.005 (−0.004, 0.014)	0.26	**−0.9 (−1.4, −0.3)**	**0.004**	0.1 (−0.3, 0.5)	0.64
Oils and fats	−0.002 (−0.008, 0.003)	0.34	0 (−0.003, 0.014)	0.85	−0.02 (−0.2, 0.2)	0.84	−0.02 (−0.15, 0.12)	0.82
Snacks	−0.001 (−0.003, 0.002)	0.48	0.001 (−0.001, 0.002)	0.3	−0.06 (−0.15, 0.02)	0.15	0.002 (−0.05, 0.06)	0.94
Coffee/tea with sugar	−0.001 (−0.011, 0.008)	0.82	−0.002 (−0.007, 0.003)	0.47	−0.1 (−0.5, 0.2)	0.37	−0.16 (−0.4, 0.08)	0.2
Soft drinks	0.005 (−0.004, 0.014)	0.27	0.002 (−0.004, 0.008)	0.51	0.3 (−0.1, 0.5)	0.14	0.1 (−0.2, 0.4)	0.58
Alcohol	−0.01 (−0.02, 0.002)	0.11	**−0.018 (−0.025, −0.01)**	**<0.001**	0.2 (−0.2, 0.5)	0.29	−0.04 (−0.39, 0.32)	0.84
Age	**0.011 (0.009, 0.014)**	**<0.001**	**0.01 (0.009, 0.012)**	**<0.001**	**−0.8 (−0.9, −0.7)**	**<0.001**	**−0.83 (−0.89, −0.76)**	**<0.001**
BMI	**0.031 (0.024, 0.038)**	**<0.001**	**0.02 (0.016, 0.024)**	**<0.001**	−0.1 (−0.4, 0.1)	0.3	−0.1 (−0.3, 0.1)	0.33
Hours of sleep	**−0.04 (−0.064, −0.016)**	**0.001**	**−0.03 (−0.04, −0.01)**	**<0.001**	−0.4 (−1.2, 0.4)	0.35	0.3 (−0.3, 0.9)	0.32

Table 5. *Cont.*

	Uric Acid			
	Male		Female	
	B	*p*	B	*p*
Meat	0.013 (−0.005, 0.03)	0.14	0.003 (−0.006, 0.013)	0.48
Fish	−0.01 (−0.04, 0.02)	0.49	−0.002 (−0.018, 0.014)	0.82
Egg	−0.004 (−0.03, 0.02)	0.77	−0.012 (−0.027, 0.003)	0.12
Soybeans	0.01 (−0.01, 0.03)	0.4	**0.013 (0.003, 0.023)**	**0.009**
Dairy products	−0.01 (−0.04, 0.02)	0.71	**−0.01 (−0.03, 0)**	**0.048**
Seaweed	−0.04 (−0.08, 0.01)	0.09	0.01 (−0.01, 0.03)	0.41
Vegetables	0.01 (−0.01, 0.03)	0.43	0.005 (−0.004, 0.015)	0.25
Fruits	−0.03 (−0.06, 0.01)	0.14	−0.012 (−0.028, 0.004)	0.15
Potatoes	0.03 (−0.02, 0.08)	0.29	0.023 (−0.001, 0.047)	0.07
Oils and fats	−0.002 (−0.02, 0.01)	0.8	**−0.01 (−0.02, −0.002)**	**0.01**
Snacks	0 (−0.008, 0.007)	0.92	−0.002 (−0.005, 0.001)	0.17
Coffee/tea with sugar	0.02 (−0.01, 0.05)	0.26	−0.002 (−0.016, 0.012)	0.79
Soft drinks	0.01 (−0.02, 0.04)	0.37	0.005 (−0.011, 0.021)	0.51
Alcohol	**0.06 (0.03, 0.09)**	**<0.001**	**0.06 (0.04, 0.08)**	**<0.001**
Age	−0.002 (−0.009, 0.005)	0.6	0.002 (−0.002, 0.006)	0.31
BMI	**0.11 (0.09, 0.13)**	**<0.001**	**0.084 (0.073, 0.096)**	**<0.001**
Hours of sleep	−0.02 (−0.09, 0.05)	0.58	−0.01 (−0.05,0.02)	0.42

The gray areas (letters in bold) indicate significance ($p < 0.05$). Abbreviations: HbA1c, glycated hemoglobin A1c; eGFR, estimated glomerular filtration.

3.6. Effects of Food Intake Frequency and Sugar-Sweetened Drink, Sweet Drink, and Alcohol Consumption on Serum Lipid Levels

Finally, we performed a multivariate analysis to determine whether food intake frequency and sugar-sweetened drinks, snacks, or alcohol consumption influenced lipid metabolism. TG levels in males were positively associated with age (1.1 (0.5, 1.7), $p < 0.001$), BMI (7.6 (5.9, 9.4), $p < 0.001$), frequency of potato intake (5 (0.9, 9), $p = 0.02$), and frequency of alcohol intake (3 (0.5, 5.4), $p = 0.02$) (Table 6). In females, TG levels were positively associated with age (1.2 (1.0, 1.4), $p < 0.001$), BMI (4.4 (3.7, 5.0), $p < 0.001$), frequency of meat intake (0.6 (0.04, 1.2), $p = 0.04$), and frequency of potato intake (1.8 (0.3, 3.2), $p = 0.02$) and negatively associated with the frequency of oil and fat intake (−0.7 (−1.2, −0.3), $p = 0.002$) (Table 6). Thus, age, BMI, and potato intake frequency were positively associated with TG levels in both men and women. In contrast, the frequency of alcohol intake was associated with TG levels only in men, whereas meat, oils, and fats were positively and negatively associated with TG levels only in women.

Table 6. Effects of food frequency on plasma lipid levels.

	TG				HDLc				non-HDLc			
	Male		Female		Male		Female		Male		Female	
	B	p	B	p	B	p	B	p	B	p	B	p
Meat	0.3 (−1.1, 1.7)	0.7	**0.6 (0.04, 1.2)**	**0.04**	0.2 (−0.01, 0.4)	0.06	−0.1 (−0.2, 0.1)	0.35	−0.1 (−0.6, 0.4)	0.65	**−0.4 (−0.6, −0.1)**	**0.02**
Fish	−1.3 (−3.5, 0.9)	0.25	0.4 (−0.5,1.4)	0.38	−0.1 (−0.4, 0.1)	0.33	0.1 (−0.2, 0.3)	0.63	−0.2 (−1.0, 0.6)	0.6	0.1 (−0.4, 0.5)	0.84
Egg	−0.3 (−2.3, 1.8)	0.8	0.8 (−0.1,1.8)	0.07	0.2 (−0.1,0.5)	0.12	0.3 (0.1, 0.5)	0.02	−0.2 (−0.9, 0.5)	0.62	**0.6 (0.1, 1.0)**	**0.02**
Soybeans	−0.7 (−2.3, 0.8)	0.36	−0.4 (−1.0, 0.2)	0.2	0.2 (−0.04, 0.4)	0.12	0.12 (−0.03, 0.26)	0.12	−0.4 (−1.0, 0.1)	0.11	**−0.3 (−0.6, −0.03)**	**0.03**
Dairy products	2.2 (−0.1, 4.5)	0.07	−0.5 (−1.3, 0.3)	0.24	0.004 (−0.3, 0.3)	0.98	−0.01 (−0.21, 0.2)	0.94	**0.9 (0.1, 1.7)**	**0.03**	0.06 (−0.4, 0.5)	0.78
Seaweed	0.2 (−3.0, 3.4)	0.9	0.3 (−0.9, 1.5)	0.67	-0.1 (−0.5,0.3)	0.65	−0.2 (−0.5, 0.1)	0.16	0.2 (−0.9, 1.3)	0.76	−0.5 (−1.1, 0.1)	0.13
Vegetables	0.3 (−1.2, 1.7)	0.73	0.1 (−0.5,0.6)	0.8	-0.2 (−0.4, 0)	0.09	0.1 (−0.04, 0.2)	0.16	0.3 (−0.3, 0.8)	0.34	0.1 (−0.2, 0.4)	0.58
Fruits	−2.2 (−4.8, 0.4)	0.1	0.6 (−0.4, 1.5)	0.27	−0.1 (−0.4, 0.3)	0.7	−0.2 (−0.5, 0.03)	0.09	−0.4 (−1.3, 0.5)	0.36	0.1 (−0.4, 0.7)	0.57
Potatoes	**5.0 (0.9, 9.0)**	**0.02**	**1.8 (0.3, 3.2)**	**0.02**	−0.1 (−0.6, 0.4)	0.71	−0.4 (−0.8, −0.04)	0.03	0.3 (−1.1, 1.7)	0.7	0.3 (−0.4, 1.0)	0.42
Oils and fats	−0.8 (−2, 0.4)	0.2	**−0.7 (−1.2, −0.3)**	**0.002**	−0.02 (−0.2, 0.1)	0.8	0.1 (−0.1, 0.2)	0.25	−0.3 (−0.7, 0.1)	0.11	0.01 (−0.2, 0.2)	0.95
Snacks	−0.2 (−0.8, 0.5)	0.63	−0.02 (−0.2, 0.2)	0.87	0.01 (−0.1, 0.1)	0.78	0.06 (0.01, 0.1)	0.02	0.1 (−0.1, 0.3)	0.27	0.06 (−0.03, 0.16)	0.21
Coffee/tea with sugar	2.2 (−0.04, 4.4)	0.054	0.3 (−0.5, 1.2)	0.43	−0.1 (−0.4, 0.1)	0.32	−0.2 (−0.4, 0.1)	0.17	0.4 (−0.4, 1.2)	0.32	−0.1 (−0.5, 0.4)	0.72
Soft drinks	1.3 (−0.8, 3.4)	0.23	0.4 (−0.6, 1.4)	0.41	−0.2 (−0.4, 0.1)	0.24	−0.04 (−0.13, 0.2)	0.78	−0.5 (−1.2, 0.3)	0.21	−0.4 (−0.9, 0.1)	0.09
Alcohol	**3 (0.5, 5.4)**	**0.02**	−0.9 (−2.1, 0.3)	0.15	**1.0 (0.7, 1.3)**	**<0.001**	**1.3 (1.0, 1.6)**	**<0.001**	−0.7 (−1.5, 0.2)	0.12	**−1.3 (−1.9, −0.7)**	**<0.001**
Age	**1.1 (0.5, 1.7)**	**<0.001**	**1.2 (1.0, 1.4)**	**<0.001**	**0.09 (0.02, 0.17)**	**0.014**	**0.12 (0.06, 0.17)**	**<0.001**	**0.8 (0.6, 1.0)**	**<0.001**	**1 (0.9)**	**<0.001**
BMI	**7.6 (5.9, 9.4)**	**<0.001**	**4.4 (3.7, 5.0)**	**<0.001**	**−1.3 (−1.5, −1.1)**	**<0.001**	**−1.2 (−1.3, −1.0)**	**<0.001**	**2.8 (2.3, 3.4)**	**<0.001**	**2.1 (1.7, 2.4)**	**<0.001**
Hours of sleep	1.8 (−3.9, 7.5)	0.53	0.4 (−1.7, 2.5)	0.7	−0.1 (−0.8, 0.7)	0.88	−0.2 (-0.7, 0.3)	0.4	**2.1 (0.2, 4.0)**	**0.04**	0.3 (−0.7, 1.4)	0.54

The gray areas (letters in bold) indicate significance ($p < 0.05$). Abbreviations: TG, triglyceride; HDLc, high-density cholesterol; non-HDLc, non-high-density cholesterol.

HDL-C in males was positively associated with age (0.09 (0.02, 0.17), $p = 0.02$) and the frequency of alcohol intake (0.067 (0.034, 0.10), $p < 0.001$) and negatively associated with BMI (−1.3 (−1.5, −1.1), $p < 0.001$) and the frequency of potato intake (−0.9 (−1.4, −0.3), $p = 0.004$) (Table 6). In females, HDL-C was positively associated with age (0.12 (0.06, 0.17), $p < 0.001$) and negatively associated with BMI (−1.2 (−1.3, −1.0), $p < 0.001$) (Table 6). Thus, sex, age, and frequency of alcohol intake were positively associated with HDL-C levels, whereas BMI was positively associated with HDL-C levels.

The non-HDL-C level in males was positively associated with age, BMI, frequency of dairy product consumption, and frequency of soft drink consumption. In females, non-HDL-C was positively associated with age (0.8 (0.6, 1.0), $p < 0.001$), BMI (2.8 (2.3, 3.4), $p < 0.001$), sleep duration (2.1 (0.2, 4.0), $p = 0.04$), frequency of dairy product intake (0.9 (0.1, 1.7), $p = 0.03$), and frequency of alcohol intake (0.06 (0.03, 0.09); $p < 0.001$) (Table 6). Non-HDL-C levels in females were positively associated with age, BMI, frequency of dairy product intake, and frequency of soft drink intake. In females, non-HDL-C was positively associated with age (1.0 (0.6, 1.0), $p < 0.001$), BMI (2.1 (1.7, 3.4), $p < 0.001$), and frequency of egg intake (0.6 (0.1, 1.0), $p = 0.02$) and negatively associated with frequency of meat intake (−0.4 (−0.6, −0.1), $p = 0.02$), frequency of soybean intake (−0.3 (−0.6, −0.03), $p = 0.03$), and frequency of alcohol intake (−1.3 (−1.9, −0.7), $p < 0.001$) (Table 6). Thus, age and BMI were positively associated with non-HDL-C levels in both men and women. In contrast, sleep duration and the frequency of dairy product intake were associated with non-HDL-C levels only in men. In women, the frequency of egg intake was positively associated with non-HDL-C levels, whereas the frequency of meat, soybean, and alcohol intake was negatively associated with non-HDL-C levels.

4. Discussion

In this study, we first examined whether the frequency of intake of 10-item foods, snacks, sugar-sweetened coffee/tea, soft drinks, and alcoholic beverages varied by age and sex in Japan. We then performed multivariate analysis in groups divided by sex to identify associations between food frequency and metabolic parameters, with special reference to age and sex differences. Consistent with the sex differences, the correlation between food frequency and metabolic phenotypes differed between males and females. Thus, since the effects of food frequency on body size and blood parameters are dependent on age and sex, dietary guidance may need to be based on sex differences in food preference.

First, we confirmed sex differences in food preferences between males and females. As expected, males preferred to eat meat, and females preferred to eat soybeans, dairy products, vegetables, and fruits. Males also preferred to drink soft drinks and alcohol, whereas females preferred to eat snacks. These results are consistent with those of previous studies [1,2]. It is interesting to observe the same differences in food preferences between men and women, regardless of race or culture. Food preferences may be based on taste rather than the type of food itself [2]. Thus, food preference is an important factor for understanding sex differences in eating habits. However, many guidelines for diabetes and dyslipidemia do not consider sex differences in food preference. Considering sex-related differences in food preferences will provide better dietary guidance to patients.

In this study, vegetables and meat were consumed daily, whereas fruits, seaweed, and potatoes were consumed less frequently. The consumption of fruits and soybeans by men and the consumption of meat and fish by women seem to be encouraged. Potatoes and seaweed are considered necessary sources of dietary fiber for both sexes. These findings suggest that awareness of the importance of green vegetable and meat consumption is widespread, but increasing awareness of the importance of the consumption of soy, fish, seaweed, fruits, and potatoes, which are rich in trace elements and vitamins, seems necessary. Moreover, dietary fiber intake and the consumption of fruits, soybeans, potatoes, and seaweed are low in Japan [26].

Aging also affects food preferences [27]. The frequency of meat and egg intake was independent of age in both males and females. In contrast, the frequency of fish, soybean, and dairy product intake increased with age in both males and females. These findings suggest that the frequency of protein intake increases with age, independent of sex. The frequency of seaweed, fruit, vegetable, and potato intake also increased with age. These findings suggest that the frequency of dietary fiber intake increases with age, independent of sex. It is likely that many individuals consider the role of food in their health during aging. Taken together, these findings indicate that dietary variety increases with age. Many healthy diets, predominantly containing nutrient-rich plant foods and limited as to red and processed meats, have been associated with lower mortality and longevity [28]. However, the frequency of seaweed, potato, and fruit intake was lower than the frequency of meat and vegetable intake. We need to educate people about the benefits of consuming seaweed, fruits, and potatoes as sources of dietary fiber.

Sleep duration was also negatively correlated with HbA1c levels independent of sex. A long sleep duration ($\geq$9 h/day) is associated with higher HbA1c levels in patients with type-2 diabetes (T2D) on glucose-lowering medications [29]. Waist circumference was also negatively associated with sleep duration, which was inconsistent with our data [30]. Thus, to increase sleep duration, it is necessary to improve the working environment and educate people on the importance of not staying late in their daily lives.

The relationships between the frequency of food intake and metabolic parameters differed between males and females. In males, meat intake was positively associated with BMI and HbA1c and negatively associated with eGFR. In contrast, the frequency of meat intake in females was correlated with waist circumference and TG levels. These findings suggest that individuals who frequently consume meat should receive dietary guidance to prevent diabetes (males) and dyslipidemia (females).

Similarly, dairy products had opposite effects on males and females. In males, dairy product intake was positively correlated with BMI, eGFR, and non-HDL-C levels. In females, dairy product intake was negatively associated with eGFR and UA levels. Consistently, some studies have reported that the risk of hyperuricemia and gout is negatively associated with the intake of dairy products or soy foods [31]. In terms of renal function, dairy products had the opposite association with eGFR in both men and women. Although no distinction was made between low-fat dairy products and regular dairy products in this study, low-fat dairy products have been reported to prevent renal dysfunction [32]. It is possible that there is a difference in the frequency of the consumption of low-fat and regular dairy products between men and women.

Fish, egg, soybean, and fruit intake were correlated with metabolic parameters only in females. Fish intake was positively correlated with BMI and eGFR. In the middle-aged to older Chinese population, higher fish and seafood consumption ($\geq$11 portions/week) was found to be associated with a greater eGFR in participants with diabetes, whereas lower fish consumption was associated with a greater eGFR in participants without diabetes [33]. However, the differences between groups, in terms of the frequency of fish consumption 0–3, 4–6, and 7–10, were not significant [33]. The participants in this study were more likely to consume fish and seafood thrice a week, and most of them did not have diabetes. Thus, the differences in the results may be due to differences in eating habits and sex.

Egg intake was positively associated with BMI, waist circumference, and non-HDL-C level only in females. Some studies have reported that, among U.S. adults, increased consumption of dietary cholesterol or eggs is significantly associated with an increased risk of incident cardiovascular disease and all-cause mortality in a dose-dependent manner [34]. In contrast, in healthy Japanese individuals, there was no association between the daily consumption of one egg and blood cholesterol levels [35]. Blood non-HDL-C levels increased to levels comparable to those in overweight and underweight women aged 50–65 years [36]. Therefore, care should be taken to avoid excessive egg consumption by women of all ages.

Soybean intake was negatively associated with BMI, waist circumference, and non-HDL-C level only in females. Soy may be a suitable food for antiobesity efforts because of its high protein and isoflavone contents [37–39]. Women who consumed more soy during adulthood had a lower BMI, but this relationship was primarily observed in Caucasian and postmenopausal women [37]. Moreover, in hypercholesterolemic postmenopausal women fed a National Cholesterol Education Program Step I diet with isolated soy protein and moderate amounts of isoflavones, non-HDL-C levels were reduced compared with those in the control group ($p < 0.05$) [38]. In Japan, a higher intake of fermented soy is associated with a lower risk of mortality [40,41]. A higher intake of total phytoestrogens, including isoflavones, lignans, and coumarins, and foods rich in these compounds was associated with a lower risk of total and cause-specific mortality in generally healthy adults in the U.S. [42]. Thus, these findings suggest that individuals who frequently consume soybeans should receive dietary guidance to prevent obesity and dyslipidemia (especially in females).

Fruit intake correlated with BMI only in females. This trend was also observed in males. Similarly, a relationship between fruit intake and BMI has also been reported [43,44]. Some studies have reported significant associations between higher fruit consumption and lower BMI among female university students [43]. Greater fruit intake is associated with a lower risk of being overweight or obese in middle-aged and older women [44]. Therefore, fruit intake may effectively prevent weight gain, particularly among women.

Sugar intake has been associated with obesity and dental caries. Sugar intake is recommended to constitute no more than 10% of total energy intake, according to the World Health Organization guidelines [45]. However, as the amount of sugar used in the diet cannot be quantified, there is no mention of quantity limits in the Japanese Dietary Intake Standards [26]. The amount of free sugar was estimated on the basis of the frequency of the consumption of snacks, sugar-sweetened coffee, tea, and other soft drinks. According to our data, the frequency of snack consumption was greater in females than in males, and the frequency of soft drink consumption was greater in males. When assessing sugar intake, particular attention should be given to the frequency of soft drink and snack consumption by men and women, respectively.

In this study, the average alcohol consumption among the participants was 1.3 times per week. However, the frequency per week significantly increased with age in both men and women. After adjusting for age and BMI, alcohol intake correlated with UA and HDL-C levels in both males and females. Many studies have reported that hyperuricemia, characterized by high UA levels, may occur due to increased UA production or reduced UA excretion [46]. A positive association between alcohol intake and HDL-C levels has also been reported by many researchers [47], but an increase in HDL-C levels is not necessarily good [48,49]. Some studies have reported that high-density lipoprotein function in binge drinkers is impaired, with lower paraoxonase activity and greater glycation [48]. In males, TG levels were associated with alcohol intake, which is consistent with previous findings [49]. Thus, drinking alcoholic beverages is harmful to UA, HDL-C, and TG levels in males.

In contrast, in females, alcohol intake was positively associated with handgrip strength and negatively associated with the HbA1c level. Several studies have shown that handgrip strength significantly increases with increased daily alcohol consumption in both sexes [50]. Our data also revealed a correlation between the frequency of alcohol consumption and handgrip strength, with a significant difference in women ($p = 0.007$) and a trend toward significance in men ($p = 0.07$). The underlying mechanism of the relationship between the frequency of alcohol consumption and grip strength is unknown, but the results are reproducible [51]. Alcohol intake was negatively associated with HbA1c levels only in females. Consistently, higher alcohol intake was associated with lower HbA1c levels, even after adjusting for confounding factors such as age, sex, and fasting glucose concentration in a nationally representative sample of Korean adults [52]. Importantly, most Japanese people drink infrequently (once per week) [53]. Thus, the frequency of alcohol consumption had a positive effect on grip strength and HbA1c levels. Therefore, although our population consumes alcohol relatively infrequently compared with the overall Japanese population, the advantages and disadvantages of drinking alcoholic beverages should be fully considered.

This study has several limitations. This was an observational study. Therefore, causality could not be demonstrated. Although it was not possible to determine a causal relationship, this study advances the previously reported relationship between diet and metabolic parameters according to sex. In addition, prospective studies are needed to determine the effectiveness of nutritional guidance in terms of sex-based differences. We did not check for information regarding the participants' menstrual cycles or lifestyle factors (exercise and smoking). Some nurses and nursing assistants walk 20,000 steps per day for their jobs, and pedometers should be used to investigate the number of steps. The sleep duration was self-reported. Another limitation of this study was the lack of information on medication use and medical history.

5. Conclusions

Sex-related differences were observed in the frequency of food intake and its effect on metabolic parameters. These findings indicate that the food restrictions in the guidelines should not be uniformly applied regardless of sex. For example, non-HDL-C was significantly positively correlated with the frequency of egg intake only in women, even though egg intake frequency was the same in men and women. Although there is no evidence that women like omelets and scrambled eggs more than men, we need to look at even the way the eggs are prepared since butter is added to scrambled eggs, and nothing is added to boiled eggs.

In contrast, the effects of alcohol intake on UA levels were similar in men and women. The frequency of potato consumption was also significantly correlated with triglycerides in both men and women. Regardless of sex, alcohol and potatoes (starch) are converted directly to uric acid and triglycerides in the body. Dietary restriction of these related foods is considered to be effective for both sexes.

We decided to conduct this study because we believe that nutrition education in the workplace can improve employee health. On the basis of these study data, our university will promote nutrition education to employees by creating cooking recipes that supplement deficient food groups (fish, soybeans, fruits, etc.) and offering cooking classes in the workplace.

Moreover, we need to test whether dietary restrictions influenced by sex have a beneficial effect on the improvement of blood markers (HbA1c, lipids, and eGFR). Prospective studies are necessary to implement nutritional guidance that considers sex-related differences.

Author Contributions: Conceptualization, K.I. and H.N.; methodology, K.I.; software, K.I.; validation, K.D. and C.U.; formal analysis, K.I.; investigation, K.Y., K.K. and Y.Y.; resources, C.U. and K.D.; writing—original draft preparation, K.I. and R.Y.-W.; writing—review and editing, K.I.; visualization, K.I.; supervision, K.I.; project administration, K.I.; funding acquisition, K.I. All authors have read and agreed to the published version of the manuscript.

Funding: This research received no external funding.

Institutional Review Board Statement: The study was conducted according to the principles of the Declaration of Helsinki and approved by the Research Ethics Committee of Fujita Health University (approval number HM23-422, 26 March 2024).

Informed Consent Statement: Written informed consent for publication has been waived since we were only dealing with anonymized information.

Data Availability Statement: The datasets used and/or analyzed during the current study will be made available by the corresponding author upon reasonable request.

Acknowledgments: We would like to thank the participants for their invaluable contributions. The authors also wish to thank Tomomi Hattori, Kumiko Furusho, Takeshi Hamashima, Shizue Ishikawa, Saori Fukuda, and Yoko Ode for their assistance with the study.

Conflicts of Interest: The authors declare no conflict of interest.

References

1. Feraco, A.; Armani, A.; Amoah, I.; Guseva, E.; Camajani, E.; Gorini, S.; Strollo, R.; Padua, E.; Caprio, M.; Lombardo, M. Assessing gender differences in food preferences and physical activity: A population-based survey. *Front. Nutr.* **2024**, *11*, 1348456. [CrossRef] [PubMed]
2. Lombardo, M.; Amoah, I.; Feraco, A.; Guseva, E.; Gorini, S.; Camajani, E.; Armani, A.; Padua, E.; Caprio, M. Gender Differences in Taste and Food Habits: Implications for Personalized Nutrition. *Biol. Life Sci. Forum* **2023**, *29*, 1. [CrossRef]
3. Kuo, C.T.; Chen, D.R.; Chan, C.C.; Yeh, Y.P.; Chen, H.H. Sex differences in the association between sugar-sweetened beverages consumption and metabolic risks among the working-age population in Taiwan. *Public Health Nutr.* **2022**, *26*, 653–660. [CrossRef]
4. Westenhoefer, J. Age and gender dependent profile of food choice. *Forum Nutr.* **2005**, *57*, 44–51. [CrossRef]
5. Chao, A.M.; Loughead, J.; Bakizada, Z.M.; Hopkins, C.M.; Geliebter, A.; Gur, R.C.; Wadden, T.A. Sex/gender differences in neural correlates of food stimuli: A systematic review of functional neuroimaging studies. *Obes. Rev.* **2017**, *18*, 687–699. [CrossRef] [PubMed]
6. Manippa, V.; Padulo, C.; van der Laan, L.N.; Brancucci, A. Gender differences in food choice: Effects of superior temporal sulcus stimulation. *Front. Hum. Neurosci.* **2017**, *11*, 597. [CrossRef]
7. Castronuovo, L.; Guarnieri, L.; Tiscornia, M.V.; Allemandi, L. Food marketing and gender among children and adolescents: A scoping review. *Nutr. J.* **2021**, *20*, 52. [CrossRef]
8. Grzymisławska, M.; Puch, E.A.; Zawada, A.; Grzymisławski, M. Do nutritional behaviors depend on biological sex and cultural gender? *Adv. Clin. Exp. Med.* **2020**, *29*, 165–172. [CrossRef]
9. Yeung, A.W.K. Sex differences in brain responses to food stimuli: A meta-analysis on neuroimaging studies. *Obes. Rev.* **2018**, *19*, 1110–1115. [CrossRef]
10. Diószegi, J.; Llanaj, E.; Ádány, R. Genetic background of taste perception, taste preferences, and its nutritional implications: A systematic review. *Front. Genet.* **2019**, *10*, 1272. [CrossRef]
11. Wardle, J.; Grilo, C.M.; De Castro, J.M. Gender differences in food choice: The contribution of health beliefs and dieting. *Ann. Behav. Med.* **2004**, *28*, 108–117. [CrossRef]
12. Yaguchi-Tanaka, Y.; Tabuchi, T. Skipping Breakfast and Subsequent Overweight/Obesity in Children: A Nationwide Prospective Study of 2.5- to 13-year-old Children in Japan. *J. Epidemiol.* **2021**, *31*, 417–425. [CrossRef] [PubMed]
13. Kojima, Y.; Murayama, N.; Suga, H. Dietary diversity score correlates with nutrient intake and monetary diet cost among Japanese adults. *Asia Pac. J. Clin. Nutr.* **2020**, *29*, 382–394. [CrossRef] [PubMed]
14. Otsuka, R.; Tange, C.; Nishita, Y.; Kato, Y.; Tomida, M.; Imai, T.; Ando, F.; Shimokata, H. Dietary Diversity and All-Cause and Cause-Specific Mortality in Japanese Community-Dwelling Older Adults. *Nutrients* **2020**, *12*, 1052. [CrossRef] [PubMed]
15. Alhusseini, N.; Ramadan, M.; Aljarayhi, S.; Arnous, W.; Abdelaal, M.; Dababo, H.; Dalati, B.; Doumani, O.A.; AlNasser, S.; Saleem, R. Added sugar intake among the saudi population. *PLoS ONE* **2023**, *18*, e0291136. [CrossRef] [PubMed]
16. Panda, A.; Booth, S.L. Nutritional Aspects of Healthy Aging. *Med. Clin. N. Am.* **2022**, *106*, 853–863. [CrossRef] [PubMed]
17. Virtanen, J.; Penttinen, M.A.; Laaksonen, M.; Erkkola, M.; Vepsäläinen, H.; Kautiainen, H.; Korhonen, P. The Relationship between Dietary Habits and Work Engagement among Female Finnish Municipal Employees. *Nutrients* **2022**, *14*, 1267. [CrossRef]
18. Kuwahara, K.; Imai, T.; Miyamoto, T.; Kochi, T.; Eguchi, M.; Nishihara, A.; Nakagawa, T.; Yamamoto, S.; Honda, T.; Kabe, I.; et al. Sleep Duration Modifies the Association of Overtime Work with Risk of Developing Type 2 Diabetes: Japan Epidemiology Collaboration on Occupational Health Study. *J. Epidemiol.* **2018**, *28*, 336–340. [CrossRef]
19. Fox, E.C.; Wang, K.; Aquino, M.; Grandner, M.A.; Xie, D.; Branas, C.C.; Gooneratne, N.S. Sleep debt at the community level: Impact of age, sex, race/ethnicity and health. *Sleep Health* **2018**, *4*, 317–324. [CrossRef]
20. Spiegel, K.; Leproult, R.; Van Cauter, E. Impact of sleep debt on metabolic and endocrine function. *Lancet* **1999**, *354*, 1435–1439. [CrossRef] [PubMed]
21. Takahashi, K. Food Frequency Questionnaire Based on Food Groups for Estimating Individual Nutrient Intake. *Jpn. J. Nutr. Diet.* **2003**, *61*, 161–169. [CrossRef]
22. Maruyama, S.; Morita, I.; Nakagaki, H. Survey on the food intake in community-dwelling elderly women. *J. Integr. Study Diet. Habits.* **2007**, *17*, 348. [CrossRef]
23. Okada, E.; Saito, A.; Takimoto, H. Association between the Portion Sizes of Traditional Japanese Seasonings—Soy Sauce and Miso—And Blood Pressure: Cross-Sectional Study Using National Health and Nutrition Survey, 2012–2016 Data. *Nutrients* **2018**, *10*, 1865. [CrossRef]
24. Oono, F.; Sakamoto, Y.; Tachi, Y.; Mabashi-Asazuma, H.; Iida, K. Effect of Cdx2 Polymorphism on the Relationship between Dietary Calcium Intake and Peak Bone Mass in Young Japanese Women. *Nutrients* **2020**, *12*, 191. [CrossRef] [PubMed]
25. Iizuka, K.; Deguchi, K.; Ushiroda, C.; Yanagi, K.; Seino, Y.; Suzuki, A.; Yabe, D.; Sasaki, H.; Sasaki, S.; Saitoh, E.; et al. A Study on the Compatibility of a Food-Recording Application with Questionnaire-Based Methods in Healthy Japanese Individuals. *Nutrients* **2024**, *16*, 1742. [CrossRef] [PubMed]
26. Dietary Reference Intakes for Japanese. Ministry of Health, Labor and Welfare. 2020. Available online: https://www.mhlw.go.jp/content/10900000/001150922.pdf (accessed on 30 June 2024).
27. Robb, C.; Carr, P.R.; Ball, J.; Owen, A.; Beilin, L.J.; Newman, A.B.; Nelson, M.R.; Reid, C.M.; Orchard, S.G.; Neumann, J.T.; et al. Association of a healthy lifestyle with mortality in older people. *BMC Geriatr.* **2023**, *23*, 646. [CrossRef]

28. Hu, F.B. Diet strategies for promoting healthy aging and longevity: An epidemiological perspective. *J. Intern. Med.* **2024**, *295*, 508–531. [CrossRef]
29. Tan, X.; Benedict, C. Sleep characteristics and HbA1c in patients with type 2 diabetes on glucose-lowering medication. *BMJ Open Diabetes Res. Care* **2020**, *8*, e001702. [CrossRef] [PubMed]
30. Sperry, S.D.; Scully, I.D.; Gramzow, R.H.; Jorgensen, R.S. Sleep Duration and Waist Circumference in Adults: A Meta-Analysis. *Sleep* **2015**, *38*, 1269–1276. [CrossRef]
31. Mena-Sánchez, G.; Babio, N.; Becerra-Tomás, N.; Martínez-González, M.Á.; Díaz-López, A.; Corella, D.; Zomeño, M.D.; Romaguera, D.; Vioque, J.; Alonso-Gómez, Á.M.; et al. Association between dairy product consumption and hyperuricemia in an elderly population with metabolic syndrome. *Nutr. Metab. Cardiovasc. Dis.* **2020**, *30*, 214–222. [CrossRef]
32. Herber-Gast, G.M.; Biesbroek, S.; Verschuren, W.M.; DA Stehouwer, C.; Gansevoort, R.T.; Bakker, S.J.; Spijkerman, A.M. Association of dietary protein and dairy intake and change in renal function: Results from the population-based longitudinal Doetinchem cohort study. *Am. J. Clin. Nutr.* **2016**, *104*, 1712–1719. [CrossRef] [PubMed]
33. Lu, T.Y.; Zhang, W.S.; Zhu, T.; Jiang, C.Q.; Zhu, F.; Jin, Y.L.; Lam, T.H.; Cheng, K.K.; Xu, L. Associations of meat, fish, and seafood consumption with kidney function in middle-aged to older Chinese: A cross-sectional study based on the Guangzhou Biobank Cohort Study. *BMJ Open* **2023**, *13*, e073738. [CrossRef] [PubMed]
34. Zhong, V.W.; Van Horn, L.; Cornelis, M.C.; Wilkins, J.T.; Ning, H.; Carnethon, M.R.; Greenland, P.; Mentz, R.J.; Tucker, K.L.; Zhao, L.; et al. Association of dietary cholesterol or egg consumption with incident Cardiovascular Disease and mortality. *JAMA* **2019**, *321*, 1081–1095. [CrossRef] [PubMed]
35. Sugano, M.; Matsuoka, R. Nutritional Viewpoints on Eggs and Cholesterol. *Foods* **2021**, *10*, 494. [CrossRef] [PubMed]
36. Iizuka, K.; Kobae, K.; Yanagi, K.; Yamada, Y.; Deguchi, K.; Ushiroda, C.; Seino, Y.; Suzuki, A.; Saitoh, E.; Naruse, H. Differing Effects of Body Size on Circulating Lipid Concentrations and Hemoglobin A1c Levels in Young and Middle-Aged Japanese Women. *Healthcare* **2024**, *12*, 465. [CrossRef]
37. Maskarinec, G.; Aylward, A.G.; Erber, E.; Takata, Y.; Kolonel, L.N. Soy intake is related to a lower body mass index in adult women. *Eur. J. Nutr.* **2008**, *47*, 138–144. [CrossRef]
38. Zhu, J.; Zhao, Q.; Qiu, Y.; Zhang, Y.; Cui, S.; Yu, Y.; Chen, B.; Zhu, M.; Wang, N.; Liu, X.; et al. Soy isoflavone intake and obesity in Chinese adults: A cross-sectional study in Shanghai, China. *Nutrients* **2021**, *13*, 2715. [CrossRef]
39. A Baum, J.; Teng, H.; Erdman, J.W., Jr.; Weigel, R.M.; Klein, B.P.; Persky, V.W.; Freels, S.; Surya, P.; Bakhit, R.M.; Ramos, E.; et al. Long-term soy protein intake improves blood lipid profiles and increases mononuclear cell low-density lipoprotein receptor messenger RNA levels in hypercholesterolemic postmenopausal women. *Am. J. Clin. Nutr.* **1998**, *68*, 545–551. [CrossRef]
40. Nagata, C.; Takatsuka, N.; Shimizu, H. Soy and Fish Oil Intake and Mortality in a Japanese Community. *Am. J. Epidemiol.* **2002**, *156*, 824–831. [CrossRef]
41. Katagiri, R.; Sawada, N.; Goto, A.; Yamaji, T.; Iwasaki, M.; Noda, M.; Iso, H.; Tsugane, S. Association of soy and fermented soy product intake with total and cause-specific mortality: A prospective cohort study. *BMJ* **2020**, *368*, m34. [CrossRef]
42. Chen, Z.; Qian, F.; Hu, Y.; Voortman, T.; Li, Y.; Rimm, E.B.; Sun, Q. Dietary phytoestrogens and total and cause-specific mortality: Results from two prospective cohort studies. *Am. J. Clin. Nutr.* **2023**, *117*, 130–140. [CrossRef] [PubMed]
43. Gholi, Z.; Rs, G.; Azadbakht, L.; Ghalaeh, R.; Bank, S.; Ss, B. Fruit and vegetable intake, body mass index, and waist circumference of young female students in Isfahan. *J. Educ. Health Promot.* **2012**, *1*, 29. [CrossRef]
44. Rautiainen, S.; Wang, L.; Lee, I.-M.; Manson, J.E.; Buring, J.E.; Sesso, H.D. Higher Intake of Fruit, but Not Vegetables or Fiber, at Baseline Is Associated with Lower Risk of Becoming Overweight or Obese in Middle-Aged and Older Women of Normal BMI at Baseline. *J. Nutr.* **2015**, *145*, 960–968. [CrossRef]
45. Guideline: Sugars Intake for Adults and Children. World Health Organization. 2015. Available online: https://www.who.int/publications/i/item/9789241549028 (accessed on 30 June 2024).
46. Nieradko-Iwanicka, B. Role of alcohol consumption in gout pathogenesis. *Crit. Rev. Food Sci. Nutr.* **2022**, *62*, 7129–7137. [CrossRef]
47. Kunutsor, S.K.; Bhattacharjee, A.; Connelly, M.A.; Bakker, S.J.L.; Dullaart, R.P.F. Alcohol Consumption, High-Density Lipoprotein Particles and Subspecies, and Risk of Cardiovascular Disease: Findings from the PREVEND Prospective Study. *Int. J. Mol. Sci.* **2024**, *25*, 2290. [CrossRef]
48. Tverdal, A.; Høiseth, G.; Magnus, P.; Næss, Ø.; Selmer, R.; Knudsen, G.P.; Mørland, J. Alcohol Consumption, HDL-Cholesterol and Incidence of Colon and Rectal Cancer: A Prospective Cohort Study Including 250,010 Participants. *Alcohol Alcohol.* **2021**, *56*, 718–725. [CrossRef] [PubMed]
49. Cho, K.H.; Nam, H.S.; Kang, D.J.; Park, M.H.; Kim, J.H. Long-term alcohol consumption causes a significant decrease in serum high-density lipoprotein (HDL)cholesterol and apolipoprotein A-I levels in middle-aged Korean women. *Int. J. Mol. Sci.* **2022**, *23*, 8623. [CrossRef] [PubMed]
50. Pownall, H.J.; Ballantyne, C.M.; Kimball, K.T.; Simpson, S.L.; Yeshurun, D.; Gotto, A.M. Effect of Moderate Alcohol Consumption on Hypertriglyceridemia: A Study in the Fasting State. *Arch. Intern. Med.* **1999**, *159*, 981–987. [CrossRef]
51. Kawamoto, R.; Ninomiya, D.; Senzaki, K.; Kumagi, T. Alcohol consumption is positively associated with handgrip strength among Japanese community-dwelling middle-aged and elderly individuals. *Int. J. Gerontol.* **2018**, *12*, 294–298. [CrossRef]

52. Hong, J.W.; Noh, J.H.; Kim, D.J. Association between Alcohol Intake and Hemoglobin A1c in the Korean Adults: The 2011–2013 Korea National Health and Nutrition Examination Survey. *PLoS ONE* **2016**, *11*, e0167210. [CrossRef]
53. Ministry of Health, Labor, and Welfare. National Health and Nutrition Survey. 2020. Available online: https://www.mhlw.go.jp/content/000711008.pdf (accessed on 9 May 2024).

MDPI AG
Grosspeteranlage 5
4052 Basel
Switzerland
Tel.: +41 61 683 77 34

Nutrients Editorial Office
E-mail: nutrients@mdpi.com
www.mdpi.com/journal/nutrients

www.ingramcontent.com/pod-product-compliance
Lightning Source LLC
Chambersburg PA
CBHW041954260926
51850CB00019B/2782
* 9 7 8 3 7 2 5 8 4 9 1 7 8 *